Reproductive Endocrinology

and Infertility

Handbook for Clinicians

2nd Edition

Dan I. Lebovic, MD
Professor
Department of Obstetrics and Gynecology
University of Wisconsin School of Medicine
Madison, WI

John David Gordon, MD
Co-Director, Dominion Fertility, Arlington, VA
Clinical Professor, Obstetrics and Gynecology
The George Washington University School of Medicine
Division Director, Reproductive Endocrinology and Infertility
Inova Fairfax Hospital

Robert N. Taylor, MD, PhD
Professor
Department of Obstetrics and Gynecology
Wake Forest School of Medicine
Winston-Salem, NC

ISBN 978-0-9645467-1-4 (pocket edition)

The opinions expressed in this book represent a broad range of opinions of the authors. These opinions are not meant to represent a "standard of care" or a "protocol" but rather a guide to common clinical conditions. Use of these guidelines is obviously influenced by local factors, varying clinical circumstances, and honest differences of opinion.

The indications and dosages of all drugs in this book have been recommended in the medical literature and conform to all the practices of the general medical community. The medications described do not necessarily have specific approval by the Food and Drug Administration for use in the diseases and dosages for which they are recommended. The package insert for each drug should be consulted for use and dosage as approved by the FDA. Because standards for usage change, it is advisable to keep abreast of revised recommendations, particularly those concerning new drugs.

Publisher: Scrub Hill Press, Inc.
Editorial Production: Scribe, Inc. Philadelphia, PA
Cover Design: Elena Antoniou

Editorial offices:
Scrub Hill Press, Inc.
46 S. Glebe Road #301
Arlington, VA 22204
e-mail: johndavidgordon@mac.com
www.scrubhillpress.com
Member of the International Association
of STM Publishers

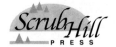

Inspiration for this book promoting 'life' comes from the lives of four special people. From my maternal grandparents I learned the value and honor of a life well-lived. From my paternal grandparents, who perished in the Holocaust, I strive to honor their memory by dedicating my life to the proliferation of life.

Dan I. Lebovic
August 2013

Two percent of the profits from the sale of this book will be donated to the Daniel Pearl Foundation (http://www.danielpearl.org).

Contents

Contributors   *vii*

Foreword: *Brad Van Voorhis, MD*   *xiii*

Preface   *xv*

1. Sexual Differentiation: From Gonad to Phallus   1
2. Puberty   17
3. Pediatric and Adolescent Gynecology   29
4. Müllerian Agenesis   37
5. Septate Uterus   41
6. Turner Syndrome   49
7. Menstrual Cycle   59
8. Abnormal Uterine Bleeding   71
9. Oral Contraceptives   81
10. Amenorrhea   105
11. Exercise-Induced Amenorrhea   113
12. Ectopic Pregnancy   117
13. Sheehan Syndrome   129
14. Premenstrual Syndrome   133
15. Chronic Pelvic Pain   143
16. Endometriosis   151
17. Fibroids   175
18. Polycystic Ovary Syndrome   183
19. Female Subfertility   209

CONTENTS

20. Male Subfertility — 229

21. Diminished Ovarian Reserve — 255

22. Assisted Reproductive Technologies — 263

23. Financially Efficient Fertility Care — 283

24. Ovarian Hyperstimulation Syndrome — 289

25. Hyperemesis in Pregnancy — 299

26. Gamete Preservation — 303

27. Luteal Phase Deficiency — 309

28. Hyperprolactinemia and Galactorrhea — 315

29. Hypothyroidism — 331

30. Recurrent Pregnancy Loss — 335

31. Management of Early Pregnancy Failure — 357

32. Primary Ovarian Insufficiency/ Primary Ovarian Failure — 365

33. Genetic Testing — 371

34. Androgen Replacement Therapy — 393

35. Postmenopausal Hormone Therapy — 403

36. Postmenopausal Osteoporosis — 421

37. Hot Flashes — 437

38. Transvaginal Ultrasound in Reproductive Endocrinology and Infertility — 445

39. Hysteroscopy — 453

40. Laparoscopy — 457

41. Journal Club Guide — 469

Chapter Key Points — 479

References — 493

Index — 539

Contributors

Editors-in-chief

Dan I. Lebovic, MD
John David Gordon, MD
Robert N. Taylor, MD, PhD

Section Editor – Chapter Summaries

Nanette F. Santoro, MD
Professor and E. Stewart Taylor Chair
Department of Obstetrics and Gynecology
University of Colorado Anschutz Medical Campus

Contributors

Arnold P. Advincula, MD
Director of Minimally Invasive Gynecologic Surgery and Fellowship
Medical Director, Florida Hospital
Orlando, FL
Chapter 15, Chronic Pelvic Pain

Sawsan As-Sanie, MD, MPH
Director of Minimally Invasive Gynecologic Surgery and Fellowship
Assistant Professor, Obstetrics and Gynecology
University of Michigan
Ann Arbor, MI
Chapter 40, Laparoscopy

Amelia P. Bailey, MD
Fellow, Reproductive Endocrinology and Infertility
Brigham and Women's Hospital
Boston, MA
Chapter 4, Müllerian Agenesis
Chapter 5, Septate Uterus

Charles L. Bormann, PhD
IVF Laboratory Director
Brigham and Women's Hospital
Boston, MA
Chapter 22, Assisted Reproductive Technologies

Pavna K. Brahma, MD
Reproductive Endocrinology and Infertility
Reproductive Biology Associates
Atlanta, GA
Chapter 8, Abnormal Uterine Bleeding

Christina E. Broadwell, MD
Assistant Professor, Reproductive Endocrinology and Infertility
University of Wisconsin
Madison, WI
Chapter 10, Amenorrhea

Colleen Casey, MD
Reproductive Endocrinology and Infertility Center for Reproductive
Medicine
Minneapolis, MN
Chapter 29, Hypothyroidism

Gregory M. Christman, MD
Professor, Obstetrics and Gynecology
University of Florida
Gainesville, FL
Chapter 17, Fibroids

Natalie A. Clark, MD
Resident, Obstetrics and Gynecology
University of Michigan
Ann Arbor, MI
Chapter 36, Postmenopausal Osteoporosis

Vanessa K. Dalton, MD, MPH
Associate Professor, Obstetrics and Gynecology
University of Michigan
Ann Arbor, MI
Chapter 31, Management of Early Pregnancy Failure

Jocelyn Davie, MS, CGC
Licensed Genetic Counselor
Good Start Genetics, Inc.
Chapter 33, Genetic Testing

Aimee D. Eyvazzadeh, MD, MPH
Reproductive Endocrinology and Infertility
San Ramon, CA
Chapter 9, Oral Contraceptives

Senait Fisseha, MD, JD
Associate Professor
Director of Reproductive Endocrinology and Infertility
University of Michigan
Ann Arbor, MI
Chapter 36, Postmenopausal Osteoporosis

Caleb B. Kallen MD, PhD
Associate Professor, Reproductive Endocrinology and Infertility
Thomas Jefferson University
Philadelphia, PA
Chapter 34, Androgen Replacement Therapy

L. April Gago, MD
Director
Gago Center for Fertility/Gago IVF
Brighton, MI
Chapter 6, Turner Syndrome

Margo C. Grady, MS, CGC
Certified Genetic Counselor, Obstetrics and Gynecology
University of Wisconsin–Madison/Meriter Hospital
Madison, WI
Chapter 33, Genetic Testing

Parviz K. Kavoussi, MD
Reproductive Urologist
Austin Fertility and Reproductive Medicine/Westlake IVF
Austin, TX
Chapter 20, Male Subfertility

Shahryar K. Kavoussi, MD, MPH
Reproductive Endocrinology and Infertility
Austin Fertility and Reproductive Medicine/Westlake IVF
Austin, TX
Chapter 26, Gamete Preservation

Kristie Keeton, MD, MPH
Maternal Fetal Medicine
Saint Joseph Mercy Health System
Ann Arbor, Michigan
Chapter 2, Puberty

Ania Kowalik, MD
Reproductive Endocrinologist
Fertility Solutions
Dedham, MA
Chapter 38, Transvaginal Ultrasound in Reproductive Endocrinology and Infertility

Jenna McCarthy, MD
South Florida Institute for Reproductive Medicine
Jupiter, FL
Chapter 32, Primary Ovarian Insufficiency/Premature Ovarian Failure

William R. Meyer, MD
Carolina Conceptions
Raleigh, NC
Chapter 11, Exercise-Induced Amenorrhea

Molly Moravek, MD, MPH
Fellow, Reproductive Endocrinology and Infertility
McGaw Medical Center of Northwestern University
Chicago, IL
Chapter 7, Menstrual Cycle

Michael D. Mueller, MD
Professor, Obstetrics and Gynecology
Director, Endometriosis Center
Frauenklinik Inselspital, University of Berne
Berne, Switzerland
Chapter 12, Ectopic Pregnancy

Ringland S. Murray, MD
Tennessee Reproductive Medicine
Chattanooga, TN
Chapter 21, Diminished Ovarian Reserve

Meghan B. Oakes, MD
Professor, Creighton University Medical Center
Reproductive Health Specialists
Omaha, NE
Chapter 14, Premenstrual Syndrome

Kenan R. Omurtag, MD
Fellow, Reproductive Endocrinology and Infertility
Washington University St Louis Department of Obstetrics and Gynecology
St. Louis, MO
Chapter 24, Ovarian Hyperstimulation Syndrome

J. Preston Parry, MD, MPH
Director of Reproductive Endocrinology and Infertility
Assistant Professor, Obstetrics and Gynecology
University of Mississippi
Jackson, MS
Chapter 23, Financially Efficient Fertility Care

Maureen Phipps, MD, MPH
Associate Professor, Obstetrics and Gynecology and Epidemiology
Warren Alpert Medical School of Brown University
Providence, RI
Chapter 40, Journal Club Guide

Elisabeth H. Quint, MD
Professor, Obstetrics and Gynecology
University of Michigan
Ann Arbor, MI
Chapter 3, Pediatric and Adolescent Gynecology

John A. Schnorr, MD
Associate Professor, Reproductive Endocrinology and Infertility
Medical University of South Carolina
Coastal Fertility Specialists
Charleston, SC
Chapter 22, Assisted Reproductive Technologies

Danny J. Schust, MD
Associate Professor, Obstetrics, Gynecology and Women's Health
University of Missouri
Columbia, MO
Chapter 27, Luteal Phase Deficiency
Chapter 30, Recurrent Pregnancy Loss

Yolanda R. Smith, MD, MPH
Professor, Reproductive Endocrinology and Infertility
University of Michigan
Ann Arbor, MI
Chapter 3, Pediatric and Adolescent Gynecology

Arleen H. Song, MD MPH
Gynecology and Laparoscopic Surgeons
Raleigh, NC
Chapter 17, Fibroids

Tony Tsai, MD
Director of Reproductive Endocrinology and Fertility
Laparoscopic and Laser Surgery, Obstetrics and Gynecology
New York Hospital Queens
Assistant Professor, Obstetrics and Gynecology
Weill Medical College of Cornell University
Chapter 39, Hysteroscopy

Mary Ellen Wechter, MD, MPH
North Florida OBGYN Division 1
Baptist Medical Center Downtown
Jacksonville, FL
Chapter 18, Polycystic Ovary Syndrome

Matthew Will, MD
Teaching Faculty, Reproductive Endocrinology and Infertility
St. Vincent Hospital
Midwest Fertility Specialists
Indianapolis, IN
Chapter 35, Postmenopausal Hormone Therapy

Jennifer A. Williams, MD
Maternal Fetal Medicine
Saint Joseph Mercy Health System
Ann Arbor, Michigan
Chapter 37, Hot Flashes

Foreword

"There is no more difficult art to acquire than the art of observation, and for some men it is quite as difficult to record an observation in brief and plain language." Sir William Osler

The authors of *Reproductive Endocrinology and Infertility: Handbook for Clinicians* have succeeded in recording the most pertinent observations and facts about the entire breadth of our field in brief and plain language. This book is remarkable in its comprehensive yet concise coverage of reproductive medicine, using notes and simple diagrams to help the reader understand the basic science underpinnings of a disease process while also imparting practical evidence based management principles. Each section notes the most critical observations on a topic and serves as a scaffold on which to build a complete understanding of gynecologic endocrinology and infertility. I think this is the perfect text for a busy resident in Obstetrics and Gynecology or Reproductive Endocrinology and Infertility fellow to study prior to an examination. The up-to-date clinical advice also makes this an invaluable resource for the practicing physician. I congratulate the authors on this second edition which is a remarkable success.

Brad Van Voorhis, MD
Professor, Obstetrics and Gynecology
Division Director, Reproductive Endocrinology
University of Iowa, Iowa City, IA

Preface

With great pleasure we present to you this second edition of *Reproductive Endocrinology and Infertility: Handbook for Clinicians* updating the inaugural edition that has become long in the tooth. As with the first edition, we wanted to offer a resource that would condense the immense literature into easily digestible essentials. This edition gives us a chance to edit and supplement every chapter with advances published since the writing of the first copy—circa 2005.

Although there are several excellent texts devoted to Reproductive Endocrinology and Infertility (REI), the present handbook was born out of a desire to provide a ready resource for clinicians to access the most important facts and figures. In order to accomplish this goal, the authors searched through textbooks, original articles and erudite colleagues' brains for answers to specific queries. This second edition, REI Handbook again strives to be a literary Occam's razor: "Among competing hypotheses, favor the simplest one" or, in this case, an amalgam of REI information distilled into a handbook.

Scientific knowledge is constantly evolving and REI is not immune to this phenomenon; this Handbook is simply a snapshot in time. The editors and authors have relied on evidence-based resources rather than tradition or dogma and references are provided along with many original or adapted figures. Opinion from experienced clinicians was obtained when rigorous trials were not available. The value of this Handbook will depend on how often the pages are turned during your training or practice. With time the images and tables may become ingrained for easier recall. Despite strong efforts from the many contributors, this Handbook should not be considered a stand-alone resource but a stepping stone to the words of Lee C. Bollinger: "You have to be willing to embarrass yourself in order to learn." Learning is not a spectator sport.

Apart from the generous contributors who offered their time to make this a better piece of work, I owe much to my teachers and colleagues and would like to acknowledge them by chronological order:

- Under the shade of the Campanile, through the arches of Sather Gate and along Strawberry Canyon at **UC Berkeley:** Dr. Russ Baldocchi, Dr. Howard Bern, Dr. Julian Boyd, Dr.

Marion Diamond, Dr. Satyabrata Nandi, Dr. Karl Nicoll and Dr. Sharon Russell.

- Amidst Foggy Bottom at George **Washington University Medical School**: Dr. Frank Allen, Dr. Isaac Ben-Or, Dr. David Levy, Dr. Vikas Mahavni and Dr. Frank Slaby.
- As a surgical intern in "Live Free or Die" **Dartmouth-Hitchcock Medical Center**: Dr. Wendy Dean, Dr. Thomas Collachio, Dr. Robert Crichlow, Dr. Horace Enriques and Dr. Paul Manganiello.
- Beside the Blue Ridge Mountains at the **University of Virginia**: Dr. Willie Andersen, Dr. John Bourgeois, Dr. Guy Harbert, Dr. James Kitchin, Dr. Lisa Kolp, Dr. Elizabeth Mandell, Dr. Howard Montgomery, Alex O'Brien, RN, Dr. Laurel Rice, Dr. Peyton Taylor and Dr. Paul Underwood.
- In the fog of **UC San Francisco**: Dr. Seth Feigenbaum, Dr. Simon Henderson, Dr. Robert Jaffe, Dr. Collin Smikle, Dr. Sae Sohn, Dr. Robert Taylor and Dr. Tony Tsai.
- Within the Big House at the **University of Michigan**: Dr. Rudi Ansbacher, Dr. Greg Christman, Dr. Steven Dominio, Dr. Dana Ohl, Dr. John Randolph, Jr., Dr. Tim Schuster, Dr. Yolanda Smith and Dr. Timothy Johnson.
- Presently, beside Camp Randall and Bucky Badger at the **University of Wisconsin**: Dr. Charles Bormann, Dr. Christina Broadwell, Dr. Jeffrey Jones, Dr. Laurel Rice and Dr. Daniel Williams.

Many thanks to Melissa Tarrao and Bill Klump at Scribe for their impeccable attention to detail and style. Danielle Lohr was a huge help in gathering all the image and figure permissions. I would like to thank my co-authors, Dr. John Gordon and Dr. Rob Taylor. I am grateful to John for his incredibly deft editing talents and allowing this project to reach prime time for a second edition. Rob was (and is) my mentor from fellowship days, who continues to inspire, entertain and comfort me beyond any imaginable call of duty. It is an honor to have trained under Dr. Taylor and now collaborate with him on this project once again. Our new feature of chapter essentials or "nuggets" has been written by Dr. Nanette Santoro to help the reader grasp some take home messages with even greater ease.

I would like to acknowledge the loving support of my wife Carol, brother Stan and my parents, Alex and Ida Lebovic. Finally, Carol and I took the messages of the first addition to heart (and to reproductive organs) as we have been blessed with the interim births of our son Henri and daughter Sophie.

Dan I. Lebovic MD
August 2013

1

Sexual Differentiation: From Gonad to Phallus

EMBRYOLOGY

- Bipotential: gonads and external genitalia (urogenital sinus; two labioscrotal swellings; genital tubercle)
- Unipotential: wolffian or müllerian ducts

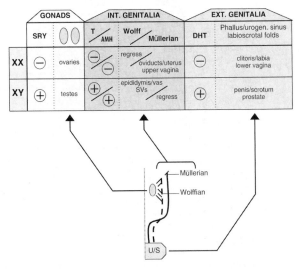

T, testosterone
AMH, anti-müllerian hormone
SVs, seminal vesicles
DHT, dihydrotestosterone
SRY, sex-determining region of the Y-chromosome
U/S, urogenital sinus

Gonads

- Formation of a testis occurs in the presence of the Y chromosome (46,XY).
- Formation of an ovary occurs in the absence of the Y chromosome and the presence of a 2nd X chromosome (46,XX).
- Gonads begin development during weeks 5–6 of gestation.

Testicular Determinants

- Sex-determining region of Y (SRY) is the gene involved in testis determination (short arm [p] of Y chromosome) (Sinclair 1990; Tilford 2001).

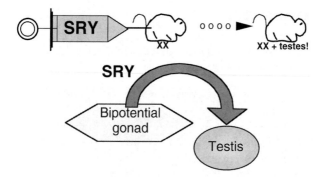

Ovarian Determinants

- Unless SRY and SOX9 are expressed, ovarian development ensues (assuming XX is present).
- **2nd X chromosome** required for normal ovarian development
- **Autosomal genes** (see diagram on page 4 regarding three facets of sexual differentiation).

Internal Genitalia

- Wolffian ducts (dependent on testosterone [T] from testes) → epididymis/vas deferens/seminal vesicles (internal genitalia)
- AMH = anti-müllerian hormone, produced by Sertoli cells
- Müllerian ducts (in absence of AMH) → fallopian tubes/ uterus/upper vagina (internal genitalia)

- Müllerian and wolffian development begin simultaneously; they are local phenomena (i.e., they occur *ipsi*laterally depending on presence/absence of T/AMH).

External Genitalia

- DHT is crucial in the development of external genitalia:
  - presence of DHT: male
  - absence of DHT: female
- DHT is produced in sufficient amounts from gestational weeks 7–8 until birth.
- Human chorionic gonadotropin (hCG) stimulates Leydig cells →↑ T
- Feminization of external genitalia completed by approximately 14 weeks.
- Masculinization of external genitalia completed by approximately 16 weeks.
- T, insulin-like 3 ligand, and its receptor (Lgr8) mediate descent of testes.

THREE FACETS OF SEXUAL DIFFERENTIATION

1. Gonadal differentiation
2. Genital differentiation
3. Behavioral differentiation
   - Sexual or gender identity:
     → Sense of oneself as man or woman
     → Established by age 2 ½ years
     → Derived through internalization of social cues based on the external genitalia
       - Patients with 5α-reductase (5αR) deficiency or 17β-hydroxysteroid dehydrogenase (17βHSD) deficiency may change from female to male gender identity at puberty; therefore, there is a *hormonal role* in sexualization of the brain.

SEXUAL DIFFERENTIATION

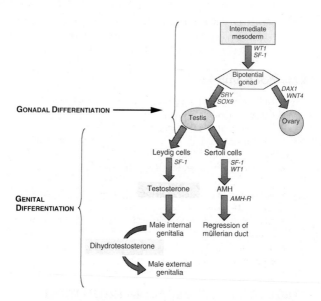

Factors involved in the determination of male sex. HOX, homeobox transcription factor; AMH-R, AMH-receptor; SF-1, steroidogenic factor 1; SOX9, SR homeobox gene (on autosomes); SRY, sex-determining region of the Y chromosome, in Y chromosome, "testis-determining factor"; WT1, Wilms' tumor 1. (Source: Adapted from Federman DD. Three facets of sexual differentiation. *N Engl J Med* 350[4]:323, 2004.)

Sexual Differentiation Timeline

Source: Reproduced with permission from White PC, Speiser PW. Congenital adrenal hyperplasia due to 21-hydroxylase deficiency. *Endocr Rev* 21:245, 2000.

SEXUAL DIFFERENTIATION GONE AWRY

46,XX: Masculinized Female

	Site of Defect
Congenital adrenal hyperplasia	21-Hydroxylase (*CYP21*) deficiency
	11β-Hydroxylase (*CYP11β1*) deficiency
	3β-Hydroxysteroid dehydrogenase (*3βHSDII*) deficiency
Maternal androgen excess	Virilizing adrenal or ovarian tumor
46,XX gonadal dysgenesis	
46,XX true hermaphroditism	

Source: Adapted from Migeon CJ, Wisniewski AB. Human sex differentiation and its abnormalities. *Best Pract Res Clin Obstet Gynaecol* 17(1):1, 2003.

Congenital Adrenal Hyperplasia

- Gonads develop into ovaries; müllerian ducts present; and wolffian ducts regress
- *21-hydroxylase (CYP21)* deficiency: 90% of congenital adrenal hyperplasia [CAH]; salt-losing form of CAH from diminished aldosterone secretion; most common cause of sexual ambiguity and most common cause of endocrine neonatal death; autosomal recessive, chromosome 6p
- *11β-hydroxylase (CYP11β1)* deficiency: 5% of CAH cases; hypertensive form of CAH from excess corticosterone and 11-deoxycorticosterone secretion
- *3β-hydroxysteroid* dehydrogenase *(3βHSDII)* deficiency: least frequent form of CAH; salt-losing form of CAH
- Mechanism of abnormal sexual differentiation: ↑ Cortisol →↑ adrenocorticotropic hormone (ACTH) →↑ adrenal androgens → virilization of external genitalia (fusion of labioscrotal folds, clitoral enlargement), normal ovaries and müllerian ducts
- Only the external genitalia are affected, because differentiation of internal genitalia is completed by the 10th week, whereas the adrenal cortex does not begin functioning until the 12th week.
- Untreated CAH:
  - Pubic hair by age 2–4, then axillary hair → body hair/beard
  - Premature epiphyseal closure
  - Male habitus
  - Acne; deep voice; primary amenorrhea and infertility

Maternal Androgen Excess

- Maternal ingestion of androgenic substances
  - Placenta is unable to aromatize synthetic androgens into estrogens.
- Androgen-producing neoplasia
  - Placenta is able to aromatize T into estrogens, therefore protecting the female fetus from masculinization.
    - → Luteomas secrete DHT, and the placenta is unable to aromatize this, so there is masculinization of female fetus.
    - → Treatment: surgical correction of abnormal external genitalia

46,XX: True Hermaphroditism

- Possess both testicular tubules and ovarian follicles (either separately or together as an **ovotestis**)

- 46,XX is the most common karyotype, although 46,XY and mosaic 45,XO/46,XY chromosome complements also are associated with true hermaphroditism.
- Etiology: unknown
- Internal genitalia depending on gonad of that side
- External genitalia masculinize to varying degrees in utero, depending on the amount of T secreted by the testicular portions of the gonads.

46,XX: Gonadal Dysgenesis (Perrault Syndrome)

- Autosomal recessive associated with sensorineural deafness
- Present as female but fail to achieve female puberty
- Elevated gonadotropins and streak gonads similar to 45,XO
- Differs from 45,XO given absence of multiple congenital malformations

	Site of Defect
Complete/partial gonadal dysgenesis	SRY, SF-1, SOX9, DMRTI/DMRT2, DAX-1, WNT4
Androgen insensitivity syndrome: Complete Partial	Androgen receptor (AR)
5α-reductase deficiency	5α-reductase-2
Leydig cell hypoplasia (Sertoli cell only syndrome)	Genes for LHRH, GnRH receptor, LH, LH receptor
Abnormalities of Leydig cell function	StAR, CYP11A, 3βHSDII, CYP17, 17βHSDII
Isolated persistence of müllerian ducts	AMH or AMH receptors I and II

GnRH, gonadotropin-releasing hormone; LH, luteinizing hormone; AMH, anti-müllerian hormone,
Source: Adapted from Migeon CJ, Wisniewski AB. Human sex differentiation and its abnormalities. *Best Pract Res Clin Obstet Gynaecol* 17(1):1, 2003.

46,XY: UNDERMASCULINIZED MALE

Gonadal Dysgenesis: Complete and Partial Deficiency

- Mutation of several transcription factors (see table above) can block the differentiation of a bipotential gonad into a testis and can result in either complete gonadal dysgenesis (Swyer syndrome, *SRY* deletion) or in partial gonadal dysgenesis.
  - Note: Must make sure there is a müllerian system present (i.e., cervix and uterus)! Otherwise, Swyer syndrome patients

(+ cervix and uterus) could instead be XY with an inactivating mutation in the luteinizing hormone (LH) receptor (also known as Leydig cell hypoplasia) and thus have no cervix/uterus due to the presence of AMH. If the patient is actually the latter, the gonadal removal will most likely benefit from the help of Urology, as these cases can be difficult.

- ○ Note: Swyer syndrome patients will also need their gonads extirpated.
- Ramifications of diminished Leydig cell and Sertoli cell development:
  - ○ **Complete:** no T, therefore, female external genitalia and persistence of müllerian ducts due to absence of Sertoli cell AMH
  - ○ **Partial:** partial masculinization of external genitalia and partial development of wolffian ducts on account of diminished testicular androgens and AMH

Androgen Insensitivity Syndrome

Complete Androgen Insensitivity Syndrome

- First termed "testicular feminization" though now the preferred term is "complete androgen insensitivity syndrome" (CAIS).
- **X-linked recessive mutation** of the AR gene located on chromosome Xq near the centromere; 40% of patients with CAIS have **no family history** of the disorder.
- Incidence: 1 in 60,000
- Bilateral testes located in the abdomen, inguinal area or even labia since testosterone among other factors normally mediates their descent; female external genitalia with blind-ending vagina; because there are normal amounts of AMH, müllerian ducts (uterus and fallopian tubes) regress, but no wolffian ducts (epididymis, vas deferens) develop since there is no ability to respond to T; absence of pubic or axillary hair, labia and clitoris slightly underdeveloped and a blind/short/absent vagina; breast development is female and may be enhanced due to unopposed androgens; average height and weight is of the male phenotype; normal female sexual orientation and generally preserved libido.
- **Gonadectomy after pubertal feminization** (>18 years old) to allow for female secondary sexual characteristics; most frequent testicular tumor = seminoma.

Diagnosis	Incidence
XO, Turner Syndrome	1:2,500
Müllerian Agenesis	1:4,000 – 1:10,000
Androgen Insensitivity (complete)	1:40,000
Swyer Syndrome	1:80,000

Partial Androgen Insensitivity Syndrome (Reifenstein's Syndrome)

- Ambiguous external genitalia with phallic development; normal male T and DHT levels and elevated LH concentrations
- Partial virilization at puberty with female-typical breasts
- The choice of sexual rearing is problematic; gender dysphoria can be seen.
- **Orchiectomy for partial androgen insensitivity syndrome (PAIS) should be done before puberty** but after breast development to prevent virilization
- Note: 17-Ketosteroid reductase deficiency can closely mimic the clinical picture of androgen insensitivity syndrome (AIS), although AIS patients have normal male level serum androgens.

5α-Reductase Deficiency

- 5αR (5α-reductase-2) deficiency = *huevos a los doce* ("eggs at twelve"; in this case, the "eggs" are actually testes)
- **Autosomal recessive**, chromosome 2p
- ↓ Conversion of T into DHT (more potent androgen) leading to undermasculinization of the external genitalia during fetal development, whereas the wolffian ducts develop normally (T dependent)
- Puberty →↑ 5αR-2 that leads to sufficient DHT and pubertal virilization (growth of the phallus, ↑ muscle mass, and deepening of the voice)
- Pseudovagina
- Erections + ejaculations from perineal urethra with normal sperm in adulthood

Leydig Cell Hypoplasia

- Sertoli cell–only syndrome
- Mutation in genes for gonadotropin-releasing hormone (GnRH), GnRH receptor, LH, LH receptor

Abnormalities of Leydig Cell Function

- Mutation in enzymes needed for the biosynthesis of T in Leydig cells (see table)
  - ↓ **Steroidogenic acute regulatory protein (StAR) or CYP11A** → no gonadal or adrenal steroids = *lipoid adrenal hyperplasia*
    - → Female external genitalia
    - → ↓ Adrenal steroids → adrenal crises at birth
  - ↓ **3βHSDII** → inability to metabolize Δ5 steroids (pregnenolone, 17-hydroxypregnenolone, dehydro-epiandrosterone) into Δ4 steroids (progesterone, 17-hydroxyprogesterone [17-OHP], androstenedione)
    - → Usually, other genes can compensate for the 3βHSDII enzyme outside of the gonads and adrenals, so female fetuses are slightly masculinized and male fetuses are markedly undermasculinized at birth.
    - → Salt-wasting due to ↓ cortisol and aldosterone
    - → Also covered in the section on CAH.
  - ↓ **CYP17** → deficient 19-carbon steroids (androgens), 18-carbon steroids (estrogens), and cortisol
    - → Adrenal crisis at birth
    - → Female external genitalia in a 46,XY subject
    - → Note: Isolated 17,20 desmolase deficiency only compromises androgen and estrogen secretion, so that 46,XY individuals present with female-appearing genitalia but no adrenal abnormality (preserved aldosterone and cortisol formation)
  - ↓ **17βHSDIII** → inability to convert androstenedione into T
    - → Lack of androgenic effects during fetal development
    - → Usually present with partial enzyme abnormality and resulting ambiguous genitalia at birth
    - → Marked pubertal masculinization if testes not removed, because several 17βHSD genes are more active at puberty than during fetal life.

Isolated Persistence of Müllerian Ducts: Hernia Uteri Inguinale

- Detected at the time of hernia repair (remnants of a uterus and fallopian tubes are found in the hernia sac)
- May be due to a mutation of *AMH* or AMH receptors
- Normal testes function and masculinized external genitalia

46,XY: True Hermaphroditism

- Possess well-defined seminiferous tubules and ovarian follicles (resulting in **ovotestis** formation)

- Wolffian duct development and degree of masculinization depend on the extent of testicular Leydig cell function.
- Müllerian duct development also depends on the level of Sertoli cell AMH production.

Abnormal Sex Chromosome Complement

- See also Chapter 6, Turner Syndrome, and Chapter 32, Genetic Testing.

Female
45,X (Turner syndrome) and variants
47,XXX ("super female")
46,XY$_p$– or 46,Xi(Y$_q$)
45,X/46,XY
Ambiguous
46,XX/46,XY
Triploidy 69,XXY/69,XYY
Male
47,XXY (Klinefelter's syndrome)
47,XYY
46,XX males

45,X: Turner Syndrome

- Absence of oocytes (streak gonads) is secondary to increased oocyte atresia, not failure of germ cell formation; normal müllerian duct system (lack of AMH) and small female external genitalia
- Incidence: 1 in 5,000 live births
- Etiology: paternal or maternal meiotic nondysjunction; curiously, 80% of liveborn 45,X individuals have lost a *paternal* sex chromosome.
- Approximately ½ of these patients have a 45,X karyotype, with the remaining individuals having a variant of this karyotype (i.e., 46,XX with variable deletions of the long or short arm of an X chromosome).
- Failure of secondary sexual development
- ↓ Estrogen and androgen; ↑ follicle-stimulating hormone (FSH) and LH
- ↑ Relative risk for diabetes, thyroid disease, and essential hypertension, and hypercholesterolemia

- Turner stigmata: growth failure, epicanthal folds, high arched palate, low nuchal hair line, webbed neck, shield-like chest, coarctation of aorta, ventriculoseptal defect, renal anomalies, pigmented nevi, lymphedema, hypoplastic nails, ptosis of the upper eyelid, cubitus valgus, inverted and widely spaced nipples, autoimmune diseases, hypertension, etc. (see Chapter 6, Turner Syndrome)

46,XYp– or 46,Xi(Yq)

- *SRY* gene is located at the tip of the short arm (p) of the Y chromosome; with its deletion, there is complete gonadal dysgenesis with female external genitalia, müllerian duct development, and no wolffian duct.

47,XXY: Seminiferous Tubule Dysgenesis (Klinefelter's Syndrome)

- 47,XXY or 46,XY/47,XXY or 46XnY
- Androgen deficiency
- Fertilization possible using testicular aspirated sperm and intracytoplasmic sperm injection (Ron-El 2000)

Other Anomalies of the Female Genitalia

Imperforate Hymen

- Results in hydrocolpos/hydrometrocolpos
- Treatment: cruciform surgical incision (Note: do not drain with needle only)

Transverse Vaginal Septum

- Incidence: 1 in 80,000 women
- Usually at junction of upper ⅓ and lower ⅔ of vagina
- May present with hydrocolpos/hydrometrocolpos
- Treatment: resection of septa with mucosal reanastomosis

Longitudinal Vaginal Septum

- Frequency: 0.2–0.5/1,000 live births
- Treatment: surgical transection

Vaginal Atresia

- Failure of urogenital sinus to form distal vagina

- Treatment: surgery if there is a cervix, uterus, and fallopian tubes; otherwise, hysterectomy necessary

Müllerian Agenesis or Hypoplasia

- No uterine corpus/cervix, upper vagina
- Treatment: surgical or nonsurgical with vaginal dilators

Incomplete Müllerian Fusion

- Unicornuate, bicornuate, didelphic, septate uteri
- The high number of ectopic pregnancies in both rudimentary horn and tube warrants the removal (laparoscopy) of the rudimentary horn and its tube when diagnosed (Heinonen 1997); unilateral renal agenesis is associated with such anomalies.

Diethylstilbestrol-Associated Anomalies

- Most common = squamous metaplasia and vaginal adenosis
- Rare = clear cell adenocarcinoma of vagina and cervix
- T-shaped endometrial cavity, uterine constrictions, bulbous dilation of lower cervical segment

DIFFERENTIAL

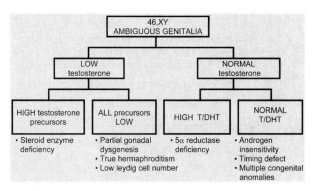

DHT, dihydrotestosterone; T, testosterone. (Source: Adapted from Migeon CJ, Wisniewski AB. Human sex differentiation and its abnormalities. *Best Pract Res Clin Obstet Gynaecol* 17[1]:1, 2003.)

- Laboratory tests
  - **Karyotype** (deletion syndromes; 46,XY; 46,XX/46,XY; 46,XX)
  - Hormone markers of testes:
    - → 3–4 months of age, T ≥ **20 ng/dL** (0.8 nmol/L); AMH ≥10 ng/mL (71.4 nmol/L)
    - → Later childhood, hCG stimulation test → T ≥ **20 ng/dL** (0.8 nmol/L)
  - T precursors:
    - → **Androstenedione, 17-OHP, 17-hydroxypregnenolone**
      - CAH can be identified via a.m. **17-OHP:**
        <200 ng/dL (6 nmol/L) → not NCAH (nonclassic adrenal hyperplasia)
        200–400 ng/dL (6–12 nmol/L) → ACTH testing
        > 400 ng/dL → NCAH
  - Abnormally **high T/DHT ratio** in peripheral blood before and/or after hCG administration to rule out 5αR deficiency
    - → *SRY* **gene** detection via fluorescence *in situ* hybridization (FISH) is a reliable way to determine the genetic sex of a child.
- Further genital evaluation:
  - hCG IM × 5 days: looking for androgen enzyme deficiency by evaluating enzyme precursor/product values
  - Short course of T ointment applied to genital tubercle: check for competency of androgen receptors
  - Send genital skin biopsy for androgen receptor studies.
- Blood/fibroblasts for DNA extraction and analysis using gene probes

MANAGEMENT STRATEGIES

- **46,XX:** usually due to CAH
  - Optimize growth and fertility.
    - → Hydrocortisone (Solu-Cortef) t.i.d. twice the normal secretion rate due to gastric metabolism
    - → Fludrocortisone (Florinef) (9α-fluroro-cortsol acetate), 0.05–0.15 mg PO q.d.
    - → Suppress excess androgens.
    - → Maintain 17-OHP between 500 and 1,000 ng/dL (15 and 30 nmol/L) and androstenedione at 10–50 ng/dL (0.3–1.5 nmol/L).

→ Monitor plasma renin activity for control of salt-water retention.

→ Dual-energy x-ray absorptiometry (DXA) scan every year

→ Monitor growth rate with stadiometer and bone-age measurement.

→ Adrenalectomy is a possible treatment option.

→ Phallus-reducing surgery should be avoided in infancy, and vaginoplasty should wait until adolescence or older.

- 46,XY
- **Female genitalia:** complete lack of masculinization (complete androgen insensitivity syndrome [CAIS], Swyer syndrome, complete T biosynthesis defect)
  - No cosmetic external genitalia surgery except for possible vaginal lengthening
  - Female sex rearing is advised.
  - Estrogen treatment for female sexual characteristics, bone preservation, and menses if uterus is present
    → Gonadectomy?

Note on gonadal tumors: Gonadal tumors are found in 30% of individuals with XY gonadal dysgenesis. These are almost always gonadoblastomas or gonadal dysgerminomas. Neoplasia occurs in patients with CAIS but rarely in those with PAIS or 5αR deficiency. In CAIS, the risk of malignant tumors is small before age 25; after age 25, the risk is approximately 2–5% (Verp and Simpson 1987) with seminomas being the most frequent tumor.

Disorder	Gonads	T Produced?	Puberty?	Gonadectomy before Age 30?
Swyer syndrome	Dysgenesis	No	No	Yes
Luteinizing hormone receptor inactivation mutation	Testes	No	No	Yes
AI	Testes	Yes	Dependent on degree of AI	Yes°

AI, androgen insensitivity.
°For complete AI, allow for pubertal feminization first. For partial AI, allow for breast development first; gonadal tumors occur late in those with AI.

- o **Ambiguous genitalia**
  - → Female sex rearing (with estrogen treatment) is recommended if there is incomplete masculinization and stretched phallus <1.9 cm.
  - → More masculinized infants may be reared as males with T treatment except those with 5αR or 17βHSD deficiency; individuals with 5αR deficiency can be fertile if reared as males.

SUMMARY

	SRY	AMH	T	Gonads	INT	EXT	
XX	—	—	—	♀	♀	♀	
XY	+	+	+	♂	♂	♂	
XO, Turner syndrome	—	—	—	undiff	♀	♀	
Swyer's	—	—	—	dysgen	♀	♀	Gonadectomy
XY-LH-R inact	+	+	—	♂	undiff	♀	Gonadectomy
AI	+	+	+	♂	mild ♂	♀	Gonadectomy after puberty
XY; 5αR def	+	+	+	♂	♂	♀	Huevos a los doce
Müllerian Agen	—	—	—	♀	undiff	♀	♀T levels; no gonadectomy

Agen, agenesis; AI, androgen insensitivity; DHT, dihydrotestosterone; dysgen, dysgenesis; EXT, external; INT, internal; LH-R inact, luteinizing hormone receptor inactivation; AMH, anti-müllerian hormone; SRY, sex determining region of Y; 5αR def, 5α-reductase deficiency; T, testosterone; undiff, undifferentiated.

2
Puberty

DEFINITION

- Puberty is the process of biologic and physical development through which sexual reproduction first becomes possible.
- Progression:
  - thelarche → adrenarche → peak growth spurt → menarche → ovulation

FACTORS AFFECTING TIME OF ONSET

- Genetics (average interval between menarche in monozygotic twins is 2.2 months compared with 8.2 months in dizygotic twins) (McDonough 1998)
- Race: African-American girls enter puberty 1.0–1.5 years before white girls (Herman-Giddens 1997)
- Nutritional status: earlier with moderate obesity; delayed with malnutrition
- General health
- Geographic location: urban, closer to the equator, lower altitudes earlier than rural, farther from the equator, higher altitudes
- Exposure to light: blind earlier than sighted
- Psychological state
- Several pathologic states influence the timing of puberty either directly or indirectly, contributing to a gaussian distribution (Palmert 2001).

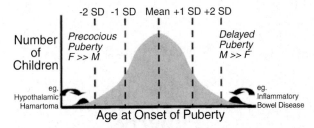

F, female; M, male; SD, standard deviation. (Source: Reproduced with permission from Palmert MR, Boepple PA. Variation in the timing of puberty: clinical spectrum and genetic investigation. *J Clin Endocrinol Metab* 86:2364, 2001.)

PHYSICAL CHANGES DURING PUBERTY

- Thelarche to menarche requires approximately 2–3 years.
  - Accelerated growth
  - Breast budding (thelarche)
  - Pubic and axillary hair growth (pubarche and adrenarche)
  - Peak growth velocity
  - Menarche
  - Ovulation (half the cycles are ovulatory approximately 1–3 years after menarche) (McDonough 1998)
- Adrenarche can precede thelarche.
  - More prevalent in girls of African descent (McDonough 1998)
- Average age of appearance of pubertal events:

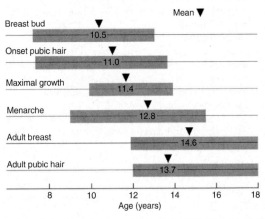

Source: Reproduced with permission from Gordon JD, Speroff L. Abnormal puberty and growth problems. In *Handbook for Clinical Gynecologic Endocrinology and Infertility* 6th ed. Philadelphia: Lippincott–Raven, 2002:199.

Classification	Description
Breast growth	
B1	Prepubertal: elevation of papilla only.
B2	Breast budding.
B3	↑ Breast with glandular tissue, without separation of breast contours.
B4	2nd mound formed by areola.
B5	Single contour of breast and areola.
Pubic hair growth	
PH1	Prepubertal: no pubic hair.
PH2	Labial hair present.
PH3	Labial hair spreads over mons pubis.
PH3	Slight lateral spread.
PH4	Further lateral spread to form inverse triangle and reach medial thighs.

B, breast; PH pubic hair.

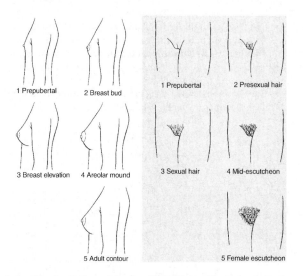

1 Prepubertal   2 Breast bud
3 Breast elevation   4 Areolar mound
5 Adult contour

1 Prepubertal   2 Presexual hair
3 Sexual hair   4 Mid-escutcheon
5 Female escutcheon

Source: Reproduced with permission from Gordon JD, Speroff L. Abnormal puberty and growth problems. In *Handbook for Clinical Gynecologic Endocrinology and Infertility* 6th ed. Philadelphia: Lippincott–Raven, 2002:205.

Pubertal Intervals	Mean ± Standard Deviation (Years)
B2 to peak height velocity	1.0 ± 0.8
B2 to menarche	2.3 ± 1.0
B2–PH5	3.1 ± 1.0
B2–B5 (average duration of puberty)	4.5 ± 2.0

B, breast; PH, pubic hair.

- Tanner staging (Marshall and Tanner 1969)
  - Developed in 1969
  - Based on cohort of 192 British children of low socioeconomic status

MECHANISMS UNDERLYING PUBERTY

- Early in puberty, the sensitivity of the gonadostat to the negative effects of low estradiol (E_2) decreases.
- Late in puberty, maturation of positive E_2 feedback → luteinizing hormone (LH) surges.
- Basal levels of follicle-stimulating hormone (FSH) and LH ↑ throughout puberty due to ↑ gonadotropin-releasing hormone (GnRH) pulse **amplitude** rather than frequency.
- GnRH is produced by less than 2,000 neurons in the brain (Ebling and Cronin 2000).
- Gonadotropin levels during prenatal and postnatal development (Delemarre-van de Waal 2002):

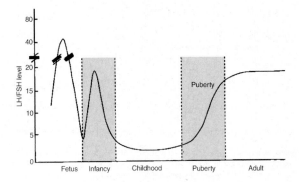

FSH, follicle-stimulating hormone; LH, luteinizing hormone. (Source: Reproduced with permission from Delemarre-van de Waal HA. Regulation of puberty. *Best Pract Res Clin Endocrinol Metab* 16:1, 2002.)

ABERRATIONS OF PUBERTAL DEVELOPMENT

Delayed or Interrupted Puberty

- Difficult to define due to wide variation in normal development (most girls should enter puberty by 13 years).

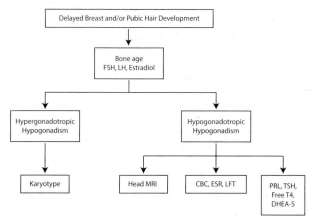

Source: Reproduced with permission from Fritz MA, Speroff L. Normal and Abnormal Growth and Pubertal Development. In Clinical *Gynecologic Endocrinology and Infertility*. 8th ed. Philadelphia: Lippincott Williams & Wilkins, 2011.

Eugonadal (Well-estrogenized [26%]) [Reindollar 1981]

- Müllerian agenesis or Mayer-Rokitansky-Kuster-Hauser syndrome (14%)
  - Second most common cause of primary amenorrhea after gonadal dysgenesis
  - Amenorrhea aside, pubertal development is normal (ovaries present).
  - 11–50% have skeletal abnormalities (scoliosis, klippel-feil anomaly)).
  - 47% have urologic abnormalities (pelvic kidney, duplicated ureters, ureteral diverticulum, bladder exstrophy)
  - Diagnosis: normal pubic hair (to differentiate from androgen insensitivity syndrome), ultrasound reveals absence of uterus and presence of ovaries
  - Treatment: counseling, creation of a neovagina (through dilators or surgery), possible assisted reproductive technology with use of a surrogate
  - Karyotype 46,XX
- Transverse vaginal septum (3%)

- Imperforate hymen (0.5%)
- Androgen insensitivity syndrome (1%)
  - Etiology: receptor absence, receptor defect, postreceptor defect
  - Complete: testes, female external genitalia, blind vaginal pouch, no müllerian derivatives
  - Incomplete (Reifenstein syndrome): partial androgen insensitivity syndrome in 46,XY men who have a predominant male phenotype and variable defects in virilization
  - Diagnosis: absent or significantly reduced pubic hair, male testosterone levels (to differentiate from müllerian agenesis), karyotype
  - Treatment: gonadectomy after breast development, estrogen therapy (ET)
  - Karyotype 46,XY
- Inappropriate positive feedback (7%): constitutional delay

Hypogonadal Hypoestrogenic (25%)

- **Hypergonadotropic hypogonadism** (FSH >30 mIU/mL) (13%)
  - Turner syndrome (45,X or mosaic) (see Chapter 6)
    → Lymphedema at birth, short stature, webbed neck, nevi and heart/kidney/skeletal/great vessel problems, streak ovaries secondary to oocyte depletion
    → Check karyotype, complete physical exam, thyroid function tests (TFTs), glucose, liver function tests, and intravenous pyelogram (IVP) or renal ultrasound.
    → Treatment: growth hormone (GH) for height, then estrogen (gradually increase to 2 × postmenopausal dose); later, progestins; counseling
  - Pure gonadal dysgenesis
    → 46,XX
      - Idiopathic
      - FSH and LH receptor mutations
      - StAR, CYP17 (congenital adrenal hyperplasia [CAH]), and CYP19 mutations
    → 46,XY
      - Swyer syndrome: point mutations in *sex-related* Y (SRY) or deletion of SRY
        ❖ No secondary sexual development, normal (or above average) height, normal but infantile female genitalia
      - Wilms' tumor suppressor gene (WT1) mutations
        ❖ Hypogonadism, nephropathy, and Wilms' tumor
      - Camptomelic dysplasia (SOX9 gene), SF-1, DAX1, Leydig cell hypoplasia

→ Treatment: estrogen, gonadectomy if XY (20–30% risk of developing a gonadal tumor)

→ Must differentiate **Swyer syndrome** (lack of SRY determined by SRY gene testing) from **LH-R mutation,** as the latter involves a more technically challenging surgery because of the lack of landmarks.

- **Hypogonadotropic hypogonadism** (LH and FSH <5 mIU/mL) (12%)
  - Physiologic or constitutional delay is most common, but it is important to exclude other causes.
  - Sustained malnutrition: gastrointestinal (GI) malabsorption, anorexia nervosa, excessive exercise
  - Endocrine disorders: hypothyroidism, Cushing's disease or syndrome, CAH, hyperprolactinemia
  - Hypothalamic-pituitary etiologies
    → Kallmann syndrome (anosmia, hypogonadism)
      - Absence of GnRH neurons in hypothalamus
      - Treatment: hormonal therapy (oral contraceptives)
      - Fertility treatment: gonadotropins or pulsatile GnRH
    → Pituitary insufficiency
    → Pituitary tumors
      - Craniopharyngioma
        ❖ Signs: headache, visual changes, growth failure, delayed puberty
        ❖ Treatment: surgical, radiation treatment

DISORDERS OF PUBERTY

Relative Frequency of Delayed Pubertal Abnormalities

Classification		
Hypergonadotropic hypogonadism	43%	
Ovarian failure, abnormal karyotype	26%	
Ovarian failure, normal karyotype	17%	
46,XX		15%
46,XY		2%
Hypogonadotropic hypogonadism	31%	
Reversible	18%	
Physiologic delay		10%
Weight loss/anorexia		3%
Primary hypothyroidism		1%

(Continues on next page)

(Continued from previous page)

Cushing's syndrome		0.5%
Prolactinomas		1.5%
Irreversible	13%	
GnRH deficiency		7%
Hypopituitarism		2%
Congenital CNS defects		0.5%
Other pituitary adenomas		0.5%
Craniopharyngioma		1%
Malignant pituitary tumor		0.5%
Eugonadism	26%	
Müllerian agenesis	14%	
Vaginal septum	3%	
Imperforate hymen	0.5%	
Androgen insensitivity syndrome	1%	
Inappropriate positive feedback	7%	

Source: Reproduced with permission from Fritz MA, Speroff L. Normal and Abnormal Growth and Pubertal Development. In *Clinical Gynecologic Endocrinology and Infertility*. 8th ed. Philadelphia: Lippincott Williams & Wilkins, 2011.

Precocious Puberty

- Distribution of diagnoses *(other than misdiagnoses)* in 80 girls referred for precocious puberty:

Diagnosis	%
Premature adrenarche	46
Premature thelarche	11
True precocious puberty	11
Early breast development	11
Pubic hair of infancy	6
Premature menses	6
No puberty	6

Source: Adapted from Kaplowitz P. Clinical characteristics of 104 children referred for evaluation of precocious puberty. *J Clin Endocrinol Metab* 89(8):3644, 2004.

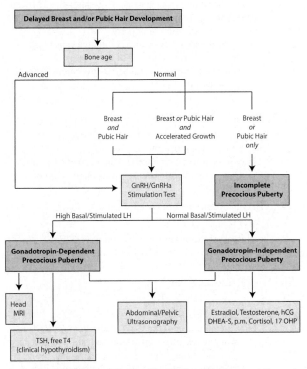

Source: Reproduced with permission from Fritz MA, Speroff L. Normal and Abnormal Growth and Pubertal Development. In *Clinical Gynecologic Endocrinology and Infertility*. 8th ed. Philadelphia: Lippincott Williams & Wilkins, 2011.

- Most patients with Tanner stage 2 breast or pubic hair can be evaluated with only a history, physical exam, and review of the growth chart, without the need for hormonal studies and an estimate of bone age, provided that growth is normal (Kaplowitz 2004).

Definitions

- Traditional precocious puberty: thelarche before 8 years, pubarche before 9 years
- Revised (Kaplowitz 1999):
  - Thelarche or pubarche before 7 years (white girls) or 6 years (African-American girls)

- Thelarche or pubarche after ages 7 (white) or 6 (African American) in conjunction with:
  - → Rapid progression of puberty
  - → Central nervous system (CNS) findings: headache, neurologic symptoms, seizures
  - → Pubertal progression that affects the emotional health of the family or girl

Central or True Precocious Puberty

- Premature stimulation by GnRH (GnRH dependent)
- Idiopathic is the most common.
- CNS tumors, infection, congenital abnormality, trauma, juvenile primary hypothyroidism, Russell-Silver syndrome

Peripheral Precocious Puberty

- GnRH independent
- Peripheral precocious puberty may result in GnRH-dependent precocious puberty if left untreated.

Isosexual Precocious Puberty

- Ovarian cysts
  - McCune-Albright syndrome
    - → Gene mutation of the G protein α-subunit (leads to hormone receptor constitutive activation in absence of the hormone); toxic multinodular goiter, pituitary gigantism, Cushing's syndrome, polyostotic fibrous dysplasia, café au lait spots
    - → Treat with testolactone or letrozole (aromatase inhibitor) (Feuillan 2007)
- Neoplasms (adrenal or gonadal); 11% of girls with precocious puberty have an ovarian tumor.
- Exogenous hormones (drugs, food)

Heterosexual Precocious Puberty

- Prepubertal production of androgens with pubarche, adrenarche, and skeletal maturation
- CAH:
  - 21-Hydroxylase deficiency (**virilizing, salt-wasting, nonclassic**)
  - 3β-Hydroxysteroid dehydrogenase (classic, **nonclassic**)
- Exogenous androgen ingestion
  - Androgen secreting tumor (i.e., adrenal masculinizing tumor)

Pseudoprecocious Puberty

- Premature thelarche
  - Early isolated breast development
  - Normal bone age
  - Close follow-up to rule out true precocious puberty
- Premature adrenarche
  - Early isolated appearance of pubic or axillary hair (polycystic ovary syndrome [PCOS] precursor?)
  - Commonly seen in African-American girls
  - May be associated with excess androgen secretion secondary to deficiencies in other enzymes

Evaluation

- Check bone age (increase in growth or bone age is more dramatic in girls with central precocious puberty or ovarian disease)
- High basal and GnRH-stimulated serum LH concentration stimulated (>6 IU/L) = gonadotropin-dependent precocious puberty

Treatment

- Incomplete precocity:
  - Premature thelarche or adrenarche → reexamine regularly
- GnRH- and gonadotropin-independent precocious puberty:
  - Tumors of adrenal or ovary → surgery
  - McCune-Albright syndrome → testolactone (aromatase inhibitor)
- Central precocious puberty:
  - GnRH-agonist–induced pituitary-gonadal suppression ± GH when growth is slowed too much:
    → Regression of secondary sexual characteristics
    → Cessation of menstrual bleeding
  - Slowing of bone growth

Classification	Female	Male
GnRH dependent (true precocity)		
Idiopathic	74%	41%
CNS problem	7%	26%
GnRH independent (precocious pseudopuberty)		
Ovarian (cyst or tumor)	11%	—
Testicular	—	10%
McCune-Albright syndrome	5%	1%
Adrenal feminizing	1%	0%
Adrenal masculinizing	1%	22%
Ectopic gonadotropin production	0.5%	0.5%

GnRH, gonadotropin-releasing hormone

Source: Reproduced with permission from Speroff L, Glass RH, Kase NG. Abnormal puberty and growth problems. In *Clinical Gynecologic Endocrinology and Infertility*. 6th ed. Philadelphia: Lippincott Williams & Wilkins, 1999.

3

Pediatric and Adolescent Gynecology

PEDIATRIC GYNECOLOGY

Physical Examination Specifics

- Weight and height → assess appropriate growth
- Breast examination → Tanner staging (see Chapter 2, Puberty, for diagram)
- External genitalia

Examination	Notes
Positioning	Frog-legged, knee-chest position (if girl takes a deep breath may actually see the cervix), mother on examination table with child, or child on mother's lap.
Pubic hair	Tanner staging (see Chapter 2, Puberty, for diagram).
Clitoris	Normal is ~3 mm × 3 mm.
Signs of estrogenization	Mucosal tissues in premenarchal child are thin and red.
Perineum	Look for hygiene.
Type of hymen	Crescent or posterior rim, annular, fimbriated or redundant, imperforate, microperforate, cribriform, septate.
Size of hymen opening	Upper limit of normal is 1 mm for each year of age, although controversy exists on method of measurement; standard → perform in prone knee-chest position with gentle traction on labia.
Vagina	Examine under anesthesia if more visualization of the vagina is needed; this allows for vaginoscopy, cultures, and biopsies as indicated.

- Rectoabdominal palpation:
  - Well tolerated if one needs to rule out a foreign body or a pelvic mass
  - Usually, only a small cervix should be palpable; ovaries should not be palpable.
  - With removal of the finger from the rectum, milk the vagina to see if there is a discharge.

Vulvovaginal Problems

Vulvovaginitis

Reasons for Susceptibility to Vulvovaginitis

- Anatomic ($\uparrow$ bacterial colonization of the vagina):
  - Lack of protective fat pads
  - Thin vulvar skin
  - Vaginal mucosa: atrophic, neutral pH
  - Proximity of the vagina to the anus
- Hygiene:
  - Poor hand-washing
  - Inadequate cleansing of the vulva after voiding or bowel movements
  - Irritants against the vulva (i.e., soaps, bubble baths, sand, dirt)
- Foreign body
- Traumatization by tight clothing, irritating materials
- Sexual abuse

Nonspecific Infection

- ~50% of infections; culture shows normal urogenital flora.

Specific Infection

- Respiratory and enteric pathogens are the most common.

Caveats

- Enteric pathogens (*Shigella* and *Yersinia*) can result in bloody discharges.
- *Candida*: very uncommon prepubertal except after antibiotics, in insulin-dependent diabetes mellitus (IDDM), and in immunocompromised states
- Sexually transmitted infections (STIs), herpes simplex virus, human papillomavirus (HPV), and *Trichomonas*:
  - Can be transmitted at birth; consider abuse

- ○ Must culture (not DNA probe) for gonorrhea and chlamydia as these will not hold up in court
- Bacterial vaginosis: usually not associated with discharge but can be associated with abuse or be present in asymptomatic children

Laboratory Tests

- If no discharge and only mild mucus/erythema → try good hygiene instructions
- If persistent discharge → wet prep, Gram's stain, and obtain cultures if suspicious for abuse
- If perianal pruritus → test for pin worms with tape test

Treatment

Specific Vaginitis

- Geared toward the causative organism

Nonspecific Vaginitis

- Initial: discuss hygiene (white cotton underwear, front-to-back wiping, urinating with legs apart), sitz baths, avoid soaps and bubble baths
- Persistent discharge for 2–3 weeks: prescribe broad-spectrum antibiotic (i.e., amoxicillin, amoxicillin/clavulanate, cephalexin, or trimethoprim/sulfamethoxazole) × 10 days; may also try estrogen cream twice daily for 2 weeks, then daily for 2 weeks to thicken the mucosa
- Persistent/recurrent discharge: consider other causes—pelvic abscess, ectopic ureters, small foreign body; consider an examination under anesthesia (EUA)

Lichen Sclerosis

- Symptoms: itching, irritation, soreness, dysuria, vaginal discharge, and bleeding
- Examination: white, atrophic, parchment-like skin; fissures; chronic ulceration or inflammation; the perianal area is often involved
- Treatment:
  - ○ Mild cases: eliminate local irritants, improve hygiene, and use protective ointments (i.e., A & D)
  - ○ More severe cases: high-dose corticosteroids (i.e., clobetasol topical) for 4 weeks with taper to milder topical steroids (although no randomized controlled trial [RCT] as yet)

Condyloma Acuminata

- If <24 months old, may have been transmitted at birth; consider sexual abuse
- Evaluation: abuse history, culture for other STDs, and occasionally EUA to determine extent of disease and to treat
- Treatment:
  - Younger children: surgical with silver sulfadiazine (Silvadene) cream and oral analgesics for postoperative care
  - Older children: may use outpatient trichloroacetic acid (TCA)

Labial Adhesions

- Consists of agglutination of the labia minora; if labia are completely adhered, there can be urinary retention or mucocolpos
- Diagnosis by inspection
- Treat if large area is agglutinated:
  - Usually estrogen cream and gentle separation of the labia while the cream is applied
  - Apply twice daily × 2 weeks → daily × 2 weeks (some need longer treatment)
  - Once open, good hygiene measures and daily application of a daily lubricant such as A & D ointment are needed; if not resolved, EUA and gentle separation may be needed

Vaginal Bleeding

- Look for signs of puberty (i.e., breast development, growth spurt).
- Vaginal bleeding with precocious puberty: see Chapter 2, Puberty
- Vaginal bleeding not associated with precocious puberty:
  - *Neonatal hormone withdrawal:* most common in first 2 weeks of life as a result of withdrawal from maternal estrogen
  - *Vaginitis:* Group A beta-hemolytic streptococcus (usually presents after an upper respiratory illness [URI]) and *Shigella* (only associated with diarrhea 25% of the time)
  - *Lichen sclerosus* (bleeding secondary to trauma)
  - *Condyloma acuminata* (bleeding secondary to trauma)
  - *Trauma:* accidental trauma (i.e., bicycles, slides, bathtub edge) may result in straddle injuries; consider sexual abuse
  - *Foreign body:* often associated with foul-smelling discharge; may try gentle outpatient vaginal irrigation

with a small Foley catheter in the vagina if the patient is cooperative; otherwise, an EUA is necessary

o *Tumors:* sarcoma botryoides

o *Urethral prolapse:* Peak incidence in children is 1:3,000 between ages 5 and 8 years; it is more common in African-American girls. Symptoms include dysuria, bleeding, and pain. Treatment includes sitz baths, topical estrogen or antibiotics, and oral antibiotics. If there is necrotic tissue, then surgery may be indicated. Resolution occurs in 1–4 weeks.

o *Precocious menarche:* cyclical vaginal bleeding without signs of puberty. May be a response to transient production of estrogen by the ovary. Sometimes associated with hypothyroidism. Usually self-limiting in approximately 2–10 months. Follow closely to confirm diagnosis.

Causes of Abnormal Uterine Bleeding in Adolescents

Cause	Notes
Anovulatory cycles	Most common cause in adolescents. Caused by anovulation secondary to an immature H-P-O axis. Maturation of the H-P-O axis takes 2–5 years (Apter 1978).
Coagulation disorders	20–40% of adolescents with heavy menstrual bleeding have coagulation disorders (most common: platelet disorders).
Pregnancy	Always rule out with β-human chorionic gonadotropin test.
Reproductive tract pathology	Rare.
Endocrine disorders	Most common: thyroid disease. PCOS may be difficult to diagnose in adolescents secondary to the relative hyperinsulinemia normally seen at this time and acne from adrenal androgens also common in adolescents. There is no randomized controlled study on the use of metformin in adolescents with PCOS.
Hypothalamic dysregulation	Eating disorders. Excessive exercise. Chronic illness. Psychological stress.

H-P-O, hypothalamic-pituitary-ovarian; PCOS, polycystic ovary syndrome.

ADOLESCENT GYNECOLOGY

Abnormal Uterine Bleeding

Evaluation

- **Complete blood count (CBC)** with platelets; coagulation profile if acute hemorrhage or hemoglobin (Hb) <10%, including a prothrombin time (PT)/partial thromboplastin time (PTT) and bleeding time; additional coagulation evaluation may be considered.
- **Von Willebrand's testing is less accurate** if the patient is taking estrogen.
- **Thyroid-stimulating hormone (TSH), prolactin, androgens**—if endocrine testing is indicated.
- **STI screening if sexually active**
- **Pelvic ultrasound** if high suspicion for anatomic abnormality and pelvic examination is not possible or inadequate.

Treatment

- If irregular bleeding neither heavy nor prolonged, may give reassurance and observe
- If more severe and vaginal bleeding (Hb 10-12 mg/dL): oral contraceptives (OCs) or cyclic progestins
- If acute severe vaginal bleeding (acute blood loss or Hb <10 mg/dL): oral, IM or IV conjugated estrogen (Premarin) or OC taper
- Iron supplementation
- Surgical dilatation and curettage (D&C) is last resort if medical therapy is unsuccessful.

Dysmenorrhea

- Most common gynecologic complaint among adolescents (Klein and Litt 1981)

Primary Dysmenorrhea

- Painful menses in the absence of anatomic pathology; believed to be caused by prostaglandins; most common type of dysmenorrhea in adolescents

Treatment

- First-line treatment is nonsteroidal anti-inflammatory drugs (NSAIDs [i.e., propionic acids, such as ibuprofen and naproxen, and fenamates such as mefenamic acid and

meclofenamate]); may have gastrointestinal (GI) or central nervous system (CNS) side effects.
- If severe dysmenorrhea, start NSAIDs the day before menses or during menses and continue for 1–3 days around the clock
- OCs if unresponsive to NSAIDs.
- If no success with either, consider causes of secondary dysmenorrhea.

Secondary Dysmenorrhea

- Painful menses in the presence of anatomic pathology

Cause	Notes
Endometriosis	See Chapter 16, Endometriosis. In adolescents, gonadotropin-releasing hormone agonists are not used without laparoscopic confirmation of the diagnosis and are generally not used until bone density is maximum (~16 years old). Endometriotic lesions are generally red or clear (early lesions). Advanced endometriosis is rare.
Ovarian cysts	Pelvic ultrasound. Most are functional and resolve spontaneously or with oral contraceptives. Often, these are actually paratubal cysts.
Sexually transmitted infections	Screen all sexually active teens.
Pelvic adhesions	History very helpful. Laparoscopy to diagnose and treat.
Congenital obstructive müllerian anomaly: duplicated uterus (didelphic or septate) with an oblique vaginal septum obstructing one of the cervices → cyclic menses with worsening, severe cyclic dysmenorrhea	In adolescents with severe pelvic pain, a pelvic ultrasound can rule out a müllerian anomaly and collection of blood behind a septum; if an ultrasound is abnormal, magnetic resonance imaging provides the best information concerning anatomy. This anomaly requires surgical correction. Do not drain with a needle, as this may introduce bacteria into the obstructed menstrual blood and result in severe infection or abscess formation. Almost always associated with absence of the kidney on the side with the obstruction.

4
Müllerian Agenesis

SYNONYMS

- Müllerian agenesis (MA)
- Mayer-Rokitansky-Küster-Hauser syndrome
- Vaginal agenesis

DEFINITION

- 46,XX with normal, functioning ovaries; lack of fallopian tubes, uterus, and upper vagina

INCIDENCE

- 1 in 5,000 to 7,000

ANATOMY *(Griffin 1976)*

- Normal external female genitalia
- Normal ovarian function; thus, normal female secondary sexual characteristics
- Absence of fallopian tubes, uterus, internal vagina → some variations in degree of müllerian structure regression; 5% have a uterus
- ⅓ of MA patients have renal anomalies (renal agenesis, malrotations, ectopic kidneys)
- Possible spinal and skeletal anomalies
- Patients usually present with primary amenorrhea; need to differentiate from those with imperforate hymen, transverse vaginal septum, or complete androgen insensitivity syndrome

ANTI-MÜLLERIAN HORMONE

- From Sertoli cells (testes) and granulosa cells (ovaries)
- Likely acts via mesenchyme
- Glycoprotein cleaved into two different protein products:
  - Embryonic testis → larger AMH protein
  - Postnatally → smaller AMH protein (function unknown)
- Target cells may contain the enzyme to cleave the AMH precursor molecule
- AMH receptor is found in SCs, fetal and postnatal granulosa cells, and the mesenchyme around müllerian ducts
- Effects exerted at 8–10 weeks of fetal life
- *Male:* smaller AMH protein elevated for several years after birth, then very low levels during puberty
- *Female:* circulating levels of AMH (large or small form) below limits of assay sensitivity until onset of puberty (but still below fetal levels); possible role in ovarian gametogenesis and useful marker for ovarian reserve in fertility patients

ETIOLOGY

- *AMH gene mutations* may lead to premature AMH production, but this cannot explain the lack of virilization, as AMH causes aromatase suppression that would lead to elevated testosterone levels in a female fetus
- *AMH-receptor gene mutations* may lead to constitutively active AMH receptor

MANAGEMENT

- Nonsurgical or surgical treatment usually delayed until patient expresses desire to initiate sexual activity
- Nonsurgical management (usually preferred) (Bach 2011)
  - Must continue to use dilators in absence of routine sexual intercourse to ensure continued patency
    → *Frank's vaginal dilation technique* (Frank 1938): increasing sizes of vaginal dilators (from 0.5-in. diameter and 4- to 5-in. length up to 1-in. diameter and 4- to 5-in. length):
      - Pressure to vaginal dimple t.i.d. × 20 minutes
        Total time: 6–8 weeks
        Normal sexual function: 76%
    → *Ingram's modified Frank's technique:* bicycle seat stool for constant perineal pressure; total daily time of 2 hours
- Estradiol (E_2) cream for vaginal epithelial transformation

- Surgical management:
  - *Abbe-McIndoe technique* with split-thickness skin graft
  - *Modifications to split-thickness skin graft:* human amnion, peritoneum, segments of colon, gracilis, rectus abdominus, myocutaneous flaps, Interceed
  - *Vecchietti operation/acrylic olive traction device:* continuous pressure to the vaginal dimple (with a plastic "olive") with strings attached laparoscopically to the suprapubic region; this traction device is tightened daily (1 cm/day)
  - Case report of *autologous vaginal tissue transplantation* in a woman with MA (Panici 2007)

5

Septate Uterus

BACKGROUND

- Congenital uterine anomalies resulting from müllerian fusion defects are the most common types of malformations of the reproductive system (Rock and Jones 1977).
- Mechanism of pregnancy loss: implantation into a poorly vascularized, fibrous septum (Fedele 1996b)
- Bicornuate uterus is not generally associated with RPL (Proctor and Haney 2003).

PREVALENCE

Prevalence (%) of Uterine Anomalies:

	General Population	Subfertile	RPL (≥3 losses)
Arcuate	3.9	1.8	6.6
Septate	**2.3**	**3**	**15.4**[a]
Bicornuate	0.4	1.1	4.7[b]
TOTAL (all types of anomalies)	5.5	8	24.5

[a] May have classified arcuate as a diagnosis of septate.
[b] May have classified septate as a diagnosis of bicornuate.
Adapted from Chan YY, Jayaprakasan K, Zamora J et al. The prevalence of congenital uterine anomalies in unselected and high-risk populations: a systematic review. *Hum Repod Update* 17(6):761-771, 2011.

- The incidence of endometriosis was found to be higher in women with a septate uterus compared to without (~26% vs. 15%) (Nawroth 2006)

EMBRYOLOGY

- Müllerian ducts develop by in-folding of the coelomic epithelium overlying the *urogenital ridge,* and, in the absence of anti-müllerian hormone (from Sertoli cells), duct growth proceeds caudally and medially, reaching the *urogenital sinus* to form the müllerian tubercle. Fusion and resorption begin at the isthmus and proceed simultaneously in both the cranial and caudal directions (Muller 1967).

- Failure of fusion → bicornuate uterus; failure of resorption → septate uterus
- Abnormal müllerian differentiation is associated with urologic/renal malformations (up to 30%) (Li 2000); however, because septum resorption usually occurs after urologic development is completed, there is no need to obtain a renal ultrasound in women with septate uteri.

HISTOLOGY

- Contrary to the conventional view that the septum consists of fibrous tissue, there may actually be more muscle fibers in the septum than previously believed (Dabirashrafi 1995).

DIAGNOSIS

Ultrasound

- Septate uterus appears as two cavities without sagittal notching and with a fundal myometrium; intercornual distance usually <4 cm.
  - If the fundal midpoint/indentation is >5 mm above a line joining both ostia → septate uterus (**see part c of diagram**) (Homer 2000).

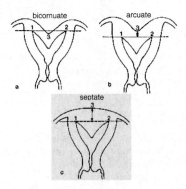

Source: Reproduced with permission from Homer HA, Li TC, Cooke ID. The septate uterus: a review of management and reproductive outcome. *Fertil Steril* 73(1):1, 2000.

Hysterosalpingogram

- Hysterosalpingogram (HSG) cannot reliably differentiate between a septate and a bicornuate/arcuate uterus (55% accuracy).
  - If the angle of divergence of the two uterine cavities seen on HSG is ≤ 75 degrees, the defect is most likely a septate uterus.
  - If the angle of divergence is >75 degrees and <105 degrees, a diagnosis cannot be made.

Magnetic Resonance Imaging

- Accurate, noninvasive means of classification and obtaining information on septal morphometry (proportion of myometrial vs. fibrous tissue) (Carrington 1990)
- If the septum extends to $\geq 30\%$ of the cavity length, it should be resected (Dr. Greg Christman, *personal communication, 2002*).

ADVERSE PREGNANCY OUTCOMES

- Septate uterus is associated with
  - 1st- and 2nd-TM loss (usually between 8–16 weeks; two-thirds in the 1st TM)
  - Premature delivery
  - Abnormal presentation
  - Intrauterine growth restriction
  - Infertility
- Reproductive performance of septate uterus:

	Spontaneous Abortion	Preterm Delivery	Live Birth
Septate	25.5%	14.5%	62.0%

Source: Adapted from Raga F, Bauset C. Reproductive impact of congenital Mullerian anomalies. *Hum Reprod* 12(10):2277, 1997.

INDICATIONS FOR SURGERY

- RCT in women with **unexplained subfertility**: One year live birth rate higher in metroplasty group, 34% vs. 19%, NNT=40 (Mollo 2008)
- RCT is underway in the Netherlands to discern any advantage to metroplasty in women with **recurrent pregnancy**

loss: TRUST (The Randomised Uterine Septum Transsection Trial).
- Consider resection if septate uterus is found in association with adverse reproductive outcome (greater than one loss) or in women >35 years old.

	Miscarriages	**Preterm Delivery**
Untreated septa (pooled data)	79%	9%

PREOPERATIVE PREPARATION

- Schedule surgery during early proliferative phase
- Gonadotropin-releasing hormone (GnRH) agonist is not essential unless there is a wide septum or septum involving the lower third of the cavity and/or cervical canal.

OPERATIVE TECHNIQUE:
RESECTOSCOPE METROPLASTY

- 0- or 12-degree lens preferred
- Dissection complete when
  - Hysteroscope can be moved freely from one cornu to the other without obstruction
  - Both ostia viewed simultaneously
  - Bleeding indicates that incision has reached the myometrium.

- Residual septum <1 cm does not seem to impair outcome (Fedele 1996a).
- Ultrasound is helpful: stop incision when distance = 1 cm between dissection and serosal surface (Querleu 1990).
- Either ultrasound or laparoscopy is necessary to guide surgeon; turn laparoscope light off and observe hysteroscopic transillumination.
- With complete septate uterus, it is recommended that the cervical portion of the septum be spared and the dissection start at the internal os to avoid cervical incompetence. Place a No. 8 Foley catheter into one cavity (prevents leakage of distending medium), inject indigo carmine into this cavity, and enter the other cavity with the resectoscope to incise the septum at the level of the isthmus (see diagram) (Romer and Lober 1997).

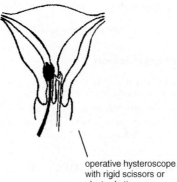

operative hysteroscope
with rigid scissors or
electrode tip

- Resection of the cervical portion may be considered, as the incidence of cervical incompetence after removal of the cervical septum is rare (1 of 43 cases [Homer 2000]; 0 of 10 cases [Nisolle and Donnez 1996]).
- Excision is rarely indicated because the septum typically retracts with incision.

POSTOPERATIVE MANAGEMENT
Hormonal Treatment

- Although, one may use 2.5 mg conjugated estrogen × 25 days and adding 10 mg medroxyprogesterone acetate for the last 10 days OR, estradiol valerate (Delestrogen), 5 mg IM: immediately postoperation
- One prospective, randomized study suggests no benefit (Dabirashrafi 1996).

Intrauterine Splint

- No. 14–16 Foley catheter
- Use 2–7 mL of sterile water for balloon
- Maintain for 5–7 days.
- Doxycycline, 100 mg PO b.i.d., for duration of catheter use
- Nonsteroidal anti-inflammatory may ↓ pain/adhesions (?)

Antibiotics

- Unnecessary unless Foley catheter is left in place

Intrauterine Device

- No role (may increase formation of synechiae)

Follow-Up Examination

- Ultrasound may be satisfactory; some prefer follow-up HSG or office hysteroscopy
- No reason to delay conception for more than two cycles
- Embryo transfer cycle within 9 weeks after resection is not inferior to waiting longer (Berkkanoglu 2008)

TRADITIONAL METROPLASTIES

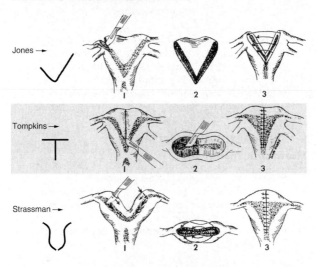

Source: Adapted from Rock JA, Zacur HA. The clinical management of repeated early pregnancy wastage. *Fertil Steril* 39(2):123, 1983.

- Jones, wedge metroplasty; Tompkins, fundal bivalve metroplasty (no excision of septum); Strassman, unification of (bicornuate or didelphic) uterine horns

APPENDIX A

American Society for Reproductive Medicine Classification of Uterine Malformations

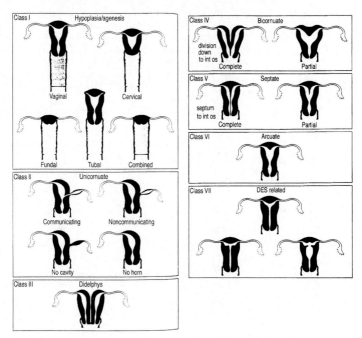

DES, diethylstilbestrol. (Source: Reproduced with permission from Gordon JD, Speroff L. Abnormal puberty and growth problems. In *Handbook for Clinical Gynecologic Endocrinology & Infertility*: Philadelphia: Lippincott-Raven, 2002.)

6

Turner Syndrome

DEFINITION AND PREVALENCE
(Ranke and Saenger 2001)

- Turner syndrome (TS; also known as *Ulrich-Turner syndrome*): combination of characteristic physical features (short stature and gonadal dysgenesis) and complete or partial absence of 2nd X chromosome
- 1 in 2,000 live births
- 1% of 45,X fetuses survive to term
- 10% of spontaneous losses have 45,X karyotype (most common aneuploid in 1st trimester [TM] loss)
- *Not* associated with advanced maternal or paternal age
- http://www.turnersyndrome.org

DIAGNOSIS *(Ranke 2001)*

- *Ultrasound findings:* ↑ nuchal translucency, cystic hygroma, coarctation of aorta ± left-sided cardiac defects, brachycephaly, renal anomalies, polyhydramnios, oligohydramnios, growth retardation
- *Karyotype (chorionic villus sampling [CVS]/amniocentesis):* necessary for diagnosis (confirm postnatally, if clinical suspicion is high and peripheral blood karyotype normal, then 2nd tissue should be checked)
- *Potential mosaic karyotypes:* 45,X/46,XX; 45,X/46,XY (mixed gonadal dysgenesis); 45,X/46,XX; 45,X/46,Xxiq (phenotype, including stature, impossible to predict with mosaics, although there is clearly a ↓ fertility rate with ↑ risk of spontaneous loss and premature ovarian failure)
  - Spontaneous menses have been reported in ~40% of 45,X/46,XX vs. only 2–10% of those with 45,X. FSH ought to be tested and repeated yearly to follow gonadal function longitudinally in mosaic individuals (Fechner 2006)

Indications for a Karyotype

- If *virilization* or *fragment of sex chromosome of unknown origin (X or Y) is present*, probe for Y chromosome (risk of gonadoblastoma → 7–10% [Gravholt 2000]; if present, recommend gonadectomy).
- Any female patient with unexplained growth failure or pubertal delay
- Newborn/infant:
  o Edema of the hands/feet, nuchal folds, left-sided cardiac anomalies, coarctation of aorta, hypoplastic left heart, low hairline, low-set ears, small mandible
- Childhood:
  o Growth velocity <10th percentile for age
  o Markedly ↑ follicle-stimulating hormone (FSH)
  o Cubitus valgus, nail hypoplasia, hyperconvex uplifted nails, multiple pigmented nevi, characteristic facies, short 4th metacarpal, high arched palate
- Adolescence:
  o No breast development by 13 years old, pubertal arrest, or primary or secondary amenorrhea with ↑ FSH
  o Unexplained short stature

PEDIATRIC MANAGEMENT *(Ranke 2001)*

Cardiac Disease

- Congenital heart defects occur in ~30%.
- Left-sided obstructive defects predominate, especially bicuspid aortic valves (30–50%)
- Coarctation of aorta (30%)
  o All TS patients should have an echocardiogram (ECHO) in childhood and repeat ECHO in adolescence (12–15 years old) if no cardiovascular malformation diagnosed earlier; MRI of the aortic arch and valve may be more sensitive than an ECHO.
  o Annual blood pressure (BP) monitoring (upper and lower extremity BPs)

Renal Disease

- Up to 30% have congenital anomalies of the urinary system (most common are horseshoe kidneys and double collecting systems).

- ↑ Risk of hypertension (HTN), urinary tract infection (UTI), hydronephrosis
  - Screening renal ultrasound and additional evaluation as indicated
  - Urine culture every 3–5 years

Thyroid

- 10–30% develop primary hypothyroidism, generally associated with antithyroid antibodies:
  - Thyroid-stimulating hormone (TSH), free thyroxine (FT_4) checked at diagnosis and every 1–2 years

Hearing

- Conductive and sensorineural hearing loss is common in girls with TS (50–90%).
- Otitis media is common and may progress to mastoiditis and/or cholesteatoma formation; typically between 1 and 6 years of age; peak incidence is at 3 years of age.
  - Aggressive treatment of otitis media is appropriate.
  - Short girls with extensive otitis media should be evaluated for TS.

Speech

- Speech problems are common in TS.
  - Referral to ear, nose, and throat (ENT) clinic and speech therapist is recommended.

Vision

- Strabismus, amblyopia, and ptosis are common in TS.
  - Ophthalmology evaluation recommended

Orthopedic

- ↑ Risk of congenital hip dislocation and may be associated with degenerative arthritis of the hips in older women
- 10% develop scoliosis, most commonly in adolescence.
  - Evaluate for orthopedic problems with annual examination.

Weight

- Predisposition for obesity

Lymphedema

- Most common in infancy but may occur at any age
  - Initiation of growth hormone (GH) or estradiol (E_2) may exacerbate; usually controlled with support stockings/ diuretics; surgery not of proven benefit

Glucose Intolerance

- Possible ↑ risk of insulin resistance, but frank diabetes rare
  - Routine glucose tolerance test (GTT) not necessary

Plastic Surgery

- High risk of keloid formation
- Even small elective procedures should be used judiciously.

SHORT STATURE *(Ranke and Saenger 2001)*

- 95% of TS; overall, ↓ final height ~20 cm below female average/ethnic group
- Comprised of mild intrauterine fetal growth retardation (IUGR), slow growth in infancy, delayed onset of childhood growth, growth failure during adolescence
- Short stature may impact socialization and academic achievement
- All girls with short stature (<3% or –2 standard deviations [SD] on growth curves) should have karyotyping if any other features of TS are present. (If –2.5 SD, even in absence of other features, karyotyping should be done.)
- Recombinant human GH and/or steroid treatment (risks/ benefits) should be discussed with the patient and family at an early age, with a goal of achieving normal height before estrogenization. Long-term effects of supraphysiologic insulin-like growth factor-I (IGF-I) are unknown.

PUBERTY MANAGEMENT *(Ranke and Saenger 2001)*

- 90% of TS patients have gonadal failure; however, 30% undergo spontaneous pubertal development and 2–10% have spontaneous menses and potential for pregnancy without medical intervention (Hovatta 1999).
- Check FSH. If it is normal, then perform ultrasound to the ovaries to assess status.
- If gonadal failure is diagnosed and estrogen treatment is required for pubertal development, the dosing and timing should attempt to mimic normal puberty.

- Goal of achieving idealized height first (±GH), followed
  by estrogen therapy slowly initiated for appropriate
  pubertal development (results in closure of epiphyses).
- Transdermal patch applied for 10 days a month leads to
  the development of secondary sexual characteristics and
  uterine growth in a gradual progress mimicking natural
  puberty (Piippo 2004).

ADULT MANAGEMENT

- Transition from pediatric care to adult at approximately
  18 years of age; care should include a gynecologist with
  expertise in fertility

Pubertal induction and maintenance estrogen therapy using transdermal estrogen: a protocol using low growth-promoting doses for 18–24 months[a]

Treatment (months)	Target E_2 (pg/mL)[b]	E_2 dose	Notes
0	3–4	0.1 µg/kg	Consider initiation of puberty at age 11–12 years if there is no breast development Cut and apply a portion of a matrix patch to deliver 0.1 µg/kg E_2. Apply in p.m. and remove in a.m.[c]
6	3–4	0.1 µg/kg	Wear a 0.1 µg/kg equivalent portion of the patch continuously. Change patch as directed (once or twice weekly). Check random E_2 level to ensure E_2 is in target range.
12	6–8	0.2 µg/kg	E_2 levels below this are believed to accelerate growth more than bone maturation.
18	~12	12.5 µg	
24	~25	25 µg	
30	~37	37.5 µg	

(Continues on next page)

(Continued from previous page)

36	~50	50 µg	Start progestin (earlier, if breakthrough bleeding occurs): 200–300 mg micronized oral progesterone for about 12 d/month qhs (causes drowsiness) or 5 mg oral medroxyprogesterone for about 12 d/month.
42	~75	75 µg	
48	50–150	100 µg	Typical adult dose; may not be high enough to protect liver, arteries, etc.

E_2, 17β-Estradiol; qhs, before bedtime.

[a] This protocol is but one of many that can be used. This specific protocol is individualized, depending on patient circumstances and desires. For example, older girls may want to be started at 25 µg.

[b] To convert picograms per milliliter to picomoles per liter, multiply by 3.671. E_2 levels should be monitored using liquid chromatography/tandem mass spectroscopy technology.

[c] Vivelle Dot, matrix transdermal patch, is small and tends to adhere well. One-sixth to one-eighth of a 25 µg patch is approximately 0.1 µg/kg dose.

Source: Adapted from Davenport ML. Approach to the patient with Turner syndrome. *J Clin Endocrinol Metab.* Apr;95(4):1487-95, 2010.

Health care checklist for individuals with TS[a]

Problems	Screening test/ referral	At Dx	Each visit	Yearly	Other
			Timing of Tests		
Hip dislocation	Physical examination (including height, weight, BP, and calculation of BMI)	X	In infancy		
Feeding problems		X	In infancy		
Strabismus		X	4 months to 5 years		
Otitis media		X	All childhood		
Growth failure		X	All childhood		
Pubertal delay		X	Adolescence		
Scoliosis/ kyphosis		X	While growing		
Dysplastic nevi		X	School-age on		
Lymphedema		X	Lifelong		
Hypertension		X	Lifelong		
Needs information/ support	Refer to TSS, other support groups	X			
Structural renal abnormalities	Renal ultrasound	X			
Cardiac abnormality[b]	Examination by cardiologist; EKG; MRI/echo	X			Every 5–10 years

(Continues on next page)

		Timing of Tests			
Problems	Screening test/ referral	At Dx	Each visit	Yearly	Other
Conductive and SNHL	Formal audiology exam	X			Every 1–3 years
Gonadal dysfunction	FSH, LH	X			At ages 0.5–3 and 10–12 years
Strabismus and hyperopia	Formal eye examination	X			At 1–1.5 years
Celiac disease	Serum IgA, TTG IgA Ab	X			q 2–5 years (begin about age 4 years)
Autoimmune thyroid disease	T_4, TSH	X			Begin about age 4 years
Developmental, educational, social problems	Developmental, educational, and/or psychosocial examination	X			Before school entry
Palatal/ occlusive abnormalities	Orthodontic evaluation				At age 7 years
Sexuality; school and/ or work plans	Counseling				Begin about age 10 years
Renal and liver dysfunction	Cr, BUN, LFTs, CBC	X			Begin about age 15 years

(Continues on next page)

Problems	Screening test/ referral	Timing of Tests			
		At Dx	Each visit	Yearly	Other
Metabolic dysfunction	Fasting BG and lipids			Begin about age 15 years	
Low BMD	DXA scan				At about age 18 years
GH action	IGF-I/IGFBP-3			During GH tx	

BG, Blood glucose; BUN, blood urea nitrogen; CBC, complete blood count; cr, creatinine; Dx, diagnosis; DXA, dual-energy x-ray absorptiometry; echo, echocardiogram; EKG, electrocardiogram; IGFBP-3, IGF binding protein-3; LFT, liver function test; SNHL, sensorineural hearing loss; TTG IgA Ab, tissue transglutaminase IgA antibodies; Q, every; tx, treatment.

[a] If the patient has a problem in one or more areas, she will generally be followed up by a specialist in those areas and evaluated more frequently.

[b] If diagnosed in infancy or early childhood, an echocardiogram may be performed. An MRI should be obtained once the child is able to undergo an MRI evaluation without sedation.

Source: Adapted from Davenport ML. Approach to the patient with Turner syndrome. *J Clin Endocrinol Metab.* Apr;95(4):1487-95, 2010.

PREPREGNANCY MANAGEMENT *(Ranke 2001)*

Turner syndrome is a relative contraindication to pregnancy; if there is a cardiac anomaly then this is an absolute contraindication to pregnancy. (ASRM 2012 97:282-4, Fertil Steril)

- Preconceptual ECHO and MRI for evaluation of aortic root, as this can pose a risk for aortic dissection during pregnancy; an aortic size index (ASI) >2 cm/m^2 identifies patients at an increased risk for dissection; the risk of death from aortic dissection/rupture during pregnancy ~2%.
- Evaluate renal function, thyroid, and glucose tolerance.
- Genetic counseling on risks of miscarriage and chromosomal anomalies in offspring
  - Out of 160 pregnancies (Tarani 1998):
    → 29%: Spontaneous loss
    → 20%: Malformed babies (TS, trisomy 21, and so forth)
    → 7%: Perinatal death

- Women with nonfunctional ovaries: adequate hormones 3–4 months before embryo transfer from donated oocytes/embryos to ↑ size and improve blood flow to uterus; ↑ dose of E_2 until endometrium ≥7 mm
- Vaginal delivery possible (if ascending ASI <2 cm/m^2), but cesarean section frequent due to narrow pelvis
- Materno-fetal outcome:
  - Chevalier 2011
    - → Only 40% of pregnancies associated with absolutely normal outcome.
    - → 37.8% incidence of pregnancy-associated hypertensive disorders
    - → 37.5% in utero growth restriction'
  - Hagman 2011
    - → Shorter gestational age but similar size at birth
    - → Chromosomal aberrations no more prevalent than for reference group

COGNITIVE AND ACADEMIC PERFORMANCE *(Ranke 2001)*

- No ↑ prevalence of mental retardation except in those with small ring X chromosome that fails to undergo inactivation
- Impaired nonverbal, visual-spatial processing; defects in social cognition (failure to appreciate subtle social cues)
- Many TS patients achieve high professional status.

7

Menstrual Cycle

CHARACTERISTICS OF THE NORMAL MENSTRUAL CYCLE

- Purpose: renewal of uterine lining to optimize embryonic implantation
- Mechanism: closely coordinated interactions between the hypothalamus, pituitary gland, and ovaries producing cyclic changes in target tissues of the reproductive tract → endometrium, cervix, and vagina
- Fast facts:
  - Mean age of **menarche** = 12.8 years old; mean age of menopause = 51 years old
  - Cycle day 1 = first day of vaginal bleeding; mean duration of flow = 4 ± 2 days
  - Cycle length:
    → Least variable between ages 20 and 40 years (gradual decrease in length)
    → 90% have menstrual cycles between **24 and 35 days;** 15% have 28-day cycles.
  - Irregular cycles: **just after menarche** (2 years); **just before menopause** (3 years)
  - Menstrual cycle phases:
    → **Follicular phase:** variable length (7–21 days); key determinant of cycle length
    → Ovulation
    → Luteal phase: more constant (≥12 days)
- Mitotic division of germ cells ceases by the 7th month of fetal life, although there are data indicating the presence of germline stem cells allowing follicular renewal in the postnatal ovary (Johnson 2004a; Tilly 2012).

- Gonadotropin-releasing hormone (GnRH) pulsatility: frequency and amplitude

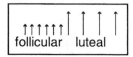

- Follicle-stimulating hormone (FSH) half-life ($t_{1/2}$) = 3 hours; luteinizing hormone (LH) $t_{1/2}$ = 20 minutes

Suggested normal limits for menstrual parameters in the mid-reproductive years

Clinical Dimensions of Menstruation and Menstrual Cycle	Descriptive Terms	Normal Limits (5th–95th Percentiles)
Frequency of menses (days)	Frequent	<24
	Normal	24–38
	Infrequent	>38
Regularity of menses (cycle to cycle variation over 12 months; in days)	Absent	—
	Regular	Variation ±2 to 20 days
	Irregular	Variation greater than 20 days
Duration of flow (days)	Normal	4.5–8.0
	Prolonged	>8.0
	Shortened	<4.5
Volume of monthly blood loss (mL)	Heavy	>80
	Normal	5–80
	Light	<5

Source: Adapted from Munro MG, Critchley HO, Fraser IS. The FIGO systems for nomenclature and classification of causes of abnormal uterine bleeding in the reproductive years: who needs them? *Am J Obstet Gynecol.* Oct;207(4):259-65, 2012.

FOLLICULAR PHASE

- Folliculogenesis occurs in waves and is actually initiated in the last few days of the preceding cycle and may begin a few cycles antecedent (Gougeon 1986).

- Small ↑ in FSH initiates follicular **recruitment,** growth, and development of a cohort of 3–30 follicles.
- Follicle development from primordial to preovulatory stage takes several months.
- **Dominant follicle is selected** from cohort, while remaining ones undergo **atresia;** follicle depletion occurs at a rate of ~1,000/month.
- In the late stages of follicle development, once antral ovarian follicle diameter increases beyond roughly 10 mm, GCs become receptive to LH stimulation, and LH becomes capable of exerting its actions on both theca cells and GCs (Filicori and Cognigni 2001).
- E_2 may not be required for follicular growth and development:

Granulosa Cells	ER-Alpha	ER-Beta
Preantral	–	+++
Antral	+	+++

ER, estradiol receptor; –, absent; +, present; +++, high levels. (Source: Adapted from Rosenfeld CS, Wagner JS, et al. Intraovarian actions of oestrogen. *Reproduction* 122(2):215, 2001.)

- If not E_2, then what is responsible for follicular growth and development?
  - Activin, inhibin, insulin-like growth factors (IGF-I, II), IGF-binding proteins

OVULATION *(Yoshimura and Wallach 1987)*

Timing

- E_2 positive feedback: E_2 (≥200 pg/mL) sustained for >50 hours constitutes the ovarian signal for initiating the midcycle gonadotropin surge, and a small increment of P_4 secreted by the preovulatory follicle is required to establish the normal dimension of the surge. Thus, P_4, although essential for creating a normal gonadotropic surge, operates by synergizing the obligatory action of E_2 (Nakai 1978; Liu and Yen 1983).
- Peak progesterone receptor expression is induced by E_2 and occurs at the time of ovulation.

- The termination of the LH surge may be related to increasing P_4 rather than an exhaustion of pituitary reserves
- Side of ovulation from cycle to cycle is random (Ecochard and Gougeon 2000).
- *Mittelschmerz:* dull, unilateral pain at time of ovulation lasting few minutes to hours; cause may be follicular expansion before ovulation

OVULATION

- *Stigma:* a small protrusion on follicular wall representing site of rupture; present well in advance of ovulation
- Follicle becomes extensively vascularized before ovulation.
- LH/HCG elicit a consistent increase in ovarian KiSS-1 mRNA levels preceding ovulation in the rat ovary (Castellano 2006)
- LH $\rightarrow \uparrow$ prostaglandin $F_2\alpha$ ($PGF_2\alpha$), prostaglandin E_2 (PGE_2), proteolytic enzymes $\rightarrow$ contractions of smooth muscle of follicular wall (therefore, avoid periovulatory prostaglandin synthetase inhibitors in patient seeking pregnancy) (Pall 2001)
- Serum LH peaks at 10-12 hours before ovulation.

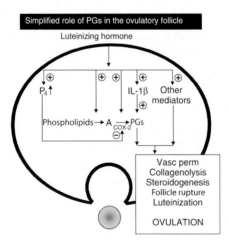

A, arachidonic acid; COX-2, cyclooxygenase-2; Foll, follicle; IL-1β, interleukin-1β; P_4, progesterone; PGs, prostaglandins; Phospholip, phospholipids; Vasc perm, vascular permeability.

LUTEAL PHASE

- Begins with expulsion of the oocyte
- Corpus luteum secretes progesterone (P_4) to prepare endometrium for conceptus; P_4 begins to rise 12 hours before the LH surge.
- P_4 peak secretion is ~1 week after LH surge (parallel ↑ in estrone [E_1], E_2, 17-OHP).
- Degeneration → corpus albicans formation
- Ovulatory women: P_4 >3 ng/mL at midluteal timeframe (Israel 1972)
- Luteoplacental shift in P_4 begins at estimated gestational age (EGA) of 6 weeks and is far advanced by the 9th week of gestation (Csapo and Pulkkinen 1978).

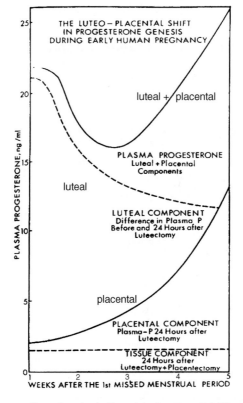

P, progesterone. (Source: Reproduced with permission from Csapo AI, Pulkkinen M. Indispensability of the human corpus luteum in the maintenance of early pregnancy. Luteectomy evidence. *Obstet Gynecol Surv* 33:69, 1978.)

- The ovarian source of P_4 is dispensable >9 weeks. If a lute-ectomy is performed before this time, P_4 replacement can be administered as follows:

Estimated Gestational Age	Progesterone Replacement (until Week 11)
<9 weeks	Crinone 8% q.h.s. per vagina
	Endometrin 100 mg q.h.s. per vagina
	Progesterone in oil 25-50 mg IM q day
	Prometrium (wet tablet per vagina) or progesterone vaginal suppository:
	Non–down-regulated cycles: 200 mg q12 hours
	Gonadotropin-releasing hormone agonist cycles: 200 mg q12 hours
≥9 weeks	None

CYCLIC CHANGES IN TARGET ORGANS

Ovary

Life History of Germ Cells

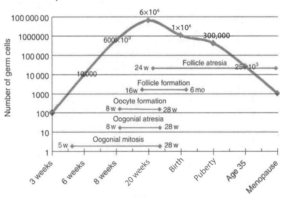

The life history of germ cells. (Source: Reproduced with permission from Oktem O, Urman B. Understanding follicle growth in vivo. *Hum Reprod* 25(12)2944-2954, 2010.)

Adult Ovary

- Each primordial follicle contains a small primary oocyte arrested in prophase of meiosis I (diplotene stage).
- Primordial follicle (50 μm) → primary follicle
  - Independent of gonadotropin control

- *Zona pellucida:* translucent "shell" of glycoproteins surrounding the oocyte; 150 μm diameter
- Within 36 hours of the onset of the LH surge, the oocyte completes the first meiotic division (reducing to 22,X chromosomes), and the first polar body is extruded.
- Second meiotic division occurs if oocyte is fertilized by a spermatozoon.
- If fertilization occurs, hCG is secreted by the developing blastocyst even before implantation (Fishel 1984).

Endometrium

- Of the two layers of the endometrium, only the basal layer is *not* shed at menstruation.
- Follicular phase: basal layer regenerates the superficial layer of compact epithelial cells and intermediate layer of spongiosa; endometrial glands proliferate in response to E_2.
- First histologic sign that ovulation has occurred is the appearance of **subnuclear intracytoplasmic glycogen vacuoles.**
- Luteal phase: glands become coiled and secretory, ↑ vascularity and edema of stroma in response to P_4; late luteal phase: stroma becomes edematous, glandular and endothelial necrosis occurs, and bleeding ensues.
- Noncoagulability of menstruum due to peak in fibrinolytic activity of endometrium (Todd 1973).

Cervix and Cervical Mucus

- $E_2 \rightarrow$ ↑ vascularity and edema of cervix leads to ↑ cervical mucus (10–30× in quantity), which becomes clear, and its elasticity (*spinnbarkeit*) increases; "palm-leaf" arborization ("ferning") becomes marked just before ovulation (secondary to NaCl).
- $P_4 \rightarrow$ mucus thickens, becomes opaque, and loses its elasticity and ability to fern.

Vagina

- Early follicular phase: thin/pale
- Late follicular phase: thickened/dusky (↑ E_2)
- Luteal phase: ↑ percentage of cornified cells; increased numbers of precornified intermediate epithelial cells and polymorphonuclear cells (↑ P_4)

OVARIAN STEROIDOGENESIS

Androgens *(Erickson 1985)*

- Androstenedione (A_4) and testosterone = 19-C steroids
- Serve as substrates for GCs and aromatization
- Major ovarian androgen = A_4; can be converted to testosterone in peripheral tissues

Estrogens *(McNatty 1979)*

- Aromatization in GCs of A-ring and androgens diffusing from theca cells
- Contain 18-C atoms
- Definition: stimulate proliferation of the endometrium

Progesterone

- Follicular phase → 2–3 mg/day
- Midluteal phase → 25–30 mg/day
- Pregnancy at term → 250–300 mg/day
- LH stimulation is required (therefore, those without pituitary function need luteal phase support for fertility).

PROTOCOL FOR HALTING VAGINAL BLEEDING IN HEMATOLOGY/ONCOLOGY/ BONE MARROW TRANSPLANT PATIENT

- Acute induction (no admission warning):
  - If not bleeding at admission:
    - → Ortho-Novum 1/35 → q.d. × 6 weeks without break
    - → GnRH agonist or GnRH antagonist to diminish LH and FSH release
    - → Note: Tell patient she may have menses-like flow after Synarel.
  - If bleeding at admission:
    - → 1st week:
      - ■ Ortho-Novum 1/35:
        - ❖ Light bleeding → 2 pills q.d.
        - ❖ Heavy bleeding → 3 pills q.d.

➔ 2nd week:
  - Taper Ortho-Novum 1/35 by one pill (if bleeding stops before end of 1st week, may go to a more rapid taper)
  - GnRH agonist or GnRH antagonist

➔ 3rd week:
  - Taper Ortho-Novum 1/35 to one pill and give continuously until week 6.
  - Continue GnRH agonist or GnRH antagonist until week 6.

- Elective consolidation or bone marrow transplant (normal blood counts with 3- to 4-week admission warning)
  - GnRH agonist or GnRH antagonist 3–4 weeks before hospitalization; doses:
    - ➔ That is, Lupron 3.75 mg IM q4 weeks; repeat dose 1–2 days after admission

APPENDIX A

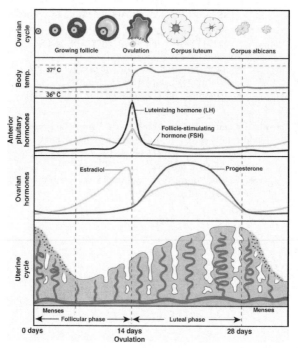

Source: Reproduced with permission from Harris-Glocker, M, McLaren, JF, Role of female pelvic anatomy in infertility. *Clin. Anat.*, 26: 89–96, 2013.

APPENDIX B

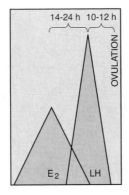

Source: Adapted from Speroff L, Glass RH, et al. Reproduction and the thyroid. In *Clinical Gynecologic Endocrinology & Infertility* (6th Ed): Philadelphia: Lippincott-Raven, 2002.

→ The rise in **serum** LH begins approximately 36 hours before ovulation.

→ The LH surge appears in **urine** 12 hours after it appears in serum.

→ Therefore, a positive urine LH-kit occurs approximately 24 hours (95% CI, 14-26 hours) before ovulation.

→ Ovulation occurs 34–46 hours after hCG administration (**mean of 36 hours**) (Andersen 1995)

APPENDIX C

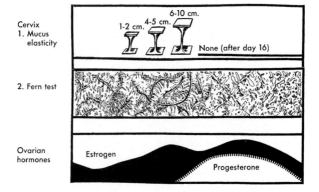

Source: Adapted from Schneeberg NG, ed. *Essentials of Clinical Endocrinology* (1st ed). St. Louis: Mosby, 1970:367.

8

Abnormal Uterine Bleeding

DEFINITION

- Abnormal menstrual volume, duration, regularity, or frequency.

CLASSIC TERMINOLOGY

Term	Menses Pattern
Oligomenorrhea	>35-day cycle length
Polymenorrhea	<21-day cycle length
Menorrhagia	↑ Flow (>80mL blood loss) or duration at regular intervals
Metrorrhagia	Bleeding between periods
Menometrorrhagia	↑ Flow or irregular intervals

PROPOSED NEWER TERMINOLOGY

Abnormal Uterine Bleeding (AUB)
- Heavy menstrual bleeding (AUB/HMB)
- Intermenstrual bleeding (AUB/IMB)

PALM: Structural Causes
Polyp (AUB-P)
Adenomyosis (AUB-A)
Leiomyoma (AUB-L)
　Submucosal myoma (AUB-L$_{SM}$)
　Other myoma (AUB-L$_{O}$)
Malignancy & hyperplasia (AUB-M)

COEIN: Nonstructural Causes
Coagulopathy (AUB-C)
Ovulatory dysfunction (AUB-O)
Endometrial (AUB-E)
Iatrogenic (AUB-I)
Not yet classified (AUB-N)

Source: Reproduced with permission from Management of acute abnormal uterine bleeding in nonpregnant reproductive-aged women. Committee Opinion No. 557. American College of Obstetricians and Gynecologists. *Obstet Gynecol* 121:891–6, 2013.

Clinical Screening for an Underlying Disorder of Hemostasis in the Patient with Excessive Bleeding

Initial screening for an underlying disorder of hemostasis in patients with excessive menstrual bleeding should be structured by medical history (positive screen comprises any of the following):*

1. Heavy Menstrual bleeding since menarche

2. One of the following:

Postpartum hemorrhage

Surgery-related bleeding

Bleeding associated with dental work

3. Two or more of the following symptoms:

Bruising one to two times per month

Epistaxis one to two times per month

Frequent gum bleeding

Family history of bleeding symptoms

*Patients with a positive screen should be considered for further evaluation, including consultation with a hermatologist and testing of von Willebrand factor and ristocetin cofactor.

Source: Reproduced with permission from Management of acute abnormal uterine bleeding in nonpregnant reproductive-aged women. Committee Opinion No. 557. American College of Obstetricians and Gynecologists. *Obstet Gynecol* 121:891–6, 2013.

ENDOMETRIAL SLOUGHING

- Intense spiral arteriole vasoconstriction (prostaglandin [PG] E_2 and $PGF_2\alpha$) precedes the onset of menses (Markee 1940).
- Two theories for the trigger of menstruation:
  1. Apoptosis, tissue regression, and release of PGs and proteases
  2. Spiral arteriole constriction and necrosis
- More than 90% of menstrual blood loss occurs during the first 3 days (Haynes 1977).
- Different hemostatic mechanisms in the endometrium compared to the rest of the body:

  ○ Initial suppression of platelet adhesion

- With ↑ blood extravasation, damaged vessels are sealed by intravascular plugs of platelets and fibrin.
- 20 hours after the onset of menses, hemostasis is achieved by further intense spiral arteriole vasoconstriction.
- 36 hours after the start of menses, tissue regeneration is initiated.

SYSTEMIC ETIOLOGIES FOR ABNORMAL UTERINE BLEEDING

Coagulation disorders

Von Willebrand's disease
Thrombocytopenia
Acute leukemia
Advanced liver disease

Endocrinopathies

Thyroid disease, hyperprolactinemia
Polycystic ovary syndrome or elevated circulating androgens
Cushing's syndrome

Anovulation or oligoovulation

Idiopathic
Stress, exercise, obesity, rapid weight changes
Polycystic ovary syndrome or endocrinopathies as above

Drugs

Contraception: oral/transdermal/vaginal contraceptive, intrauterine device, medroxyprogesterone acetate (Depo-Provera)
Anticoagulants
Antipsychotics
Chemotherapy
Drugs related to dopamine metabolism: tricyclic antidepressants, phenothiazines, antipsychotic drugs

Trauma

Sexual intercourse
Sexual abuse
Foreign bodies
Pelvic trauma

Other

Urinary system disorders: urethritis, cystitis, bladder cancer
Inflammatory bowel disease, hemorrhoids

GENITAL TRACT DISORDERS LEADING TO ABNORMAL UTERINE BLEEDING

	Uterus	**Cervix**	**Vagina**	**Vulva**
Infection	Endometritis	Cervicitis	Bacterial vaginosis, STIs, atrophic vaginitis	STI
Benign	Polyps, endometrial hyperplasia, adenomyosis, leiomyomas	Polyps, ectropion, endometriosis	Gartner's duct cysts, polyps, adenomyosis	Skin tags, condylomata, angiokeratoma
Cancer	Adenocarcinoma, sarcoma	Invasive or metastatic cancer	Vaginal cancer	Vulvar cancer

STI, sexually transmitted infection

CAUSES OF ABNORMAL UTERINE BLEEDING BY AGE GROUP

- Neonates:
  - Estrogen withdrawal

- Premenarchal:
  - Foreign body
  - Adenomyosis
  - Trauma, abuse
  - Vulvovaginitis
  - Cancer (i.e., sarcoma botryoides)
  - Precocious puberty

- Early postmenarche:
  - Anovulation: hypothalamic immaturity (>90% of cases)
  - Stress: exercise induced
  - Pregnancy
  - Infection
  - Coagulation disorder

- Reproductive age:
  - Anovulation
  - Pregnancy
  - Endocrine disorder
  - Polyps/fibroids/adenomyosis
  - Medication related (oral contraceptives)
  - Infection

- o Sarcoma, ovarian
- o Coagulation disorder
- Perimenopausal:
  - o Anovulation leading to unopposed estrogen and hyperplasia
  - o Polyp/fibroid/adenomyosis
  - o Cancer
- Postmenopausal:
  - o Atrophy
  - o Cancer/polyp
  - o Estrogen therapy
  - o Selective estrogen receptor modulators (SERMs)

INITIAL EVALUATION

History

- Timing: frequency, temporal pattern, last menstrual period
- Nature of bleeding: duration, postcoital, quantity, temporal pattern
- Associated symptoms: pain, fever, vaginal discharge, changes in bowel/bladder function
- Pertinent medical history, history of bleeding disorders (family history as well), and medication history
- Changes in weight, excessive exercise, chronic illness, stress

Physical Examination

- General: signs of systemic illness, ecchymosis, thyromegaly, evidence of hyperandrogenism (hirsutism, acne, male pattern balding), acanthosis nigricans
- Pelvic: determine site of bleeding; assess contour, size, and tenderness of the uterus; any suspicious lesions or tumors

Laboratory Testing

- Urine pregnancy test to rule out pregnancy-related bleeding
  - o Serum β-human chorionic gonadotropin (βhCG) if there has been a recent pregnancy (rule out trophoblastic disease)
- Pap smear
- Complete blood count (CBC) and platelets (PLTs)
- Thyroid-stimulating hormone (TSH) to exclude hypothyroidism
- If history of heavy menstrual bleeding since onset of menses, mucocutaneous bleeding, or family history of coagulopathy (Kouides 2000), check prothrombin time (PT)/ partial thromboplastin time (PTT), factor VIII, and von Willebrand's factor antigen (especially in adolescents).

- Liver function tests (LFTs) in those with chronic liver or renal disease
- Determine ovulatory status (see also Chapter 26, Luteal Phase Deficiency)
  - Menstrual cycle charting: >10 days of variance from one cycle to the next suggests anovulatory cycles.
  - Normal menstrual cycle length: 21–35 days
  - Luteinizing hormone (LH) urine predictor kit: False positives include premature ovarian failure, menopause, and polycystic ovary syndrome (on occasion).

Endometrial Biopsy

- See algorithms on pages 79-80 for when to perform an endometrial biopsy.
- Perform in women with unopposed estrogen exposure, regardless of age
- Risk factors for endometrial hyperplasia:
  - Obesity, chronic anovulation, history of breast cancer, SERM (tamoxifen) use
  - Family history of endometrial, ovarian, breast, or colon cancer (Farquhar 1999)
- In a postmenopausal woman, a biopsy is **not necessary** if (a) the lining is ≤ 4 mm or (b) there is no bleeding but a thick endometrial echo is discovered incidentally; however, evaluate all patients on a case-by-case basis (Goldstein 2010)

Summary of Initial Evaluation

History and physical
Pregnancy tests: exclude pregnancy or trophoblastic disease
Pap smear
CBC/PLTs
TSH
LFTs, BUN/Creatinine (those with chronic liver or renal disease)
PT/PTT, factor VIII, von Willebrand's factor antigen (if suspicious history)

Ovulatory status
  Menstrual charting
  Luteal phase length (21–35 days)
  LH urine predictor kits

Transvaginal ultrasound (possible sonohysterogram or hysteroscopy)
Endometrial biopsy based on alogrithms presented on page 79-80.

SECONDARY EVALUATION

- **Transvaginal ultrasound** (TVS) evaluates for structural lesions in the setting of abnormal pelvic examination or normal endometrial biopsy.
  - Can demonstrate a thickened endometrial lining; cannot reliably distinguish between submucous fibroids, polyps, adenomyosis, and neoplastic change
  - Utility of TVS in excluding endometrial abnormalities is more reliable in postmenopausal women.
  - In premenopausal women, TVS should be performed on cycle days 4–6; if returns with an endometrial stripe >5 mm → obtain sonohysterogram.
    - → However, consider sonohysterograms in all women since in 200 premenopausal women with AUB, 16 of 80 women (20%) with an endometrial stripe <5 mm had an endometrial polyp or submucosal fibroid seen on sonohysterogram (Breitkopf 2004).

- **Sonohysterography** allows for careful evaluation of cavity by infusing sterile saline into the endometrial cavity and monitoring by TVS.
  - Can better detect smaller lesions such as polyps or small submucosal fibroids
  - Advantage: higher sensitivity in detecting polyps than TVS alone (94% vs. 75%, respectively) (Kamel 2000)
  - Disadvantage: no tissue for histologic diagnosis

- **Hysteroscopy:** direct visualization of the endometrial cavity
  - Considered the gold standard for the diagnosis of AUB
  - Can biopsy or excise lesions identified

TREATMENT

Acute Vaginal Bleeding

- Attempt oral, intramuscular and, if needed, intravenous 25 mg conjugated equine estrogen
- 30-cc Foley balloon catheter (tamponade) until medical or surgical therapy can be performed
- Resuscitate with blood transfusion as needed
- Surgical: if persistent heavy vaginal bleeding, may consider dilatation and curettage (D&C)

Chronic Menorrhagia

Medical Options

	↓ **Blood Flow (%)**	**Comments**
Oral contraceptives	50	Continuous or cyclic°
Levonorgestrel intra-uterine device	80–90	May induce amenorrhea
Nonsteroidal anti-inflammatory drugs	20–50	Effective in ovulatory women
Cyclic progestin	—	Particularly in anovulatory bleeding
Antifibrinolytics (tranexamic acid, 650 mg, 2 tablets PO t.i.d. during menses, maximum x 5 days	50	Side effects: nausea, leg cramps, potential deep venous thrombosis risk
Gonadotropin-releasing hormone agonists and antagonists	—	Hypoestrogenemia side effects: hot flashes, osteopenia; limit use to 6 months

°May need an oral contraceptive with a more estrogenic progestin, such as ethynodiol diacetate; if the endometrium is thick on oral contraceptives, then a higher dose of progestin (1 mg norethindrone) may be necessary. Could use such an oral contraceptive 3 times a day for a week followed by one pill for the next 3 weeks.

- Tranexamic acid:
    - 650 mg, 2 tablets PO taken 3-times a day (3,900 mg/day) for a maximum of 5 days during monthly menstruation.
    - FDA approved for the treatment of heavy menstrual bleeding.
    - Occupies the lysine binding site of plasmin thus preventing binding to fibrin and preserving/stabilizing fibrin's matrix structure. This leads to maintaining the integrity of the clot.
    - Contraindicated in a woman with increased risk of thromboembolism; should not be used concomitantly with oral contraceptives unless absolutely necessary.

Failed Medical Therapy or Known Surgical Indication

- Hysteroscopy/D&C
- Endometrial ablation
- Approximately 20% of patients require further surgery, with 10% needing hysterectomy.
- Hysterectomy: definitive surgery

Diagnostic Algorithm for Premenopausal Bleeding

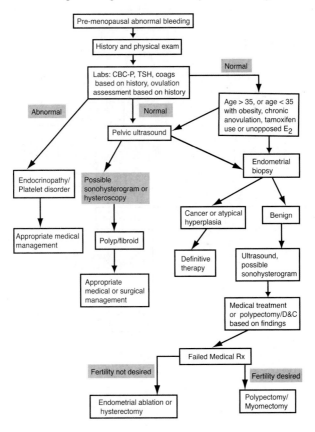

CBC-P, complete blood count/platelets; coags, coagulation disorders; D&C, dilatation and curettage; E$_2$, estradiol; Rx, treatment; TSH, thyroid-stimulating hormone.

Diagnostic Algorithm for Postmenopausal Bleeding

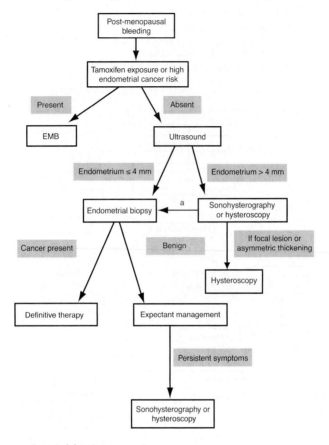

a. >3 mm single layer (premenopause)
   >2 mm single layer (postmenopause)
EMB, endometrial biopsy.

9

Oral Contraceptives

STEROID COMPONENTS OF ORAL CONTRACEPTIVES

Estrogen Component

- Peak serum levels in 1.2–1.7 hours
- **Estradiol** (E_2) is the most potent natural estrogen (E) and the major E secreted by the ovaries. An ethinyl group at the C-17 position makes E_2 orally active. All current oral contraceptives (OCs) use ethinyl estradiol (EE), estradiol valerate or mestranol.
- Physiologic effects:
  - Potentiates the action of the progestogenic component by ↑ progesterone (P_4) receptors
  - Stabilizes the endometrium to minimize breakthrough bleeding (BTB) and irregular shedding

Progestin Component

- Peak serum levels in 2 hours

Synthetic Progestins

- Physiologic effects:
  - Contraception but not an absolute anovulatory effect (with current lower EE doses)
    - → Ovulation still occurs in approximately 3% of cycles (Teichmann 1995).
  - Turbidity of cervical mucus
  - Inhibit *spinnbarkeit*
  - Suppression of endometrial gland maturation → decidualized

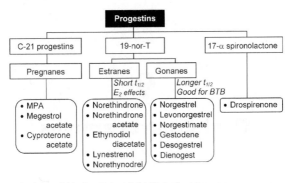

BTB, breakthrough bleeding; E_2, estradiol; MPA, medroxyprogesterone acetate; $t_{1/2}$, terminal half-life.

Generation Terminology

- 1st generation: ≥ 50 μg E
- 2nd generation: <50 μg E and any progestin except norgestimate, desogestrel, or gestodene
- 3rd generation: <50 μg E and progestin of a levonorgestrel derivative (norgestimate, desogestrel, or gestodene)

Potency

- Potency varies depending on the target organ and endpoint being studied.
  - The biologic effect of the various progestational components in current low-dose OCs is approximately the same.

Multiphasic Formulations

- The aim is to alter steroid levels to ↓ metabolic effects and ↓ BTB/amenorrhea.

Mechanism of Action

- E and progestin are given every day for 3 of 4 weeks.
- Contraception efficacy derived from the negative feedback actions of progestins
- Bleeding is controlled by the E component.
- P_4 inhibits luteinizing hormone (LH).
- E inhibits follicle-stimulating hormone (FSH) and LH.
- E minimizes irregular shedding of endometrium and BTB.
- E potentiates the action of progestin via ↑ progestin receptors (thus allowing ↓ progestin dose).

- Efficacy of OCs at inhibiting ovulation based on when OC use was initiated: (Baerwald 2006)
  - follcile diameter of 10 mm, 0/16 ovulations
  - follicle diameter 14 mm, 4/14
  - follicle diameter 18 mm, 14/15

Efficacy

- Annual failure rate = 0.1% (with typical use, 3.0% in 1st year)

PATIENT MANAGEMENT

Practice Guidelines for Oral Contraceptive (OC) Selection: Summary

1 = first choice; combination formulation contains 30–35 µg of ethinyl estradiol except where noted. See footnotes.

2 = second choice; combination formulation contains 30–35 µg of ethinyl estradiol except where noted. See footnotes.

Patient Characteristics	Progestin Androgenic Activity		
	Low	*Medium*	*High*
	Norgestimate Desogestrel Norethindrone 0.4–0.5 mg monophasic	Levonorgestrel triphasic Norethindrone 1 mg monophasic or triphasic Norethindrone acetate 1 mg Ethynodiol diacetate 1 mg	Norgestrel 0.3 mg Norethindrone acetate 1.5–2.5 mg Levonorgestrel 0.15 mg
General Formulation Selections for Women Initiating OC Use			
New start	1	2	
Adolescent	1	2	
Perimenopause	1	2	
Postpartum (lactating)	If no supplemental feedings and no menses, conception unlikely for 2–3 months; if OC desired, progestin-only pill recommended 6 weeks after delivery. Replace with combination pill when supplemental feeding introduced.		
Postpartum (non-lactating) (start at 2 weeks)	1	2	

(Continues on next page)

(Continued from previous page)

Formulation selections in minimizing or managing unwanted OC side effects

Breakthrough bleeding	1[a]	1[a]
Weight gain	1	2
Acne/hirsutism	1	2
Headaches/ common migraine	1[b, c]	2
Nausea	1[b, d]	2
Breast tenderness	1[b, d]	2
Mood change	1[b]	2

Formulation selections in minimizing or managing OC adverse effects

Adverse lipid/ lipoprotein effects (except hypertriglyceridemia)	1	2
Adverse carbohydrate effects	No current formulations have a clinically significant effect on glucose metabolism.	
Adverse thrombotic effects	Thrombotic effects are primarily related to the dose of the estrogen component; use OC containing <50 µg estrogen or other method.	

[a]The lowest incidence of breakthrough bleeding appears to be with formulations containing either levonorgestrel, norgestimate, or desogestrel. If breakthrough bleeding persists after switching from one such formulation to another—and if poor compliance, infection, and other potential problems have been ruled out—placement of the patient on a preparation containing 50 µg estrogen may be considered.

[b]A formulation containing a progestin with low androgenic activity remains the agent of choice, but evidence for a clear advantage in this parameter is lacking; if the problem persists, switching to a pill containing a different type of progestin may be beneficial in some individuals.

[c]If headache occurs exclusively during the pill-free interval, use daily, continuous, combined OCs to avoid cyclicity.

[d]This effect is largely estrogenic and infrequent with low-estrogen-dose OCs. If the problem persists, a 20-µg ethinyl estradiol formulation may be tried.

Practice Guidelines for Oral Contraceptive (OC) Selection: Summary

1 = first choice; combination formulation contains 30–35 µg of ethinyl estradiol except where noted. See footnotes.

2 = second choice; combination formulation contains 30–35 µg of ethinyl estradiol except where noted. See footnotes.

Patient Characteristics	Progestin Androgenic Activity		
	Low	Medium	High
	Norgestimate Desogestrel Norethindrone 0.4–0.5 mg monophasic	Levonorgestrel triphasic Norethindrone 1 mg monophasic or triphasic Norethindrone acetate 1 mg Ethynodiol diacetate 1 mg	Norgestrel 0.3 mg Norethindrone acetate 1.5–2.5 mg Levonorgestrel 0.15 mg

Formulation selections for women with medical conditions

Acne/hirsutism	1	2	
Obesity	1	2	
History of vascular disease (e.g., thromboembolism, coronary artery disease)	Contraindication		
Hypertension (uncontrolled)	Contraindication		
Hypertension (controlled or history of pregnancy-induced)	1	2	
Hypercholesterolemia	1,	2	
Hypertriglyceridemia	OCs contraindicated above 350–600 mg/dL, depending on panel member's view and presence/absence of other factors (e.g., low HDL); with mild elevations, a norgestimate-containing OC may be preferred.		

(Continues on next page)

(Continued from previous page)

Smoker >35 years of age		Contraindication
Smoker 30–35 years of age	1[a]	1 (<50 µg estrogen)
Heavy smoker <30 years of age	1[a]	1 (<50 µg estrogen)
Family history of coronary heart disease	1	2
Classic migraine		Contraindication
Common migraine	1[b]	2
Depression	1[b]	2
Family history of breast cancer	1[b, c]	2
Personal history of breast cancer		Contraindication
Benign breast disease	1[b, d]	2
Diabetes/gestational diabetes	1[b]	2
Antiepileptic drug use	Formulation containing 50 µg estrogen may be preferable.	
Family history of ovarian cancer	1	2
Sickle cell	1	2
Prosthetic heart valve	1	2
Anticoagulant use	1	2
Mitral valve prolapse	1	2

[a]There is no epidemiologic evidence indicating that there is a difference in risk of venous thrombosis in 20-µg ethinyl estradiol and 30–35-µg ethinyl estradiol OCs in smokers as well as nonsmokers.

(Continues on next page)

(Continued from previous page)

[b]A formulation containing a progestin with low androgenic activity remains the agent of choice, but evidence for a clear advantage in this parameter is lacking; if the problem persists, switching to a pill containing a different type of progestin may be beneficial in some individuals.

[c]A formulation containing a progestin with low androgenic activity remains the agent of choice, but there is no evidence that any particular OC formulation is preferable in women with a family history of breast cancer.

[d]OCs generally protect against the development of benign breast disease; a formulation containing a progestin with low androgenic activity remains the agent of first choice.

Practice Guidelines for Oral Contraceptive (OC) Selection: Summary

1 = first choice; combination formulation contains 30–35 µg of ethinyl estradiol except where noted. See footnotes.

2 = second choice; combination formulation contains 30–35 µg of ethinyl estradiol except where noted. See footnotes.

Patient Characteristics	Progestin Androgenic Activity		
	Low	*Medium*	*High*
	Norgestimate Desogestrel Norethindrone 0.4–0.5 mg monophasic	Levonorgestrel triphasic Norethindrone 1 mg monophasic or triphasic Norethindrone acetate 1 mg Ethynodiol diacetate 1 mg	Norgestrel 0.3 mg Norethindrone acetate 1.5–2.5 mg Levonorgestrel 0.15 mg

Formulation Selections in Women for Whom OCs Are Being Considered in Some Measure for Therapeutic Purposes

	Low	Medium	High
Ovulatory dysfunctional uterine bleeding	1	2	
Persistent anovulation	1	2	
Premature ovarian failure	1	2	
Dysmenorrhea	1[a, b]	1[a, b]	
Functional ovarian cysts	1 (monophasic only)		2 (monophasic only)
Mittelschmerz	1[a]	2	

(Continues on next page)

(Continued from previous page)

Endometriosis (pain)	1 (monophasic continuous)	2 (monophasic continuous)
Bleeding with blood dyscrasias	1 (continuous)	2 (continuous)

[a]A formulation containing a progestin with low androgenic activity remains the agent of choice, but evidence for a clear advantage in this parameter is lacking; if the problem persists, switching to a pill containing a different type of progestin may be beneficial in some individuals.

[b]A formulation containing a progestin with low androgenic activity remains the agent of first choice and may be used in combination with a prostaglandin synthetase inhibitor. If dysmenorrhea persists, options include the use of an agent with higher androgenic activity plus a prostaglandin synthetase inhibitor or diagnostic tests to rule out endometriosis.

Source: Adapted from Mishell DR, Darney PD, et al. Practice guidelines for OC selection: update. *Dialogues Contracept* 5(4):7, 1997.

METABOLIC EFFECTS OF ORAL CONTRACEPTIVES

Myocardial Infarction

- 2nd-generation OCs ↑ risk of myocardial infarction by approximately twofold among users even after controlling for cardiovascular risk factors (Tanis 2001)
- Major mortality risk in smokers >35 years of age

Ischemic Stroke

- Risk of ischemic stroke is not significantly different in women with simple migraine (no aura) compared to those with classic migraine (with aura) (Curtis 2002).
- OCs should not be used for women with visual changes or focal neurologic deficits associated with migraines.

Hemorrhagic Stroke *(Farley 1999)*

- <35 years old → no increased risk for OC users
- >35 years old → 2.2-fold higher risk for users (95% confidence interval [CI], 1.5–3.3)

Venous Thromboembolism

- Minimal risk of thrombosis associated with OCs (perhaps on the order of 3 out of 10,000 woman-years vs. 8 out of

10,000 woman-years in pregnancy); most VTE are asymptomatic and never diagnosed making estimates suspect at best.

- If a woman has a known inherited or acquired thrombophilia, or personal history of idiopathic VTE, she should not take an estrogen-containing OC; there is no justification to screen for prothrombotic mutations with a family history of venous thromboembolism (Grimes 2012).

Hypertension

- No ↑ incidence of clinically significant hypertension (HTN) has been reported to date.
- Hormonal contraception can safely be provided based on careful review of medical history and blood pressure (BP) measurement; for most women, no further evaluation is necessary (Stewart 2001).

Carbohydrate Metabolism

- Insulin resistance and glucose changes with low-dose monophasic and multiphasic OCs are so minimal that it is now believed that they are of no clinical significance.
- OCs do not increase risk of diabetes mellitus (DM).

Other Effects

- Minimally ↑ risk of gallbladder disease (secondary to change in composition of bile due to ↑ cholesterol from E), although low-dose OCs have yet to be tested.
- OCs contraindicated in acute or chronic cholestatic liver disease.
- Nausea and breast discomfort are most intense within first few months and usually disappear (lower incidence with low-dose pills).
- No causal association between OCs and weight gain (Gupta 2000).
- ↑ Erythrocyte sedimentation rate (ESR)/total Fe-binding capacity; ↓ prothrombin time (PT)
- Telangiectasia; melasma
- Thick cervical mucus (leukorrhea)
- Rarely → depression/↓ libido
- Progestin-associated side effects: mood swings, depression, fatigue, ↓ libido, weight gain

ORAL CONTRACEPTIVES AND CANCER
Breast Cancer

- After 2 years of use, there is a 40% reduction in fibrocystic disease.
- There are conflicting data, but epidemiologic studies have generally not demonstrated a strong association between OC use and breast cancer. (Lancet 1996)
  - Small increase in relative risk of localized breast cancer if <35 yo associated with current OC use (RR = 1.24; 95% CI, 1.15–1.33) (Lancet 1996).
  - Small increase if <35 yo with past OC use within 1 to 4 years (RR = 1.16; 95% CI, 1.08–1.23) compared with controls.
  - Risk declines after stopping use and disappears within 10 years
  - No difference in risk of breast cancer in ever-users and controls by age 50
- A case-control study on a total of 4,575 women aged 35–64 years found current or former OC use was not associated with a significant ↑ risk of breast cancer: odds ratio (OR), 1.0 (0.8–1.3) (Marchbanks 2002).

Cervical Cancer

- Risk for dysplasia and carcinoma *in situ* ↑ with use of OCs for >1 year; invasive cancer may be ↑ after 5 years of use, reaching a twofold ↑ after 10 years; ↑ risk for both adeno-carcinoma and squamous cell carcinoma (Smith 2003; Green 2003)
- Risk seems to ↓ after discontinuation of OCs.
- Risk in human papillomavirus (HPV)-positive OC users may be related to the 16α-hydroxyestrone metabolite of E_2, which can act as a cofactor with oncogenic HPV to promote cell proliferation (Newfield 1998).
- There are many confounding variables, and the conclusions regarding cervical cancer are not definite.

Endometrial Cancer

- ↓ Cancer risk (adenocarcinoma, adenosquamous carci-noma, and adenoacanthoma) by 56%, 67%, and 72% with use of combined OCs for 4, 8, and 12 years (Schlesselman and Collins 1999).

- Protection persists for up to 20 years after discontinuation (Schlesselman and Collins 1999).
- Lower dose (30–35 µg) OCs provide comparable protection (Weiderpass 1999).

Ovarian Cancer *(Ness 2000; Royar 2001)*

- ↓ Cancer risk (serous, endometrioid, mucinous, and clear cell) by 41%, 54%, and 61% with use of OCs for 4, 8, and 12 years (Schlesselman and Collins 1999).
- Protection persists for up to 20 years after discontinuation (Schlesselman and Collins 1999).
- There may not be a protective effect for those with *BRCA1* or *BRCA2* mutation (Modan 2001), although a case-control study found a 50% ↓ in risk in past OC users with *BRCA* mutations compared with OC nonusers with the same mutations (Narod 1998).

Colorectal Cancer

- OCs may protect women from developing colorectal cancer:
  - Relative risk (RR) of colon cancer in OC users: 0.82 (95% confidence interval [CI], 0.74–0.92) (Fernandez 2001)

Tumors of the Liver

- Evidence for an association between OC use and hepatic adenoma is good, while the evidence for an association with focal nodular hyperplasia and/or hepatocellular carcinoma is inconclusive.

Summary of Oral Contraceptives and Cancer

Form of Cancer	Risk with Oral Contraceptives (OCs)
Breast	Small increase in RR in women under 35 (risk goes from 1/1,000 to 1.24/1,000) but this risk declines after stopping OCs and disappears within 10 years; no increased risk in women over 35 who were current or former users of OCs. Data are inconsistent on the risk of breast cancer associated with OC use in BRCA mutation carriers. (Cibula 2011)
Cervical	OCs used for <5 years did not increase the risk of cervcial cancer but use for 5 to 9 years showed ↑ risk (OR=2.82; 95% CI, 1.46-5.42).
Endometrial	OCs ↓ endometrial cancer by 56%, 67% and 72% with OC use for 4, 8 and 12 years, respectively
Ovarian	OCs ↓ ovarian cancer by 41%, 54% and 61% with OC use for 4, 8 and 12 years, respectively. Protective effects start after just 3 to 6 months of use and continue for up to 20 years after discontinuation. There are protective benefits for women at risk for hereditary ovarian cancer (BRCA1 and BRCA2)

Source: Adapted from Practice Committee of American Society for Reproductive Medicine. Hormonal contraception: recent advances and controversies. *Fertil Steril.* Nov;90(5 Suppl):S103-13, 2008.

ENDOCRINE EFFECTS

Adrenal Gland

- ↑ Free and active cortisol levels but still within normal limits
- Normal pit-adrenal reaction to stress in women taking OCs

Thyroid Gland

- No change in free thyroxine

ORAL CONTRACEPTIVES AND REPRODUCTION

Inadvertent Use while Pregnant

- Initial reports linking OCs to congenital malformations have not been substantiated.
- Risk of a significant congenital anomaly is no greater than the general rate of 2–3%.

Subsequent Fertility

- 98.9% incidence of spontaneous menses or pregnancy within 90 days; median time to return to menses = 32 days (Davis 2008)
- Spontaneous loss: Prospective case-control study revealed that use of OCs for ≥2 years could be associated with a higher risk of miscarriage, or 2.56 (95% CI, 1.16–5.67) (Garcia-Enguidanos 2005).
- Pregnancy outcome: ↑ dizygotic twinning (1.6% vs. 1.0%) in women who conceive soon after cessation of OCs.
- Conception rates at 12 months following discontinuation of various contraceptives.

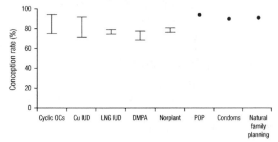

12-month conception rates following discontinuation of various contraceptive methods.

Source: Reproduced with permission from Barnhart K, Schreiber C. Return to fertility following discontinuation of oral contraceptives. *Fertil Steril* 91(3)659-63, 2009.

Oral Contraceptives and Breast-Feeding

- ↓ Quantity and quality of lactation (no matter the starting month), although no impairment of infant growth
- ↓ Lactation at 3.7 months vs. 4.6 months for controls
- It has been argued that the threshold for ovulation suppression is ≥5 feedings for ≥ 65 minutes/day of suckling duration.
- Amenorrheic women who exclusively breast feed at regular intervals, including nighttime, during the first 6 months have the contraceptive protection equivalent to that provided by OCs; with menstruation or after 6 months, the risk of ovulation increases.
- The progestin-only pill has no negative impact on breast milk, and some studies show ↑ milk production.

Initiation of Oral Contraceptives in Postpartum Period

- Rule of 3s for postpartum (pp) contraception:
  - Full breast-feeding → begin OCs *3 months* pp
  - Partial or no breast-feeding → begin in *3rd week* pp

Postpill Amenorrhea

- No evidence that OCs cause secondary amenorrhea
- Women who have not resumed menstrual function within 6 months should be evaluated as any other patient with secondary amenorrhea.

ORAL CONTRACEPTIVES AND INFECTION

Bacterial Sexually Transmitted Infections

- After 12 months of OC use women are protected against pelvic inflammatory disease; mechanism is unknown:
  - Cervical mucus thickening?
  - Decreased menstruum?

Viral Sexually Transmitted Diseases

- No proven association between OCs and human immunodeficiency virus (HIV)/HPV/hepatitis B virus (HBV)

PATIENT MANAGEMENT

Absolute Contraindications

Thrombophlebitis
Markedly impaired liver function
Breast cancer (see table below)
Undiagnosed vaginal bleeding
Pregnancy
Smokers >35 years old
Vascular disease associated with lupus (use progesterone-only pill or intrauterine device)
Current or past deep vein thrombosis or pulmonary embolus

Relative Contraindications

Migraines: ↑ risk stroke vs. improvement
Hypertension in those >35 years old (see table below)
Diabetes mellitus: benefits of contraception outweigh the small risk in diabetic women <35 years old.
Elective surgery: probably less important with today's low-dose pill.
Antiepileptic drugs may ↓ effectiveness of OCs.
Sickle cell disease or sickle C: protection warrants use of low-dose pill.
Gallbladder disease.

American College of Obstetricians and Gynecologists Guidelines	Comment
Smoker >35 years old	Risk unacceptable
Hypertension	
BP controlled	Risk acceptable
BP uncontrolled	Risk unacceptable
History of stroke, ischemic heart disease, or venous thromboembolism	Risk unacceptable
Diabetes	Risk acceptable if no other CV risk factors and no end-organ damage
Hypercholesterolemia	Risk acceptable if low-density lipoprotein <160 mg/dL and no other risk factors
Multiple CV risk factors	Not addressed
Migraine headache	
<35 years old	Risk acceptable
>35 years old	Risk outweighs benefit
With aura	Risk unacceptable
Breast cancer	
Current disease	Risk unacceptable
Past disease, no active disease for 5 years	Risk unacceptable
Family history of breast or ovarian cancer	Risk acceptable

BP, blood pressure; CV, cardiovascular.

Note: Progestin-only pill or intrauterine devices are preferable for those with a prior stroke, diabetes with vascular disease, diabetes and >35 years old, or hypertensive with vascular disease.

Source: Adapted from ACOG Committee on Practice Bulletins-Gynecology. ACOG practice bulletin. No. 73: Use of hormonal contraception in women with coexisting medical conditions. *Obstet Gynecol.* Jun;107(6):1453-72, 2006.

Surveillance

- Monitor blood pressure yearly all other health surveillance as per health recommendations

Proper Pill Taking

- Immediate initiation of the pill ("Quick Start" protocol) improves short-term continuation and compliance in adolescents (Lara-Torre 2002; Westhoff 2007).
- Effective contraception is present during the first cycle of pill use, provided the pills are started ≤5th day of cycle; Sunday starts usually avoid weekend bleeding.
- Postponing a period can be achieved by omitting the 7-day hormone-free interval.
- Missed pills:
  - 1 Missed pill → take 1 pill as soon as possible, then resume.
  - 2 Missed pills (in first 2 weeks) → take 2 pills × 2 days with backup × 7 days.
  - 3 Missed pills (in 3rd week or more than 2 anytime) → backup × 7 days

CLINICAL PROBLEMS

Breakthrough Bleeding

- Most frequently occurs in first few months of use (10–30% in 1st month, 1–10% in 3rd month).
- Occurs due to tissue breakdown as the endometrium adjusts its architecture.
- Take the pill at the same time every day.
- If BTB just before end of pill cycle → stop pills, wait 7 days, and start new cycle.
- Control of BTB: estradiol valerate, 5 mg IM × 1 dose.
- There is no evidence that any specific formulation is significantly superior to any other in terms of the rate of BTB; in general, pills with higher doses of E and lower doses of P_4 have the lowest rates of BTB.
- Try switching from an estrane to a gonane.

Amenorrhea

- There is no harmful, permanent consequence of developing amenorrhea while taking OCs.

- Incidence: 1st year = 1%; several years = 5%

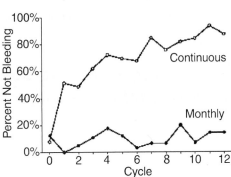

Rates of amenorrhea for continuous vs. monthly oral contraceptives. (Source: Reproduced with permission from Miller L, Hughes JP. Continuous combination oral contraceptive pills to eliminate withdrawal bleeding: a randomized trial. *Obstet Gynecol* 101[4]:653, 2003.)

Weight Gain

- No association between OCs and weight gain

Acne

- Improvement shown (even with 20-μg-EE OCs) (Thorney-croft 1999)
  - $E_2 \rightarrow \downarrow$ gonadotropins + $\uparrow$ sex hormone–binding globulin (SHBG) to bind T
  - Progestins $\rightarrow \downarrow$ gonadotropins + $\uparrow$ T metabolism + $\downarrow$ 5α-reductase

Ovarian Cysts

- OCs do not hasten resolution of functional ovarian cysts; surgery would be warranted if persistent beyond 2–3 cycles (Grimes 2011)
- Functional ovarian cysts occur less frequently in women taking higher-dose OCs.

Drugs Possibly Decreasing Oral Contraceptive Efficacy

- Rifampin/phenobarbital/phenytoin (Dilantin)/primidone/carbamazepine (Tegretol)

Alternative Route of Administration

- One pill per vagina every day if patient has significant nausea/vomiting with the oral route (Coutinho 1993); equivalent efficacy

SUMMARY OF ORAL CONTRACEPTIVE BENEFITS

Control of Menstrual Cycle Symptoms

- ↓ Dysmenorrhea
- ↓ Menorrhagia
- ↓ *Mittelschmerz*
- ↓ Anemia
- Possible ↓ in premenstrual syndrome (PMS)

Beneficial Effects on the Breasts

- ↓ Benign breast disease

Cancer Prevention

- ↓ Endometrial cancer
- ↓ Ovarian cancer

Reduction in Gynecologic Conditions

- ↓ Ectopic pregnancies
- ↓ Endometriosis
- Possibly ↓ fibroids

Other Benefits

- Treatment of androgen excess disorders
- ↑ Bone density
- Possibly ↓ rheumatoid arthritis

PROGESTIN-ONLY PILL

- Ovrette: Neogest: 0.075 mg norgestrel
- Micronor, NOR-QD: 0.35 mg norethindrone

Mechanism of Action

- Endometrium involutes and becomes hostile to implantation; cervical mucus becomes thick and impermeable (within 2–4 hours).

- ~40% ovulate normally.
- Because of the low dose, the minipill must be taken q.d. at the same time of day.
- Immediate return to fertility on discontinuation

Efficacy

- In *motivated women*, the failure rate = that of combination pills.

Pill Taking

- Start on day 1 of menses with 7-day backup.
- If ≥2 missed pills and there is no menstrual bleeding in 4–6 weeks → pregnancy test
- If >3 hours late in taking pill → use backup × 48 hours

Problems

- Bleeding:
  - 40% → normal ovulatory cycles
  - 40% → short, irregular cycles
  - 20% → irregular bleeding/spotting/amenorrhea

Clinical Decisions

- Progestin-only pills are a good choice for
  - Lactating women
  - Women >40 years old
  - Women for whom E is contraindicated (uncontrolled hypertension, nausea with combined oral contraceptives, smokers > 35 years)
  - Women who complain of gastrointestinal (GI) upset/breast tenderness/headaches with OCs
  - Women who have migraines
  - Women with a history of thromboembolic disease.

POSTCOITAL EMERGENCY CONTRACEPTION

- Single act of intercourse 1–2 days before ovulation is associated with the following pregnancy rate:
  - Fertile couples = 8% (Wilcox 1995)
  - Women 19–26 years old = 50% (Dunson 2002)

- The next menses after treatment usually occurs within 1 week before or after the expected date.

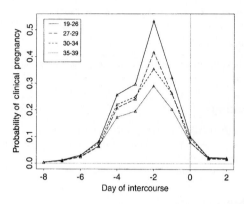

Source: Reproduced with permission from Dunson DB, Colombo M, Baird DD. Changes with age in the level and duration of fertility in the menstrual cycle. *Hum Reprod* 17:1399, 2002.

Product	Estrogen (µg)	Progestin (mg)	Pills per Dose
Ella	–	ulipristal acetate (PR modulator)	1[a]
Next Choice	–	0.75 mg LNG	1[b]
Plan B	–	0.75 mg LNG	1[b]

[a]Treatment consists of two separate doses taken 12 hours apart.
[b]Treatment only once within 5 days of unprotected sex.
PR, progesterone receptor; LNG, levonorgestrel

Intrauterine Device Method

- Copper intrauterine device (IUD) (progestin IUD not studied as yet) may be placed within 5 days of unprotected intercourse.
- Mechanism of action:
  o Toxic to sperm
  o Inflammatory response initiated
- <1% failure rate
- Contraindications: multiple partners, active pelvic infection, victim of sexual assault

ORAL CONTRACEPTIVES FOR OLDER WOMEN (>40 YEARS OLD)

- Pregnancy-related mortality ratios among women ≥40 years of age are five times those of women betwen 25–29 years of age (Kaunitz 2008).
- Healthy, lean, nonsmoking women ≥40 years old can safely use combination oral contraceptives.
- Use low-dose OCs or progestin-only pill
- Note: The E dose in even the low-dose OCs is at least four times greater than necessary for postmenopausal treatment. Hormonal therapy for postmenopausal women (~5–10 µg ethinyl estradiol) is inadequate to prevent ovulation (Gebbie 1995).
- Summary of benefits of OCs in perimenopausal women:
  - Effective contraception
  - Treatment of irregular menses/dysfunctional uterine bleeding (DUB), menorrhagia, and/or dysmenorrhea
  - ↓ Vasomotor symptoms
  - High bone density/fewer fractures (Michaëlsson 1999)
  - Prevention of ovarian and endometrial cancers
  - Treatment of acne

WHEN TO CHANGE TO HORMONE THERAPY FOR POSTMENOPAUSAL WOMEN

- Menopause diagnosis while on OCs: day 8 of pill-free interval (Creinin 1996) → menopausal **if:**
  - FSH:LH >1, or
  - E_2 <20 pg/mL
- Can also empirically switch to hormone therapy (HT) when patient enters mid-50s

OTHER METHODS OF HORMONAL CONTRACEPTION

Levonorgestrel Intrauterine System: Mirena/Skyla

- 52 mg (initial release rate of 20 µg/day) levonorgestrel; approved for up to five years of use
- Effective treatment for heavy menstrual bleeding
- Intrauterine systems (IUS) do not increase the risk of infertility, STI or ectopic pregnancy.

- Women with no current STI and if not engaged in risky sexual behaviors are appropriate candidates for IUS, **regardless of age, parity or history of ectopic pregnancy.**
- ~90% Decreased menstrual blood loss by 1 year
- 5-year pregnancy rate: 0.71/100 women; ectopic rate: 0.02/100 women years
- Immediate insertion following 1st-trimester uterine aspiration resulted in higher rates of IUS use at 6 months without increased risk of complications (Bednarek 2011).
- A low-dose (13.5 mg) levonorgestrel-releasing intrauterine device (Skyla) became available in 2013. It is smaller in size than the Mirena and may be easier to insert in nulliparous women. It is approved for up to three years of use.

Vaginal Ring: NuvaRing

- Progestin: etonogestrel, 120 µg/day (serum: ~1,500 pg/mL), and EE, 15 µg/day (serum: ~20 pg/mL)
- Worn for 3 of 4 weeks and, although off-label (extended-cycle use is under study), if the ring is left for longer than 3 weeks, the user is likely still protected from pregnancy for up to 35 days from the same ring.
- The vaginal ring contraceptive carries the same risks as other combined hormonal contraceptives.

Transdermal

- The transdermal contraceptive patch (Ortho Evra) provides continuous sustained release of 20 µg of ethinyl estradiol and 150 µg of norelgestromin daily; a new patch is applied weekly.
- The risks of the patch are similar to those with combined OCs, except the patch may be associated with more estrogen-related adverse events, including venous thromboembolism since the systemic ethinyl estradiol values are higher with the patch than with a 30 µg pill.
- Possible increased risk of failure in women weighing more than 200 pounds

Implant

- Single-rod subdermal implants containing 68 mg of etonorgestrel include Implanon System and Nexplanon (same as Implanon but in a radiopaque form)
- Placed subdermally in the inner upper arm; good for 3 years

CURRENTLY AVAILABLE ORAL CONTRACEPTIVES

Type (Progestin/estrogen)	Product	Progestin (mg)	Estrogen (µg)	Active tablets
COMBINATION EXTENDED CYCLE Levonorgestrel/EE	Introvale	0.15	30	peach
	Jolessa	0.15	30	pink
	LoSeasonique	0.1	20	84 orange
		—	10	7 yellow
	Lybrel	0.09	20	yellow
	Seasonale	0.15	30	Pink
	Seasonique	0.15	30	84 light blue-green
		—	10	7 yellow
COMBINATION MONOPHASIC Norethindrone/EE	Balziva	0.4	35	light peach
	Brevicon	0.5	35	blue
	Junel 21 1/20	1*	20	yellow
	Junel Fe 1/20	1*	20	yellow
	Junel 21 1.5/30	1.5*	30	pink
	Juenl Fe 1.5/30	1.5*	30	pink
	Loestrin 1/20	1*	20	white
	Loestrin Fe 1/20	1*	20	white
	Loestrin 24 Fe	1*	20	white
	Loestrin 1.5/30	1.5*	30	green
	Loestrin Fe 1.5/30	1.5*	30	green
	Lo Loestrin Fe	1*	10	24 blue
		—	10	2 white
	Norinyl 1 + 35	1	35	yellow-green
	Nortrel 0.5/35	0.5	35	light yellow
	Nortrel 1/35	1	35	yellow
	Ortho-Novum 1/35	1	35	peach
	Ovcon 35 Fe	0.4	35	peach
	Femcon Fe	0.4	35	white
*as norethindrone acetate	Ovcon 50	1	50	yellow
Levonorgestre/EEI	Altavera	0.15	30	peach
	Aviane	0.1	20	orange
	Lessina	0.1	20	pink
	Levien	0.15	30	light orange
	Levlite	0.1	20	pink
	Nordette	0.15	30	light orange
	Portia	0.15	30	pink
Norgestrel/EE	Cryselle	0.3	30	white
	Lo/ovral	0.3	30	white
Ethynodiol diacetate/EE	Kelnor 1/35	1	35	light yellow
Norethindrone/mestranol	Norinylw 1 + 50	1	50	white
	Ortho-Novum 1/50	1	50	yellow
Desogestrel/EE	Apri	0.15	30	rose
	Desogen	0.15	30	white
	Ortho-cepi	0.15	30	orange
Drospirenone/EE	Ocella	3	30	yellow
	Yasmin	3	30	yellow
	Yaz	3	20	light pink
Norgestimate/EE	Ortho-Cyclen	0.25	35	blue
	Sprintec	0.25	35	blue
COMBINATION MONOPHASIC w. FOLATE Drospirenone/EE/levomefolate calcium (as Metafolin) 451 µg plus levomefolate calcium (as Metafolin) 451 µg only (4 light orange tabs)	Beyaz	3	20	24 pink
Drospirenone/EE/levomefolate calcium 451µg plus levomefolate calcium 451 µg only (7 light orange tabs	Safyral	3	30	21 orange

EE = ethinyl estradiol (Rev. 5/2011)

Type (Progestin/estrogen)	Product	Progestin (mg)	Estrogen (µg)	Active tablets
COMBINATION BIPHASIC	Ortho-Novum 10/11	0.5	35	10 white
Norethindrone/EE		1	35	11 peach
Desogestrel/EE	Kariva	0.15	20	21 white
		—	10	5 light blue
	Mircette	0.15	20	21 white
		—	10	5 light blue
COMBINATION TRIPHASIC	Cyclessa	0.1	25	7 light orange
Desogestrel/EE		0.125	25	7 orange
		0.15	25	7 red
	Velivet	0.1	25	7 beige
		0.125	25	7 orange
		0.15	25	7 pink
Norethindrone/EE	Aranelle	0.5	35	7 light yellow
		1	35	9 white
		0.5	35	5 light yellow
	Nortrel 7/7/7	0.5	35	7 light yellow
		0.75	35	7 blue
		1	35	7 peach
	Ortho-Novum 7/7/7	0.5	35	7 white
		0.75	35	7 light peach
		1	35	7 peach
	Tri-Norinyl	0.5	35	7 blue
		1	35	9 yellow-green
		0.5	35	5 blue
Norgestimate/EE	Ortho Tri-Cyclen	0.18	35	7 white
		0.215	35	7 light blue
		0.25	35	7 blue
	Ortho Tri-Cyclen Lo	0.18	25	7 white
		0.215	25	7 light blue
		0.25	25	7 dark blue
	Ti-Previfern	0.18	35	7 white
		0.215	35	7 light blue
		0.25	35	7 blue
	Tri-Sprintec	0.18	35	7 gray
		0.215	35	7 light blue
		0.25	35	7 blue
Levonorgestrel/EE	Enpresse	0.05	30	6 pink
		0.075	40	5 white
		0.125	30	10 orange
	Tri-Levlen	0.05	30	6 brown
		0.075	40	5 white
		0.125	30	10 light yellow
COMBINATION MULTIPHASIC	Natazia	—	3,000	2 dark yellow
Dienogest/Estradiol valerate		2	2,000	5 medium red
		3	2,000	17 light yellow
		—	1,000	2 dark red
COMBINATION ESTROPHASIC	Estrostep Fe	1	20	5 white triangle
Norethindrone acetate/EE		1	30	7 white square
		1	35	9 white round
	Tilia Fe	1	20	5 white triangle
		1	30	7 white square
		1	35	9 white round
	Tri-Legest Fe	1	20	5 light pink round
		1	30	7 light yellow round
		1	35	9 light blue round
PROGESTIN-ONLY	Camila	0.35	none	light pink
Norethindrone	Errin	0.35	none	yellow
	Micronor	0.35	none	lime green
	Nor-QD	0.35	none	yellow

10

Amenorrhea

DEFINITION

- No menses by age 14 in absence of 2° sexual characteristics (primary)
- No menses by age 16 despite 2° sexual characteristics (primary)
- No menses in 3 cycles or 6 months (secondary)

PHYSIOLOGIC AMENORRHEA

- Prepubertal (menarche range, 9–17 years old)
- During lactation and pregnancy
  - When amenorrhea is present in a woman of child-bearing age, must first rule out pregnancy
- Postmenopausal

ETIOLOGY

Primary

- 43% Gonadal failure
- 14% Congenital absence of the vagina
- 10% Constitutional delay

Secondary

- 39% Chronic anovulation
- 20% Hypothyroidism/hyperprolactinemia
- 16% Weight loss/anorexia

DIAGNOSTIC ALGORITHM FOR
AMENORRHEA *(see algorithms in the appendices)*

- Majority of cases accounted for by polycystic ovary syndrome (PCOS), hypothalamic amenorrhea, hyperprolactinemia, and ovarian failure.

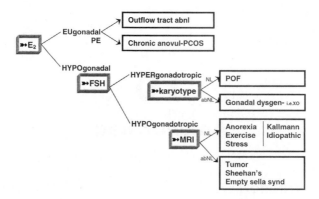

abnl, abnormal; E$_2$, estradiol; FSH, follicle-stimulating hormone; MRI, magnetic resonance imaging; NL, normal; PCOS, polycystic ovary syndrome; PE, pelvic examination; POF, primary ovarian failure; synd, syndrome.

- β-Human chorionic gonadotropin (β-hCG), prolactin (PRL), thyroid-stimulating hormone (TSH), follicle-stimulating hormone (FSH), estradiol (E$_2$)
  → If there is gonadal failure, check karyotype.
  → If PRL is elevated, check insulin-like growth factor I (IGF-I) (rule out growth hormone microadenoma) and magnetic resonance imaging (MRI).
- Genital examination:
  → Blind or absent vagina with breast development usually indicates müllerian agenesis, transverse vaginal septum, or androgen insensitivity syndrome.

Vaginal Agenesis vs. Androgen Insensitivity Syndrome

	Mayer-Rokitansky-Kuster-Hauser Syndrome	Complete Androgen Insensitivity Syndrome
Vagina	Absent	Absent
Pubic hair	Present	Absent
Breasts	Present	Present
Gonads	Ovaries	Testes
Uterus	Absent	Absent
Karyotype	46,XX	46,XY
Other anomalies (renal, cardiac)	Increased	Not increased

DISTRIBUTION OF CAUSES OF PRIMARY AMENORRHEA

Primary Amenorrhea

Definition

- Absence of menses by 16 years old in the presence of normal secondary sexual development (breasts)
- Menarche within 5 years after breast development if that occurs before age 10

Category	Frequency (%)
No breast development: high FSH	**43**
45,X and variants	27
46,XX	14
46,XY	2
Breast development (eugonadal)	**30**
Müllerian agenesis	15
PCOS	7
Vaginal septum	3
Cushing and thyroid disease	2
Imperforate hymen	1
Androgen insensitivity	1
CAH	1
No breast development: low FSH	**27**
Constitutional delay	14
Prolactinomas	5
Kallmann syndrome	5
Stress, weight loss, anorexia	2
Other central nervous system disorder	1

FSH, follicle-stimulating hormone.
Source: Adapted from Reindollar RH, Byrd JR, McDonough PG. Delayed sexual development: a study of 252 patients. *Am J Obstet Gynecol* 140(4):371, 1981.

Mnemonic for Primary Amenorrhea Differential: XMAS

Diagnosis	Incidence
XO, Turner Syndrome	1:2,500
Müllerian Agenesis	1:4,000 – 1:10,000
Androgen Insensitivity (complete)	1:40,000
Swyer Syndrome	1:80,000

DISTRIBUTION OF CAUSES OF SECONDARY AMENORRHEA

Secondary Amenorrhea

Definition

- Absence of menses for 3 cycles or months
- Oligomenorrhea <9 cycles/year
- Most commonly → PCOS, hypothalamic amenorrhea, hyperprolactinemia, and ovarian failure

Category	Frequency (%)
Low or normal FSH	**67.5**
Chronic anovulation (PCOS)	28
Nonspecific hypothalamic	18
Weight loss/anorexia/stress	15.5
Pituitary tumor/empty sella	2
Hypothyroidism	1.5
Sheehan syndrome	1.5
Cushing syndrome	1
High prolactin	**13**
High FSH: Gonadal failure	**10.5**
46,XX	10
Abnormal karyotype	0.5
Anatomic	**7**
Asherman syndrome	7
Hyperandrogenic states	**2**
Ovarian tumor	1
Nonclassic CAH	0.5
Undiagnosed	0.5

Source: Adapted from Reindollar RH, Novak M, Thos SP, et al: Adult-onset amenorrhea: a study of 262 patients. *Am J Obstet Gynecol* 155(3):531, 1986.

Intrauterine Synechiae (Asherman Syndrome)

- Ovarian function is normal. Amenorrhea is caused by intrauterine adhesions that obliterate the uterine cavity. Adhesions usually secondary to an induced abortion or postpartum curettage complicated by endometritis and intrauterine scarification. More common after pregnancy due to ↓ estrogen. Those with normal-appearing endometrium above the level of obstruction on transvaginal ultrasound are likely to have successful hysteroscopic treatment and resumption of menses (Schlaff and Hurst 1995).
- Four out of seven patients undergoing uterine artery embolization were subsequently found to have intrauterine adhesions (Honda 2003).
- American Society of Reproductive Medicine (ASRM) classification of intrauterine adhesions (see page 112).

Causes of Intrauterine Adhesions

%	Antecedent Event
46	Hysteroscopic resection of multiple fibroids
40	Retained products of conception
39	Recurrent miscarriage
31	Late (fibrotic villi and no blood vessels) spontaneous miscarriage D&C
31	Hysteroscopic resection of single fibroid
23	Postpartum D&C (2nd–4th week)
13	Elective abortion D&C
7	Infertility
7	Hysteroscopic metroplasty
6	Early (villi contain blood vessels) spontaneous abortion D&C
4	Postpartum D&C (anytime)
3	Post-cesarean delivery
2	Secondary amenorrhea

Source: Adapted from March CM. Asherman's syndrome. *Semin Reprod Med.* Mar;29(2):83-94, 2011.

Incidence after a D&C following "X" spontaneous losses

%	Number
16	One
14	Two
32	Three or more

Source: Adapted from Friedler S, Margalioth EJ, Kafka I, et al. Incidence of post-abortion intra-uterine adhesions evaluated by hysteroscopy—a prospective study. *Hum Reprod.* Mar;8(3):442-4, 1993.

PROGESTIN WITHDRAWAL TEST

- Indirectly reflects hypothalamic-pituitary-ovarian activity. Patients with adequate endogenous estrogen bleed within 3–5 days after medication, indicating adequate endogenous estrogen stimulation of the endometrium. However, this is an inaccurate test, as there may be enough extragonadal estrogen present to allow for endometrial growth and, hence, withdrawal bleed. High false-positive (Rarick 1990) and false-negative (Nakamura 1996) rates.

APPENDIX A

Algorithm for Amenorrhea

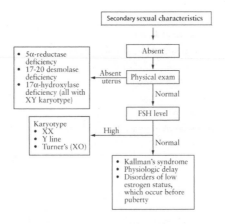

Source: Adapted from Schillings WJ, McClamrock HD, Amenorrhea. In *Berek & Novak's Gynecology. 14th ed.* Berek JS, ed. Philadelphia: Lippincott Williams & Wilkins, 2007.

APPENDIX B

Algorithm for Amenorrhea

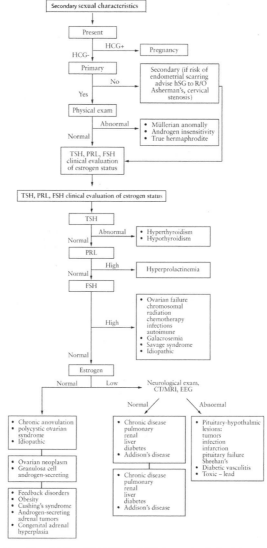

Source: Adapted from Schillings WJ, McClamrock HD, Amenorrhea. In *Berek & Novak's Gynecology. 14th ed.* Berek JS, ed. Philadelphia: Lippincott Williams & Wilkins, 2007.

APPENDIX C

American Society for Reproductive Medicine Classification of Intrauterine Adhesions

Patient's Name _____ Date _____ Chart # _____

Age _____ G _____ P _____ Sp Ab _____ VTP _____ Ectopic _____ Infertile Yes _____ No _____

Other Significant History (i.e. surgery, infection, etc.) _____

HSG _____ Sonography _____ Photography _____ Laparoscopy _____ Laparotomy _____

Extent of Cavity Involved	<1/3	1/3 - 2/3	>2/3
	1	2	4
Type of Adhesions	Filmy	Filmy & Dense	Dense
	1	2	4
Menstrual Pattern	Normal	Hypomenorrhea	Amenorrhea
	0	2	4

Prognostic Classification

	HSG* Score	Hysteroscopy Score
Stage I (Mild) 1-4	_____	_____
Stage II (Moderate) 5-8	_____	_____
Stage III (Severe) 9-12	_____	_____

*All adhesions should be considered dense

Additional Findings: _____

_____

_____

_____

Treatment (Surgical Procedures): _____

_____

_____

_____

Prognosis for Conception & Subsequent Viable Infant*

_____ Excellent (> 75%)

_____ Good (50-75%)

_____ Fair (25%-50%)

_____ Poor (< 25%)

*Physician's judgment based upon tubal patency

Recommended Followup Treatment: _____

_____

_____

DRAWING

HSG Findings

Hysteroscopy Findings

Source: Reproduced with permission from The American Fertility Society classifications of adnexal adhesions, distal tubal occlusion, tubal occlusion secondary to tubal ligation, tubal pregnancies, mullerian anomalies and intrauterine adhesions. *Fertil Steril* 49(6):944, 1988.

11

Exercise-Induced Amenorrhea

DEFINITION

- Hypothalamic amenorrhea arising from a combination of energy drain, caloric deprivation, and/or exercise intensity

PATHOPHYSIOLOGY

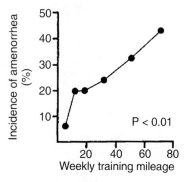

Correlation between training mileage and amenorrhea (Source: Reproduced with permission from Feicht CB, Johnson TS, et al. Secondary amenorrhoea in athletes. *Lancet* 2[8100]:1145, 1978.)

- Hypogonadotropic hypoestrogenemia is often associated with the "female athlete triad" (Otis 1997).
- Amenorrhea may persist in up to 30% despite improved BMI and diminished exercise.
- The percentage contribution of weight loss and dietary restrictions to the syndrome of exercise-induced amenorrhea (EIA) is controversial:
  - EIA may occur with a relative caloric deficiency due to ↓ nutritional intake for the amount of energy expended (Laughlin and Yen 1996).
  - A disrupted energy balance, accompanied by ↓ triiodothyronine (T_3) levels and loss of diurnal release of leptin from adipose cells, may lead to EIA (Laughlin and Yen 1997).

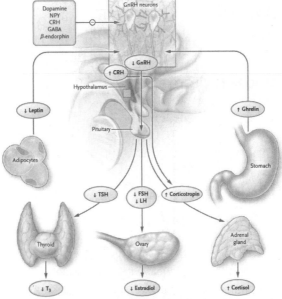

Source: Reproduced with permission from Gordon CM. Clinical practice. Functional hypothalamic amenorrhea. *N Engl J Med.* Jul 22;363(4):365-71, 2010.

- High-intensity exercise shifts estrogen metabolism from 16α to C-2 hydroxylation, which forms catecholestrogens that disrupt gonadotropin-releasing hormone (GnRH) pulsatility (i.e., ↓ GnRH secretion).

- Likelihood of developing EIA:

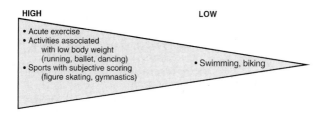

- Swimmers tend to have higher body weight and increased luteinizing hormone (LH) and dehydroepiandrosterone sulfate (DHEA-S) secretion (more polycystic ovary syndrome [PCOS]-like).
- In women who exercise at recreational levels (i.e., running ~12–15 miles/week): 16% prevalence of anovulatory cycles despite regular (26–32 days) intervals of menses (De Souza 1998).

CONSEQUENCES

- Menstrual disturbances
- Infertility
- Vaginal and breast atrophy
- ↓ Bone mineral density (lumbar spine)
- ↑ Total cholesterol

EVALUATION

- Diagnosis of exclusion
- Similar workup as for primary and/or secondary amenorrhea: human chorionic gonadotropin (hCG), prolactin (PRL), thyroid-stimulating hormone (TSH), and free thyroxine to rule out both primary and central hypothyroidism, follicle-stimulating hormone (FSH), estradiol, free testosterone and dehydroepiandrosterone sulfate to rule out hyperandrogenism, anatomic evaluation, dual-energy x-ray absorptiometry (DXA) scan—use a Z-score when examining the BMD (a Z-score ≤1.0 in an athlete requires evaluation as they tend to have higher BMD (by 5–15%).
- MRI of the brain is not necessary in women with presumed hypothalamic amenorrhea and absence of neurological symptoms.

TREATMENT

General

1. ↓ Exercise
2. ↑ Caloric intake (generally need to gain 4.4 lbs higher than the weight at which menses was lost); >45 kcal/kg of lean body mass/day may be required to increase BMD; protein intake should be at least 1 g/kg of body weight.
3. Estrogen therapy (i.e., oral contraceptives [OCs]) (estradiol [E_2] will ↓ bone resorption) (Rickenlund 2004) although several RCTs did not show a significant increase in bone density (Gordon 2010) likely due to the persistent energy imbalance.
4. Calcium: 1,000–1,500 mg/day (diet + 1 g supplemental calcium)
5. Vitamin D: 400–800 IU/day
6. Vitamin K: 60–90 µg/day

- Although estrogen deficiency is the basis for the amenorrhea in EIA, nutritional factors may contribute. No randomized controlled study of estrogen treatment in athletes has been published.
- Recalcitrant low bone remodeling rate may explain the suboptimal response to antiresorptive agents such as estrogen and bisphosphonates (not recommended due to the unknown effects on a fetus from bisphosphonates which reside in the bone for 10 years).

Infertility

1. ↓ Exercise
2. ↑ Caloric intake
3. Exogenous gonadotropins (FSH + LH)

- Clomiphene citrate or aromatase inhibitors tend to be ineffective due to a baseline hypoestrogenic state.

12
Ectopic Pregnancy

INCIDENCE *(Lipscomb 2000)*

- 2% of pregnancies (1992); 9% of pregnancy-related deaths (5/10,000)
- Recurrence risk: approximately 15%

ETIOLOGY

- Tubal disease
  - In histologic sections of ectopic sites, there was a 45% incidence of pelvic inflammatory disease.
- Gonadotropin therapy
- Ratio of ectopic pregnancies (EPs) to all pregnancies:
  - All women—1:50
  - Copper intrauterine device (IUD)—1:16
  - Levonorgestrel IUD—1:2

DIAGNOSIS *(extrauterine pregnancy)*

- Signs and symptoms of eccyesis: severe abdominal pain (90%), vaginal spotting (80%), amenorrhea (80%), pelvic mass on examination (50%) (Pisarska 1998)
- Most common location: ampullary region of tube (80%), isthmic (12%), fimbria (6%)

Human Chorionic Gonadotropin

- 0.79 mIU human chorionic gonadotropin (hCG) per cell per day approximately 2 weeks after fertilization (Braunstein 1973)
- hCG produced 8–9 days after ovulation by cytotrophoblasts (for corpus luteum rescue)
- βhCG normally 100 mIU/mL at time of missed menses

- Levels rise in curvilinear fashion until plateau at 100,000 mIU/mL by 10 weeks.
- βhCG 1,000 mIU/mL at term

Gestational Age	↑ β-Human Chorionic Gonadotropin over 48 Hours
<41 days	103%
41–56 days	33%
57–65 days	5%

- Linear increase early in pregnancy: mean doubling time for viable intrauterine pregnancy (IUP) = 48 hours (only ⅓ of EPs)
- hCG half-life (t½) = 1 day
- 90% of EPs have βhCG <6500 mIU/mL.
- Normal IUP should show at least 53% βhCG in 48 hours (Barnhart 2004b); the rate of increase in hCG is similar in multiple and single gestations.
- If hCG >3,000 mIU/mL then one should use ultrasound findings and not hCG curves.
- With suspected miscarriages, a rate of decline **<21% after 2 days** or 60% after 7 days suggests retained trophoblasts or an EP (Barnhart 2004a).
- If βhCG <1,000 mIU/mL → 88% of abnormal pregnancies (regardless of location) resolve without methotrexate (MTX).
- Note: Beware of the false-positive serum hCG due to heterophile antibodies (Cole 1998).
- Of 18 brands, **First Response, Early Result** is the test most likely to detect a pregnancy at the time of the missed menses (best to include faintly discernible results and at extended reading time of 10 minutes) (Cole 2004).

Progesterone (McCord 1996)

- Serum progesterone (P_4) stays relatively constant from the 5th to 10th week of pregnancy, then ↑ (Tulchinsky and Hobel 1973).
- Single serum P_4 can be used as a screen for EP; it cannot be used to rule out an EP, however.

Progesterone (ng/mL)	Intrauterine Pregnancy (%)	Spontaneous Abortion (%)	Ectopic Pregnancy (%)
>25	—	—	2
20.0–24.9	—	—	4
<5.0	**0.16**	85	14
<2.5	0	—	—

Source: Adapted from McCord ML, Muram D, Buster JE, et al. Single serum progesterone as a screen for ectopic pregnancy: exchanging specificity and sensitivity to obtain optimal test performance. *Fertil Steril* 66:513, 1996.

ULTRASOUND

GS = 2 mm	4 weeks estimated gestation age
GS ≥10 mm	+ Embryo
GS ≥17 mm	+ Fetal cardiac activity (5 weeks)

GS, gestational sac.

- Discriminatory βhCG value for transvaginal sonography (TVS) → >2,000 mIU/mL
- Nonviability if (–) fetal cardiac activity associated with:
  - GS >17 mm or βhCG >30,000 mIU/mL
  - Presence of visible adnexal mass cannot be considered diagnostic of EP if βhCG <2,000 mIU/mL unless a yolk sac, fetal pole, or FCA can be seen; otherwise, may just be a corpus luteum cyst.

Dilatation and Curettage

- If βhCG <2,000 mIU/mL and abnormal βhCG rise, dilatation and curettage (D&C) eliminates the possibility of administering MTX unnecessarily to a patient with a nonviable IUP (Ailawadi 2005).
- Rising or plateau of βhCG values 12–24 hours after D&C or manual vacuum aspiration is diagnostic of an EP; minimal hCG drop one would expect is ↓20% 12–24 hours later

Laparoscopy

- More of a therapeutic tool (linear salpingostomy vs. salpingectomy) than diagnostic

MEDICAL TREATMENT *(Buster and Pisarska 1999)*

- MTX-folate antagonist that inactivates dihydrofolate reductase leading to ↓ tetrahydrofolate (essential cofactor in DNA and RNA synthesis during cell division).
- Single-dose MTX: 91.5% success (although ~20% require more than one course of treatment)
- History of a previous EP is an independent risk factor for failure (18.6%) of systemic MTX, but failure is not affected by previous treatment modality (salpingectomy, salpingostomy, MTX) (Lipscomb 2004).
- Dose: MTX, 50 mg × m^2; m^2 = body surface area (BSA) (http://www.halls.md/body-surface-area/bsa.htm)
- 24% of patients using the single-dose MTX approach receive ≥2 doses (Lipscomb 2005).
- Indications/contraindications to MTX:

Indications

Unruptured

Ectopic mass <3.5 cm (exceptions noted)

No FCA (exceptions noted)

β-Human chorionic gonadotropin <5,000 mIU/mL (exceptions noted)

Contraindications

Abnormal labs (creatinine [>1.3 mg/dL], liver function tests [>50 IU/L])

Alcoholism, alcoholic liver disease, chronic liver disease

Preexisting blood dyscrasias

Active pulmonary disease

Peptic ulcer disease

Hepatic, renal, or hematologic dysfunction

Height	Surface area	Weight
cm 200 — 79 in	⌐ 2.80 m²	kg 150 ⌐ 330 lb
78		145 — 320
195 — 77	— 2.70	140 — 310
76		135 — 300
190 — 75	— 2.60	130 — 290
74	— 2.50	125 — 280
185 — 73		— 270
72	— 2.40	120 — 260
180 — 71	— 2.30	115 — 250
70		
175 — 69	— 2.20	110 — 240
68		105 — 230
170 — 67	— 2.10	100 — 220
66		
165 — 65	— 2.00	95 — 210
64	— 1.95	90 — 200
160 — 63	— 1.90	
62	— 1.85	85 — 190
155 — 61	— 1.80	— 180
60	— 1.75	80 — 170
150 — 59	— 1.70	75 —
58	— 1.65	— 160
145 — 57	— 1.60	70 — 150
56	— 1.55	
140 — 55	— 1.50	65 — 140
54	— 1.45	
135 — 53	— 1.40	60 — 130
52	— 1.35	
130 — 51	— 1.30	55 — 120
50		
125 — 49	— 1.25	50 — 110
48	— 1.20	— 105
120 — 47	— 1.15	45 — 100
46	— 1.10	— 95
115 — 45		— 90
44	— 1.05	40 — 85
110 — 43	— 1.00	— 80
42	— 0.95	35 — 75
105 — 41		— 70
40	— 0.90	
cm 100 — 39 in	⌐ 0.85 m²	kg 30 — 66 lb

Body surface area nomogram. (Source: Reproduced with permission from DiSaia PJ and Creasman WT. Epithelial ovarian cancer. In *Clinical Gynecologic Oncology*. St. Louis: Mosby Year Book, 1997:529.)

- Single dose protocol (stop prenatal vitamins [PNVs] and folate):

Day 1: MTX, 50 mg/m²	βhCG, ALT, Cr, CBC, type and screen	Rho(D) immune globulin (RhoGAM; 300 μg IM) if Rh negative.
Day 4	βhCG	Usually > than day 1 βhCG[a]
Day 7	βhCG, ALT, Cr, CBC	If not ↓ by 15% from day 4, give 2nd MTX dose (50 mg/m²) or laparoscopy.
Weekly	βhCG	Continue until <5 mIU/mL[b]

ALT, alanine aminotransferase; βhCG, β-human chorionic gonadotropin; CBC, complete blood count; Cr, creatinine; MTX, methotrexate.
[a]Decreasing hCG levels between days 1–4 are a reliable predictor of success Nguyen Q, Kapitz M, Downes K, Silva C. Are early human chorionic gonadotropin levels after methotrexate therapy a predictor of response in ectopic pregnancy? *Am J Obstet Gynecol.* Jun;202(6):630, 2010.
[b]If <15% decline in any follow-up week, protocol is repeated.

- Two-dose protocol (stop PNVs and folate) (Barnhart 2007):

Day 0: MTX, 50 mg/m² IM	βhCG, ALT, Cr, CBC, type and screen	Rho(D) immune globulin (RhoGAM; 300 μ IM) if Rh negative
Day 4: MTX, 50 mg/m² IM	βhCG	
Day 7	βhCG, ALT, Cr, CBC	If not ↓ by 15% from day 4, administer 3rd and 4th doses of MTX, 50 mg/m² IM on day 7 and 11. If >15% decline from day 4, check hCG weekly until <5 mIU/mL
Day 11	βhCG	If not ↓ by 15% from day 7, consider surgical treatment. If >15% decline from day 7, check hCG weekly until <5 mIU/mL

ALT, alanine aminotransferase; βhCG, β-human chorionic gonadotropin; CBC, complete blood count; Cr, creatinine; MTX, methotrexate.
If follow-up hCG value plateau or rise, consider surgical intervention.

- Multidose protocol (stop PNVs and folate):

Day 1: MTX, 1 mg/kg IM	βhCG, ALT, Cr, CBC, type and screen	RhoGAM (300 µg IM) if Rh negative
Day 2: LEU, 0.1 mg/kg IM	—	—
Day 3: MTX	βhCG	If not ↓ by 15% from day 1, give 2nd MTX dose
Day 4: LEU	—	—
Day 5: MTX	βhCG	If not ↓ by 15% from day 3, give 3rd MTX dose
Day 6: LEU	—	—
Day 7: MTX	βhCG, ALT, Cr, CBC	If not ↓ by 15% from day 5, give 4th MTX dose
Day 8: LEU	—	—
Weekly	βhCG	Continue until <5 mIU/mL

ALT, alanine aminotransferase; βhCG, β-human chorionic gonadotropin; CBC, complete blood count; Cr, creatinine; LEU, leucovorin; MTX, methotrexate; RhoGAM, Rho(D) immune globulin.

- For details on the above protocols refer to the ACOG Practice Bulletin No. 94, Medical Management of Ectopic Pregnancy (*Obstet Gynecol* 111(6):1479-1485, 2008)
- Average time to resolution (βhCG <15 mIU/mL) for those successfully treated with MTX = approximately 35 days, although it can take up to 109 days (Lipscomb 1998).
- Longest interval between initial treatment and rupture = 42 days (Lipscomb 2000)
- Pretreatment βhCG level is the only significant prognosticator of failure (Lipscomb 1999a).
- Previous EP appears to be an independent risk factor for MTX failure (failure rate of 18.6% in those with a prior EP compared to a 6.8% failure rate for first-time EP) (Lipscomb 2004).

β-Human Chorionic Gonadotropin Level (mIU/mL)	Failure Rate (%)
<1,000	1.7
1,000–9,999	7–13
10,000–14,999	18
>15,000	**32**

Source: Adapted from Lipscomb GH, McCord ML, Stovall TG, et al. Predictors of success of methotrexate treatment in women with tubal ectopic pregnancies. *N Engl J Med* 341:1974, 1999.

- If the initial βhCG <1,000 mIU/mL, 88% resolve without MTX (this is equivalent to MTX efficiency) (Trio 1995) yet follow hCG till <15 mIU/mL.
- After MTX, 56% of the masses increase in size (not necessarily treatment failures, but hematomas) (Brown 1991).
- MTX complications:
  - Impaired liver function, stomatitis, gastritis-enteritis, bone marrow suppression
  - MTX leads to abdominal pain (tubal abortion or hematoma stretching tube-T11,12 [umbilical]).
    - → Treat with ibuprofen, 800 mg q6 hours.
    - → Presence of blood in pelvis is not considered an absolute indication for surgical intervention if hemodynamically stable (Lipscomb 1999a).
  - Use of MTX after IVF does not seem to compromise future IVF cycle success (Oriol 2008)

SURGICAL TREATMENT

- Linear salpingostomy reserved for nonisthmic first-time EPs <5 cm in diameter (DeCherney AH, 1985).
  - **Ampullary** EPs usually grow within the cavity of the lumen; postoperative patency expected.
  - Isthmic EPs usually invade the muscularis layer and usually destroy the tubal mucosa; segmental resection is the treatment of choice.
- 5–15% chance of retained trophoblasts after surgery; some surgeons give one dose of MTX at time of surgery although the NNT is 8 (Farquhar 2005); more common with laparoscopic approach vs. laparotomy (Seifer 1993)

- Use of hydrodissection to flush conceptus out the tube preferred to piecemeal removal
- There is an approximately 30% chance that a contralateral, patent tube will pick up an egg ovulated from the other ovary (Ross 2013)

PROGNOSIS

- Risk of persistent EP after laparotomy = 5%, laparoscopy = 15%
- Intrauterine conception rate similar for surgery vs. MTX (51% vs. 63%, $P = .37$) (Strobelt 2000)
- Subsequent intrauterine pregnancy rates are higher for salpingostomy compared with salpingectomy (73% vs. 57%) but the rates of subsequent EP are higher (15% vs. 10%).
- Subsequent rate of EP for laparoscopic and laparotomy salpingostomy: 7% and 14%, respectively (Yao and Tulandi 1997)
- Recurrent EP: ~15% salpingostomy vs. ~8% salpingectomy (Yao and Tulandi 1997). Others note equal recurrent EP rates (Bateman and Taylor 1991).
- After two EPs, the risk of a subsequent EP ↑ by tenfold.

Systemic MTX vs. laparoscopic salpingostomy:

Outcome Measure	Relative Risk (Confidence Interval)
Primary treatment success—ND	1.20 (0.93–1.40)
Tubal preservation—ND	0.98 (0.87–1.10)
Tubal patency—ND	0.93 (0.64–1.40)
Spontaneous IUP—ND	0.89 (0.42–1.90)
Spontaneous repeat ectopic—ND	0.77 (0.17–3.40)
Cumulative spontaneous IUP rates at 18 months, 36% vs. 43%	

IUP, intrauterine pregnancy; ND, no difference.
Bottom line: Treatment with systemic methotrexate is not superior to laparoscopy based on effectiveness, side effects, burden to patients, and costs to society.
Source: Adapted from Dias Pereira G, Hajenius PJ, et al. Fertility outcome after systemic methotrexate and laparoscopic salpingostomy for tubal pregnancy. *Lancet* 353(9154):724, 1999.

APPENDIX A

Cornual vs. Angular vs. Interstitial

Pregnancy *(Jansen and Elliott 1983; Moawad 2010)*

- **Cornual:** a pregnancy in one horn of a bicornuate uterus or in lateral half of a septate or subseptate uterus
- **Angular:** implantation just medial to the uterotubal junction, in the lateral angle of the uterine cavity; round ligament (*) is reflected upward and outward (see figure below); may be managed conservatively (i.e., expectant management) if there is no rupture or bleeding noted; on ultrasound, the intrauterine angular pregnancy will be surrounded on all sides by at least 5 mm of myometrium
- **Interstitial:** implantation within interstitial portion of the tube reflecting the round ligament (*) medially so that the swelling is lateral to the round ligament (see figure below); conservative treatment option includes MTX (local and systemic).

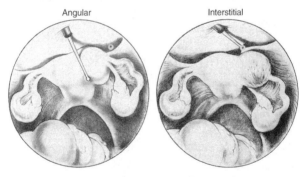

Angular   Interstitial

Source: Reproduced with permission from Jansen R, Elliott P. Angular intrauterine pregnancy. *Obstet Gynaecol* 58:167, 1981.

APPENDIX B

Approach to False-Positive Human Chorionic Gonadotropin Results

- Frequency of false-positive βhCG: between 1 in 10,000 and 1 in 100,000 tests
- False-positive βhCG is usually <150 mIU/mL.
- Most false positives are due to interference by non-hCG substances (i.e., anti–animal immunoglobulin antibodies).
- Characteristically, the serum is positive, but the urine is negative because the heterophilic antibodies are usually immunoglobulins G with a molecular weight of ~160,000 daltons and are not easily filtered through the renal glomeruli. In addition, serial dilutions of serum are not parallel to the hCG standard.

Causes of False-Positive Serum hCG

Interference by non-hCG substances
  Anti–animal heterophilic immunoglobulin antibodies
  hLH or hLHβ-subunit
  Rheumatoid factor
  Nonspecific serum factors

Injection of exogenous hCG

Pituitary hCG-like substance (hCG increases with age and the postmenopausal cutoff is 15 mIU/mL) (Snyder 2005)

Assay contaminants

hCG, human chorionic gonadotropin; hLH, human luteinizing hormone.

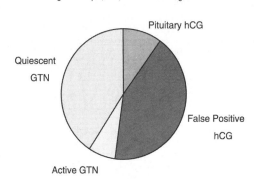

Graph representing causes of human chorionic gonadotropin (hCG) elevation outside of pregnancy. Of 170 patients, 10% had pituitary hCG, 42% had false-positive hCG, 41% had quiescent gestational trophoblastic neoplasia (GTN), and 7.6% had active GTN. (Source: Adapted from Khanlian SA, Cole LA. Management of gestational trophoblastic disease and other cases with low serum levels of human chorionic gonadotropin. *J Reprod Med.* Oct;51(10):812-8, 2006.)

127

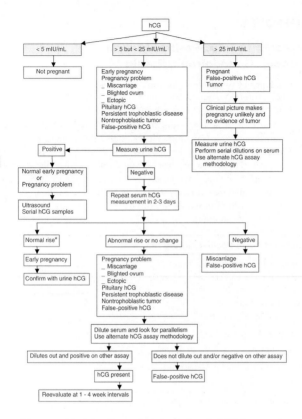

*Slowest or minimal rise of human chorionic gonadotropin (hCG) for a normal pregnancy: 1 day = 24%; 2 days = 53% (Barnhart 2004a). (Source: Adapted from Braunstein, GD. False-positive serum human chorionic gonadotropin results: causes, characteristics, and recognition. *Am J Obstet Gynecol* 187[1]:217, 2002.)

1 3

Sheehan Syndrome

INCIDENCE

- 1/10,000 deliveries
- Hemorrhagic infarction usually occurs in the presence of a pituitary tumor.
- Ischemic infarction may occur after obstetric hemorrhage (Sheehan syndrome).

DEFINITIONS

- Postpartum pituitary necrosis is preceded by a history of massive obstetric hemorrhage, resulting in severe circulatory collapse, hypotension, and shock.
- Clinical manifestations may range from partial deficiency to panhypopituitarism (PRL, GH, LH, FSH, ACTH, TSH).
- The posterior pituitary is usually spared.
- Return of normal fertility has been documented.

ETIOLOGY

- Anterior pituitary grows during pregnancy due to estrogenic stimulation, resulting in hyperplasia and hypertrophy of pituitary lactotropes: 500 mg → 1,000 mg.
- Anterior pituitary insufficiency occurs when >75% of the gland has been destroyed.
- Severity of hemorrhage and occurrence of Sheehan syndrome may not correlate.
- Severe hypotension, in a setting of low portal vein pressure, leads to occlusive spasm of the arteries that supply the anterior pituitary and the stalk; when arteriospasm relaxes, blood flows into the damaged vessels, resulting in vascular congestion and thrombosis.

- Infarction with hemorrhage and edema may cause rapid expansion of the lesion, compressing surrounding structures with neurologic (visual) manifestations.
- With modern fluid resuscitation and blood product replacement, Sheehan syndrome is very uncommon (Feinberg 2005).

COURSE

- Classic progression of deficits:
  - Prolactin (PRL; 67–100%), growth hormone (GH; 88%), gonadotropins (58–76%), adrenocorticotropic hormone (ACTH; 66%), thyroid-stimulating hormone (TSH; 42–53%), diabetes insipidus (2%)

Acute form

Hypotension
Tachycardia
Failure to lactate (breast involution)
Hypoglycemia
Extreme fatigue
Nausea and vomiting
Failure to regrow shaved pubic hair

Chronic form

Light headedness
Fatigue and cold intolerance
Failure to lactate
Scanty or absent menses
↓ **Body hair**
Skin: dry, pale, and waxy
Nausea and vomiting
↓Melanin → **pale areolae**
↓Libido

- ↓ ACTH signs and symptoms: fatigue, hypotension, poor tolerance to stress and infection, hypoglycemia, loss of pubic and axillary hair, ↓ body hair, ↓ pigment in skin, waxy skin
- ↓ TSH signs and symptoms: fatigue, slow speech, slow movements, cold intolerance, dry skin, constipation

DIAGNOSIS

- Magnetic resonance imaging (MRI) assesses the hemorrhage extension and need for ophthalmologic examination.
- Diagnostic tests:

- ○ Serum a.m. cortisol, ACTH, TSH, thyroxine (T_4), PRL, luteinizing hormone (LH), follicle-stimulating hormone (FSH), estradiol (E_2), insulin-like growth factor (IGF)-I
  - ○ Metyrapone stimulation test: Metyrapone (2 g PO at 11 p.m.) blocks 11-deoxycorticosterone (DOC) → cortisol, which leads to ↑ ACTH (>100 pg/mL) and ↑ precursor 11-DOC (>7 µg/dL).
- Hormone deficits may be transient; therefore, function should be reevaluated several months after the event.
- May require pituitary reserve testing: draw blood (serum) samples at −30, 0, 30, and 60 minutes, through an indwelling IV catheter; at time 0, give IV:
  1. Thyroid-releasing hormone (TRH), 200 µg → stimulates TSH and PRL release
  2. Gonadotropin-releasing hormone (GnRH), 100 µg → stimulates LH and FSH release
  3. Corticotropin-releasing hormone (CRH), 50 µg → stimulates ACTH release
  4. Growth hormone–releasing hormone (GHRH), 50 µg → stimulates GH release
  - ○ **Interpretation of results**: All hormones should at least double above mean baseline values; pulsatile secretion necessitates several baseline values.
- No test for antidiuretic hormone (ADH) deficiency: urine specific gravity <1.005; symptoms are polyuria and polydipsia.
- After a full-term pregnancy without lactation, it takes 4 weeks for the FSH pulsatility to return to normal (Liu 1983).

TREATMENT

- Appropriate replacement of target hormones when needed (corticoid, thyroid, sex steroids, desmopressin acetate [DDAVP])
- Corticosteroids (usually aldosterone production is sufficient in the absence of ACTH, unlike in Addison disease): dexamethasone, 2 mg q6 hours
- Use oral contraceptives (OCs) if necessary.

PROGNOSIS

- Overall: excellent with correct diagnosis and treatment
- Fertility: Pregnancy can occur spontaneously in partial cases. Otherwise, human menopausal gonadotropin (hMG) induction of ovulation is necessary; if pregnancy ensues, hypoglycemia may occur due to ↓ GH and ACTH reserves.

14

Premenstrual Syndrome

HISTORY

- Dr. Frank at Mt. Sinai Hospital in New York City first defined premenstrual syndrome (PMS) in 1931 as a "Feeling of indescribable tension from 10 to 7 days preceding menstruation which in most instances continues until the time that the menstrual flow occurs" (Frank 1931).
- Drs. Greene and Dalton first used the phrase *premenstrual syndrome* in 1953 in a report of 84 cases (Greene and Dalton 1953).

DEFINITIONS

- **PMS:** both physical and behavioral symptoms that occur repetitively in the 2nd ½ of the menstrual cycle to interfere with a woman's life followed by a period of time free of symptoms.
- **Premenstrual dysphoric disorder (PMDD):** American Psychiatric Association's *Diagnostic and Statistical Manual of Mental Disorders*, 5th Edition (*DSM-V*), designation with prominence of anger, irritability, and internal tension; presumably the most severe form of PMS, although this designation is nonfunctional.

PREVALENCE *(Rivera-Tovar and Frank 1990; Raja 1992)*

- Mild PMS: up to 80% in women with regular cycles, moderate to severe PMS affects 20–40% and severe PMDD affects 3–8%
- No correlation with ethnicity
- Higher concordance rate in monozygotic twins compared with dizygotic twins (Condon 1993), although role of genetic factors is far from certain (Glick 1993)

PATHOGENESIS

Neurotransmitters

- Cyclic changes in ovarian steroids may influence central neurotransmitters (opioid, γ-aminobutyric acid, serotonin).
  - Women with PMS may be biochemically supersensitive to biologic challenges of the serotonergic system (Halbreich and Tworek 1993).
  - PMS patients have lower serotonin and higher levels of serotonin metabolites during the luteal phase (Taylor 1984; Steege 1992).
  - Serotonin antagonist administration to women with PMDD $\rightarrow$ recrudescence of symptoms (Roca 2002).
  - PMS symptoms improved with serotonin agonists (Brzezinski 1990) or serotonin reuptake inhibitors (e.g., fluoxetine).

Ovarian Steroids

- Gonadotropin-releasing hormone agonists used to induce hypoestrogenemia led to resolution of PMS symptoms (Muse 1984).
  - The addition of estradiol (E_2) or progesterone (P_4) led to a recurrence of symptoms (Schmidt 1998); however, the addition of a placebo in lieu of steroids also led to a return of symptoms.
- Luteal phase free E_2 was significantly lower and SHBG concentrations were significantly higher in PMDD than those without PMDD (Thys-Jacobs 2008).
- P_4 antagonist RU-486 did not ameliorate PMS symptoms (Chan 1994).

Vitamins and Minerals

- No deficiencies in vitamin A, B_6, or E in women with PMS (Chuong 1990a; Chuong 1990b)
- One controlled study showed improved symptoms with magnesium pyrrolidone carboxylic acid (360 mg t.i.d.) given in the luteal phase (Facchinetti 1991).

Psychosocial Factors

- Stress has little influence on PMS severity (Beck 1990).

SYMPTOMS

- Symptoms worsen 6 days before and peak ~2 days before menses begins; anger and irritability are the most severe and start earlier than other symptoms.

- By definition there must be a symptom-free interval before ovulation
- 22 symptoms documented by Mortola in 1990, occurring in the last 7–10 days of the cycle:

Symptom	Frequency (% of Cycles)
Fatigue	92
Irritability	91
Bloating	90
Anxiety/tension	89
Breast tenderness	85
Mood lability	81
Depression	80
Food cravings	78
Acne	71
↑ Appetite	70
Oversensitivity	69
Swelling	67
Expressed anger	67
Crying easily	65
Feeling of isolation	65
Headache	60
Forgetfulness	56
Gastrointestinal symptoms	48
Poor concentration	47
Hot flashes	18
Heart palpitations	14
Dizziness	14

Source: Adapted from Mortola JF, Girton L, Beck L, et al. Diagnosis of premenstrual syndrome by a simple, prospective, and reliable instrument: the calendar of premenstrual experiences. *Obstet Gynecol* 76(2):302, 1990.

DIAGNOSIS

- Symptoms, severity of symptoms, temporal relationship to luteal phase, absence of external factors (i.e., drugs) or other diagnoses
- Two established guidelines for diagnosing PMDD:

1. *DSM-V* criteria

DSM-V Premenstrual Dysphoric Disorder Diagnostic Criteria

A. In the majority of cycles, at least five symptoms must be present in the final week before the onset of menses, start to *improve* within a few days after the onset of menses, and become *minimal* or absent in the week postmenses.

B. One (or more) of the following symptoms must be present:

   1. Marked affective liability (e.g., mood swings; feeling suddenly sad or tearful, or increased sensitivity to rejection).
   2. Marked irritability or anger or increased interpersonal conflicts.
   3. Marked depressed mood, feelings of hopelessness, or self-deprecating thoughts.
   4. Marked anxiety, tension, and/or feelings of being keyed up or on edge.

C. One (or more) of the following symptoms must additionally be present, to reach a total of *five* symptoms when combined with symptoms from Criterion B above.

   1. Decreased interest in usual activities (e.g., work, school, friends, hobbies).
   2. Subjective difficulty in concentration.
   3. Lethargy, easy fatigability, or marked lack of energy.
   4. Marked change in appetite; overeating; or specific food cravings.
   5. Hypersomnia or insomnia.
   6. A sense of being overwhelmed or out of control.
   7. Physical symptoms such as breast tenderness or swelling, joint or muscle pain, a sensation of "bloating," weight gain.

   Note: The symptoms in Criteria A-C must have been met for most menstrual cycles that occurred in the preceding year.

D. The symptoms are associated with clinically significant distress or interference with work, school, usual social activities, or relationships with others (e.g., avoidance of social activities; decreased productivity and efficiency at work, school, or home).

E. The disturbance is not merely an exacerbation of the symptoms of another disorder, such as major depressive disorder, panic disorder, persistent depressive disorder (dysthymia), or a personality disorder (although it may co-occur with any of these disorders).

F. Criterion A, should be confirmed by prospective daily ratings during at least two symptomatic cycles. (**Note:** The diagnosis may be made provisionally prior to this confirmation.)

G. The symptoms are not attributed to the physiological effects of a substance (e.g., a drug of abuse, a medication, or other treatment) or another medical condition (e.g., hyperthyroidism).

Source: Reproduced with permission from American Psychiatric Association. Diagnostic and Statistical Manual of Mental Disorders (5th ed). Washington, DC: American Psychiatric Association, 2013.

2. **National Institute of Mental Health guidelines** (Osofsky and Blumenthal 1985):
   o Diagnosis requires the documentation of ≥30% ↓ severity of symptoms in the 5 days after menses (follicular phase) compared with the 5 days before menses (luteal phase) within a single cycle (using Prospective Record of the Severity of Menstruation [PRISM]).
   o Calendar of premenstrual experiences: **PRISM**
     → Before recording in the calendar, the physician identifies the patient's chief complaints and the symptoms to be followed throughout treatment.
     → Scores for the symptoms of interest are added for 5 follicular days (cycle days 7–11) and 5 luteal days (–6 to –2), and these total phase scores are then compared.
     → Within-cycle % change is calculated as follows:

$$\frac{\text{Luteal score} - \text{Follicular score}}{\text{Luteal score}} \times 100$$

PRISM Calendar Instructions

1. Prepare the calendar on the first day of menses. Considering the first day of bleeding as day 1 of your menstrual cycle, enter the corresponding calendar date for each day in the space provided.

   e.g., Day of menstrual cycle. Month: _____ Date: _____

2. Each evening, at about the same time, complete the calendar column for that day as described below:

   Bleeding: Indicate if you have had bleeding by shading the box above that day's date; for spotting, use an (x).

   Symptoms: If you do not experience any symptoms, leave the corresponding square blank. If present, indicate the severity by entering a number from 1 (mild) to 7 (severe).

   Lifestyle impact: If the listed phrase applies to you that day, enter an (x).

   Life events: If you experienced one of these events that day, enter an (x).

   Experiences: For positive (happy) or negative (sad/disappointing) experiences unrelated to your symptoms, specify the nature of the events on the back of this form.

   Social activities: This implies such events as a special dinner, show, or party, etc., involving family or friends.

   Vigorous exercise: This implies participation in a sporting event or exercise program lasting >30 minutes.

   Medication: In the bottom five rows, list medication used, if any, and indicate days when they were taken by entering an (x).

   Study number: _____ Baseline weight on Day 1 _____ lb or kg. (circle one)

Source: Reproduced with permission from Reid RL. Premenstrual syndrome. *Curr Probl Obstet Gynecol Fertil* 8:1–57, 1985.

Study Number [ ][ ][ ][ ]

Baseline weight on Day 1 _____ lbs. or kg. (circle one)

Day of Menstrual Cycle Month: Date:	Bleeding	1	2	3	4	5	6	7	8	9	10	11	12	13	14	15	16	17	18	19	20	21	22	23	24	25	26	27	28	29	30	31	32	33	34	35
SYMPTOMS
Irritable
Fatigue
Inward anger
Labile mood (crying)
Depressed
Restless
Anxious
Insomnia
Lack of control
Edema or rings tight
Breast tenderness
Abdominal bloating
Bowels: const. (c) loose (l)
Appetite: up ^ down ˅
Sex drive: up ^ down ˅
Chills (C)/sweats (S)
Headaches
Crave: sweets, salt
Feel unattractive
Guilty
Unreasonable behavior
Low self-image
Nausea
Menstrual cramps
LIFESTYLE IMPACT
Aggressive towards others — Physically
Aggressive towards others — Verbally
Wish to be alone
Neglect housework
Time off work
Disorganized, distractible
Accident prone/clumsy
Uneasy about driving
Suicidal thoughts
Stayed at home
Increased use of alcohol
LIFE EVENTS
Negative experience
Positive experience
Social activities
Vigorous exercise
MEDICATIONS

PRISM survey. (Source: Reproduced with permission from Reid RL. Premenstrual syndrome. *Curr Probl Obstet Gynecol Fertil* 8:1–57, 1985.)

- Fine distinction between PMDD and PMS:
  - Women with PMDD meet criteria for PMDD by *DSM-V* criteria.
  - Women with PMS do not meet all *DSM-V* criteria for PMDD but do demonstrate symptom exacerbation premenstrually as calculated above.
  - In all practicality, this is a distinction that is best left in research papers, as either PMDD or PMS is a debilitating life stressor.

DIFFERENTIAL DIAGNOSIS

- Psychiatric disorders: major depression, anxiety disorders
- Perimenopause
- Medical disorders: migraine, irritable bowel syndrome, hyper- or hypothyroidism

DIAGNOSTIC TESTS

- History and physical examination (including past psychiatric history)
- Complete blood count, thyroid-stimulating hormone
- Record symptoms for 3 months with a menstrual calendar (PRISM).

TREATMENT

Serotonin Reuptake Inhibitors

- Fluoxetine (Prozac): 20 mg/day (Steiner 1995) for at least two cycles
  - U.S. Food and Drug Administration approved for PMDD
  - Approximately 75% overall response rate within 2–3 months (Steiner 2001)
  - Effect is maintained for many years (Pearlstein and Stone 1994).
  - Some women may find that use is only required on cycle day 14 until menses (Halbreich and Smoller 1997).
  - Side effects (15% incidence): headache, anxiety, nausea, anorgasmia
- Sertraline (Zoloft): 50–150 mg/day
- Paroxetine (Paxil): 10–30 mg/day
- Citalopram (Celexa): 20–30 mg/day
- Venlafaxine (Effexor): 50–200 mg/day

- Buspirone (BuSpar): 5 mg t.i.d. or 7.5 mg b.i.d., with maximum of 20 mg t.i.d. or 30 mg b.i.d. daily (12 days before menses)
- Sumatriptan (85 mg) and naproxen (500 mg) combination treatment for menstrual migraines—maintained for up to 48 hrs in RCTs (Mannix 2009).

Alprazolam (Xanax)

- 0.25 mg t.i.d. or q.i.d. in luteal phase only due to risk of dependence
- 2nd-line therapy

Ovulation Suppression

Gonadotropin-Releasing Hormone Agonists

- Limited efficacy with many disadvantages due to hypoestrogenemia
- May be more effective for behavioral and physical symptoms and less effective for psychological symptoms
  - Leuprolide (Lupron): 3.75 mg IM each month
  - Nafarelin acetate (Synarel): 2 mg/mL daily, intranasally
  - Appropriate add-back regimen: 0.5 mg estradiol gel daily with 14 days of 400 mg vaginal progesterone once daily every third month (Segebladh 2009).

Oral Contraceptives

- Most studies reveal ineffectiveness (Joffe 2003).
- Possible utility as continuous oral contraceptives with drospirenone-containing (a progestin that is a spironolactone analog) contraceptive Yasmin or drospirenone and ethinyl estradiol (Freeman 2001)

MENSTRUAL MIGRAINES

- Treatment: 0.1-mg E_2 patch/day before menses

Debatable Treatment Approaches

- Magnesium: 360 mg/day, 14 days before menses (small trials) (Facchinetti 1991; Walker 1998)
- Calcium: 1 g/day (Thys-Jacobs 1989)

- Regular exercise, relaxation, vitamin and mineral supplements, changes in work or recreation, changes in diet (small, frequent complex-carbohydrate meals; ↓ tobacco, chocolate, caffeine, alcohol, salt)

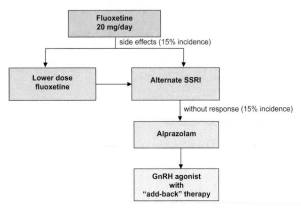

Treatment plan. GnRH, gonadotropin-releasing hormone; SSRI, selective serotonin reuptake inhibitor. (Source: Adapted from Casper RF. Treatment of premenstrual dysphoric disorder. UpToDate Patient Information Web site: http://www.utdol.com. Accessed February 2005.)

15
Chronic Pelvic Pain

DEFINITION

ACOG: Non-cyclic pain of 6 or more months duration that localizes to the anatomic pelvis, anterior abdominal wall at or below the umbilicus, the lumbosacral back, or the buttocks and is of sufficient severity to cause functional disability or lead to medical disability

INCIDENCE

- Affects 15% of women in the United States (9 million)
- Accounts for 10% of gynecologist visits
- Accounts for 40% of laparoscopies
- Accounts for ~12% of hysterectomies

HISTORY

- Menses with dysmenorrhea
- Dyspareunia (superficial suggests inflammatory process or introital muscle control; deep suggests endometriosis or pelvic adhesive disease)
- Sexually transmitted infections (STIs); abnormal Pap smear
- Obstetric history
- Detailed social and family history
- Gastrointestinal (GI), urologic, and musculoskeletal review of symptoms (ROS)
- Past surgical history (abdominal or pelvic) → review old operative reports
- Past and current state of mental health
- History of sexual abuse; depression

Pain Inquiry

- Character
- Radiation

- Intensity
- Duration
- Location
- Associated events

Symptoms Suggestive of Irritable Bowel Syndrome

- Alternating constipation/diarrhea, abdominal distention, mucus per rectum, improvement in pain after a bowel movement, sensation of incomplete evacuation after defecation (Manning 1978)

PHYSICAL EXAMINATION

- Observe posture and gait
- Back
- Skin
- Abdominal wall (single finger pointing by patient and examiner)
  - Evaluation with the patient's head raised off the table and rectus muscles tensed: Visceral origin pain usually diminishes with this, whereas myofascial pain or trigger points exacerbate.
- Pelvic (Gyang 2013):
  - Vulva: focal tenderness of the posterior vestibule may indicate vestibulodynia
  - Vagina, cervix, and paracervical tissues
  - Unimanual (single digit) followed by a bimanual examination: finger rotated anteriorly to palpate the anterior vaginal wall and base of the bladder; exquisitely painful bladder with interstitial cystitis

History	Examination Findings	Disease State
Progressively worsening dysmenorrhea; deep dyspareunia	Tenderness in implant areas; uterosacral ligament nodularity	Endometriosis
Symptom onset 3–6 months after surgery; tugging and pulling sensation in abdomen or pelvis	Diminished mobility of the pelvic viscera	Pelvic adhesive disease

(Continues on next page)

(Continued from previous page)

Abnormal uterine bleeding; dysmenorrhea	Enlarged, firm, irregular uterus	Leiomyoma or andenomyosis
Buttocks pain on arising, climbing stairs, driving car	Ipsilateral foot is found to be externally rotated in supine position; tenderness on palpation transvaginally or externally over the piriformis attachment to greater trochanter	Piriformis muscle spasm
Frequency and urgency; urethral or bladder pain	Bladder tender to palpation	Interstitial cystitis

LABORATORY AND DIAGNOSTIC STUDIES

- Urine analysis (UA)/culture and sensitivity (C&S)
- Ultrasound
- Wet prep (saline and potassium hydroxide [KOH])
- Laparoscopy (pain mapping)
- Pelvic cultures (gonococcus [GC] and chlamydia)
- Cystoscopy and colonoscopy
- Psychometric screening questions
- Trigger point injections

PROCEDURES

- Laparoscopic findings (for chronic pelvic pain [CPP]) in a community survey (n = 1318):

Finding	%
No pathology	39
Endometriosis	28
Adhesions	25
Chronic pelvic inflammatory disease	6
Ovarian cyst	3
Leiomyomata	<1
Pelvic varicosities	<1
Other	4

Source: Adapted from Howard FM. The role of laparoscopy in chronic pelvic pain: promise and pitfalls. *Obstet Gynecol Surv* 48:357, 1993.

CAUSES OF CHRONIC PELVIC PAIN

Gynecologic

- Extrauterine
  - Adhesions
  - Endometriosis
  - Residual ovary syndrome
- Uterine
  - Adenomyosis
  - Chronic endometritis
  - Leiomyomata
  - Intrauterine contraceptive device
  - Pelvic congestion
  - Pelvic support defects
  - Polyps

Urologic

- Chronic urinary tract infection
- Detrusor overactivity
- Interstitial cystitis
- Urolithiasis
- Suburethral diverticulitis
- Urethral syndrome

Gastrointestinal

- Cholelithiasis
- Chronic appendicitis
- Constipation
- Diverticular disease
- Enterocolitis
- Gastric/duodenal ulcer
- Inflammatory bowel disease (Crohn's disease, ulcerative colitis)
- Irritable bowel syndrome
- Neoplasia

Musculoskeletal

- Coccydynia
- Disk problems
- Degenerative joint disease
- Fibromyositis
- Hernias

- Herpes zoster (shingles)
- Low back pain
- Levator ani syndrome (spasm of pelvic floor)
- Myofascial pain (trigger points, spasms)
- Nerve entrapment syndromes
- Osteoporosis (fractures)
- Poor posture
- Scoliosis/lordosis/kyphosis (typical pelvic pain posture)
- Strains/sprains

Other

- Abuse (physical or sexual, prior or current)
- Heavy metal poisoning (lead, mercury)
- Hyperparathyroidism
- Porphyria
- Psychiatric disorders (depression, bipolar disorders, inadequate personality disorder)
- Psychosocial stress (marital discord, work stress)
- Sickle cell disease
- Sleep disturbances
- Somatoform disorders
- Substance use (especially cocaine)
- Sympathetic dystrophy
- Tabes dorsalis (third-degree syphilis)

Source: Reproduced with permission from ACOG technical bulletin. Chronic pelvic pain. Number 223. *Int J Gynaecol Obstet.* Jul;54(1):59-68, 1996.

DYSMENORRHEA

Primary Dysmenorrhea: No Pelvic Pathology Evident

- Caused by the release of prostaglandins $F_{2\alpha}$ and E_2
- Other associated factors include family history, early menarche, increased duration of menses, and smoking
- Usually begins 6–12 months after menarche at the initiation of ovulatory cycles
- Antiinflammatories: dosing for primary dysmenorrhea:
  - Nonsteroidal anti-inflammatory drugs (NSAIDs):
    - → Ibuprofen, 400–800 mg PO q6–8 hours
    - → Naproxen sodium, 275–500 mg PO q6–8 hours
    - → Mefenamic acid, 250–500 mg PO q6–8 hours
  - Another option (off label): Tranexamic acid, 1,300 mg PO t.i.d. during menses (max: x5 days)

Secondary Dysmenorrhea: Pelvic Pathology Present

- Common causes include endometriosis, pelvic infections, cervical stenosis, adenomyosis, leiomyomas, congenital malformations (i.e., imperforate hymen), or intrauterine device (IUD).
- First-line medical management: oral contraceptives (and NSAIDs)

Residual Ovary Syndrome

- Occurs in 3% of women who have undergone hysterectomy with ovarian conservation
- Perioophoritis with a thickened ovarian capsule leading to pain from cyclical expansion of the ovary encased in adhesions

Ovarian Remnant Syndrome

- Follicle-stimulating hormone (FSH) in *pre*menopausal range
- Clomiphene citrate can assist in ultrasound diagnosis as well as surgical identification (100 mg/day for 7–10 days before the day of surgery; last dose, 1–2 days before surgery)

Vulvodynia

- Vulvar vestibulitis patients typically present with dyspareunia on entry, persistent yeast infection, soreness, burning, or rawness
- Tight clothing, prolonged sitting, or exercise may exacerbate these symptoms (itching is rarely a symptom).
- Treatment recommendations: Avoid soaps, douches, creams, or synthetic underwear; topical vegetable oil or zinc oxide or local anesthetic; low-dose tricyclic antidepressants or anticonvulsant, gabapentin (100 mg at bedtime, increasing by 100 mg every 2 days to 3 g/day in divided doses); surgical vestibulectomy may be effective in recalcitrant cases.

TREATMENT

- Integrated either by an individual or an interdisciplinary/ multispecialty team
- Set expectations early on.

- Medical and/or surgical management
- Low threshold for referral
- See respective entities in this manual (e.g., Chapter 16, Endometriosis; Chapter 17, Fibroids).
- Narcotics used in chronic pain management:

Drug	Usual Dose Range	Side Effects
Hydrocodone bitartrate with acetaminophen (all are scored tablets) Lorcet 10/650 Lorcet Plus 7.5/650 Lortab 2.5/500, 5/500, or 7.5/500 Vicodin 5/750	5–10 mg hydrocodone either q6 hours or q8 hours Can use additional acetaminophen between doses to potentiate effect	Lightheadedness, dizziness, sedation, nausea, vomiting, and constipation (these are all common side effects of all narcotics)
Oxycodone hydrochloride Percocet, 5 mg with 325 mg acetaminophen Percodan, 4.5 mg with 325 mg aspirin (also contains 0.38 mg oxycodone terephthalate)	1 tablet q6 hours or q8 hours Additional acetaminophen between doses may serve to potentiate effect	Common effects (see above)
Oxycodone controlled release OxyContin	10–40 mg q12 hours	Common effects (see above)
Methadone hydrochloride Dolophine, 5 or 10 mg scored tablets	2.5 mg q8 hours to 10 mg q6 hours Commonly 15–20 mg q.d.	Common effects; lower extremity edema or joint swelling may occur and require discontinuation; cautious use in patients taking monoamine oxidase inhibitors

Coninues on next page

(Continued from previous page)

Acetaminophen with codeine Tylenol No. 3, 300 mg acetaminophen with 30 mg codeine	1–2 tablets q6–8 hours	Common effects. Constipation likely. Nausea and vomiting more common than with other narcotics. More common allergy rash.
Morphine sulfate MS Contin or Oramorph	15–60 mg q12 hours; controlled-release tablets	Common effects. Higher doses increase risk of respiratory depression.
Fentanyl transdermal system Duragesic	25-µg patch, one q72 hours; also available in 50 or 75 µg Always start with lowest dose	Common effects. Patch must be kept from heat sources, or dose may be increased. Extreme caution in patients taking other central nervous system medicines. Respiratory depression can result.
Tramadol	50–100 mg q4–6 hours	Common effects: Dizziness, nausea, constipation, headache, somnolence, vomiting.

Source: Reproduced with permission from Steege JF. Chronic pelvic pain. In Curtis MG, Hopkins MP, eds. *Glass's Office Gynecology*. 4th ed. Philadelphia: Lippincott Williams & Wilkins, 1999:330.

16

Endometriosis

DEFINITION

- Presence of functioning endometrial glands and stroma outside the usual location of the uterine cavity
- First described in 1860 by the Viennese pathologist Karl von Rokitansky
- Visual inspection at the time of laparoscopy is sufficient; in fact, negative histology does not exclude a diagnosis of endometriosis (Kennedy 2005).

PREVALENCE

- 11% of reproductive-age group
- 25–35% of infertile women
- 70% of women with pelvic pain
- Average age at diagnosis: 25–29 years; similar rates in the various races and socioeconomic backgrounds
- 7 million U.S. women are affected.
- Visualizing endometriosis:
  - 70% of women with pelvic pain (Koninckx 1991)
  - 84% of women with pain and infertility (Koninckx 1991)
  - 45% of women with no symptoms (Balasch 1996)
  - 6% of biopsies of normal peritoneum in normal pelvis show microscopic lesions (Balasch 1996)
  - 11–25% of biopsies of normal peritoneum in endometriosis patients (Murphy 1986; Balasch 1996)

Positive Histology for Endometriosis Based on Site of Lesion Biopsied During Surgery:

Site of Lesion	Positive Histology (%)
Bladder/uterovesical	50
Cul-de-sac	67
Ovarian	77
Overlying ureter	100
Uterosacral ligament	79

Source: Adapted from El Bishry G, Tselos V, Pathi A. Correlation between laparoscopic and histological diagnosis in patients with endometriosis. *J Obstet Gynaecol.* Jul;28(5):511-5, 2008.

RISKS OF CANCER

Cancer	Incidence Ratio	95% Confidence Interval
Overall	1.0	1.00–1.07
Brain	1.2	1.04–1.41
Ovarian	1.4	1.19–1.71
Ovarian cancer with history of endometrioma	1.8	1.38–2.24
Non-Hodgkin's lymphoma	1.2	1.02–1.49

Source: Adapted from Melin A, Sparén P, et al. Endometriosis and the risk of cancer with special emphasis on ovarian cancer. *Hum Reprod* 21(5):1237-1242, 2006.

- Malignant neoplasms can arise in endometriotic tissue of the ovary. Distribution by type:
  - Endometrioid: 57%
  - Other epithelial: 22.4%
  - Clear cell: 10%
  - Serous: 7%
- The overall lifetime probability of ovarian cancer is quite small: general population ~1%; women with endometriosis ~1.5%.

RISKS OF AUTOIMMUNE DISORDERS

Autoimmune Disorder	Prevalence in Women with Endometriosis vs. General U.S. Female Population (%)
Hypothyroidism	9.6 vs. 1.50
Fibromyalgia	5.9 vs. 3.40
Chronic fatigue syndrome	4.6 vs. 0.03
Rheumatoid arthritis	1.8 vs. 1.20
Systemic lupus erythematosus	0.8 vs. 0.04
Sjögren's syndrome	0.6 vs. 0.03
Multiple sclerosis	0.5 vs. 0.07

Source: Adapted from Sinaii N, Cleary SD, et al. Autoimmune and related diseases among women with endometriosis: a survey analysis. *Fertil Steril* 77[Suppl 1]:S7, 2002.

- Women with endometriosis may have a high rate of concomitant interstitial cystitis (66%); symptoms include urinary frequency, urgency, and nocturia (Paulson 2007).

PATHOGENESIS

Transplantation Theory *(Sampson 1927)*

- Retrograde menstruation seeds the abdominal cavity.
- Prevalence of retrograde menstruation: 70–90%
- Higher incidence associated with outflow obstruction, shorter cycles, menorrhagia, delayed child-bearing
- A disease of menstruation; delaying childbirth has increased number of menstrual cycles (~450 cycles/lifetime).
- The sigmoid colon and filmy adhesions that frequently cover the left adnexa create an area isolated from the rest of the peritoneal cavity and, therefore, may be less exposed to the peritoneal current and thus clearance by the immune system. Cells regurgitated through the right tube are more exposed to the clockwise peritoneal current and may be removed by the macrophage disposal system (Rosenheim 1979).

Coelomic Metaplasia

- Peritoneal mesothelium (from which the müllerian duct is derived) undergoes metaplastic transformation into endometrial tissue.

- This could explain how endometriosis is formed in men treated with high doses of estrogens.
- Probable etiology of rectovaginal (RV) endometriotic nodules (Donnez 1996)
  - Lower mitotic activity
  - Smooth muscle and glandular elements
  - Decreased vimentin, estrogen, and progesterone receptors

Induction Theory

- Unknown biochemical substances (from shed endometrium?) induce undifferentiated peritoneal cells to form endometriotic tissue.

Immunologic Theory (Halme 1987; Lebovic 2001b; Reis 2013)

- Alterations in cell-mediated immunity: natural killer (NK), macrophage, T- and B-cells
- Abnormal autoantibodies?
- Altered immune response → inhibited clearance of viable endometrial cells via immunosurveillance evasion:
  - Modification of human leukocyte antigen (HLA) class I antigen expression (related to immune recognition) (Semino 1995)
  - ↑ Soluble HLA or intercellular adhesion molecule (ICAM)-I that competes with surface antigens critical to immune recognition (Somigliana 1996; De Placido 1998)
  - ↑ Growth factors/cytokines that inhibit specific immune population functions (i.e., soluble tumor necrosis factor [TNF] receptor) (Hirata 1994; Somigliana 1996; Koga 2000)
  - Induction of apoptosis in immune cells via Fas-mediated mechanisms (Garcia-Velasco 1999)
  - ↑ Antiapoptotic factors (i.e., osteoprotegerin, Bcl-2 family) (Harada 2004; Nishida 2005)
  - Resistance to interferon (IFN)-γ–induced apoptosis (Nishida 2005)
  - NK cell defect (D'Hooghe 1995)

GENETIC PREDISPOSITION
Familial Disposition

- The risk to 1st degree relatives of women with endometriosis is 4–8 times that of the general population (Simpson JL 1980; Moen MH 1993; Stefansson H 2002)
- Multifactorial inheritance

Other

- Dioxin? The environmental pollutant dioxin was found in 18% of women with endometriosis vs. 3% of the controls (P <.05) (Mayani 1997).
- Peritoneal, ovarian, and RV endometriotic lesions may be considered as three separate entities with different pathogeneses: (a) peritoneal = retrograde effluent; (b) endometriomas = coelomic metaplasia; and (c) RV = müllerian remnants (Nisolle and Donnez 1997).
- Up-regulation of enzymes involved in E_2 activation and P_4 inactivation seen in endometriomas (Smuc 2008).
- Alternate mechanism of endometrioma formation: nonresorbed bleeding corpus luteum incorporates some retrograde endomaterial cells that then populate and lead to adherence of the corpus luteum to the pelvic sidewall (Vercellini 2009).

CLINICAL PRESENTATION
Pain

- Dysmenorrhea with premenstrual intensification
- Dyspareunia
- Chronic pelvic pain (>6 months):
  - Peritoneum is richly supplied with afferent nerve fibers (Ottinger 1974).

Infertility *(de Ziegler 2010)*

- Biased predilection for laparoscopy in infertile patients may overestimate the incidence of endometriosis in this group.
  - Prevalence in subfertile women vs. fertile women: 50% vs. 5–10% (D'Hooghe 2003)
- Severe endometriosis: adhesions adhesions leading to tubal disease
- Mild endometriosis is associated with a lower fecundity rate:
  - Prospective double-blinded study in women with azoospermic partners undergoing donor insemination (Matorras 2010):

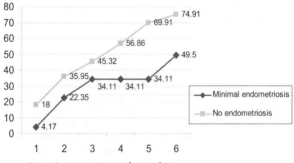

Donor insemination cycle number

The per-woman pregnancy rate was 40% lower for women with minimal endometriosis although not enough patients recruited to obtain statistical significance. (Source: Reproduced with permission from Matorras R, Corcóstegui B, Esteban J, et al. Fertility in women with minimal endometriosis compared with normal women was assessed by means of a donor insemination program in unstimulated cycles. *Am J Obstet Gynecol.* Oct;203(4):345, 2010.)

- Cumulative pregnancy rate (carried beyond 20 weeks) without fertility treatment for minimal-mild endometriosis vs. unexplained subfertility: 15.7% (0.72; 95% confidence interval [CI], 0.45–1.17) vs. 23.6% (Berube 1998)
- Probability of pregnancy 3 years (untreated) after diagnostic laparoscopy for minimal-mild endometriosis vs. unexplained subfertility: 36% vs. 55% ($P < .05$) (Akande 2004)
- Probability of live birth 3 years (untreated) after diagnostic laparoscopy for minimal-mild endometriosis vs. unexplained subfertility: 33% vs. 48% (not significant [NS], although type II error) (Akande 2004)

- o Fertility for minimal-mild endometriosis vs. unexplained subfertility (Sung 1997; Jensen 1998; Hammond 1986; Toma 1992; Omland 1998; Nuojua-Huttunen 1999):

	Monthly Fecundity Rate after Expectant Management (%)	Monthly Fecundity Rate after Intra-uterine Insemination (%)	Monthly Fecundity Rate after Therapeutic Donor Insemination (%)	Pregnancy Rate after Donor Oocyte (In Vitro Fertilization) (%)[a]
Minimal-mild endometriosis	2.5	9	4	28
Unexplained subfertility	3.5 NS[b]	19 $P < .01$	16 $P < .01$	29 NS

NS, not significant.

[a]Data in this column from Diaz I, Navarro J, Blasco L, et al. Impact of stage III-IV endometriosis on recipients of sibling oocytes: matched case-control study. Fertil Steril 74(1):31, 2000.

[b]Two caveats: (a) women with red/white/vesicular lesions considered as controls (may have lowered control group outcome); (b) underpowered to show smaller difference (Berube 1998).

- Proposed mechanism of reduced fecundity for minimal-mild endometriosis:
  - o ↑ Prostaglandins (PGs), cytokines, oligoovulation, luteal phase defect, ↑ complement C3 and ↓ $\alpha_v\beta_3$ integrin, glycodelin A, osteopontin, lysophosphatidic acid receptor 3 and HOXA10 expression in endometrium in mid-secretory phase (Khorram 2002; Wei 2008) autoimmune reaction
  - o Inhibitory effect of peritoneal fluid from women with moderate-severe endometriosis on sperm motility (Oral 1996) adverse effect on sperm capacitation by macrophage migration inhibitory factor (Carli 2007)
  - o Cumulative pregnancy rate after 5 years without therapy: 90% (minimal disease) (D'Hooghe 2003)
- Comparison of pregnancy outcome after in vitro fertilization (IVF)/intra-cyloplasmic sperm injection (ICSI) for endometriosis (stage I) vs. unexplained subfertility (Omland 2005):
  - o ↓ 1st cycle pregnancy rate (48.6% endometriosis vs. 58.8% unexplained; $P < .05$)
  - o ↓ Live birth rate (66% endometriosis vs. 78.8% unexplained; $P < .05$)

- ○ ↑ Spontaneous abortion < 6 weeks estimated gestational age (19.3% endometriosis vs. 11.7% unexplained; $P < .05$)
- Women with stage III/IV endometriosis have diminished ovarian reserve (lower anti-müllerian hormone [AMH]) compared to age-matched controls undergoing IVF for male factor (Shebl 2009).

Menstrual Irregularities *(Vercellini 1997)*

- Premenstrual spotting (15–20%)
- Heavy menstrual bleeding more common

Gastrointestinal Involvement *(Weed and Ray 1987)*

- ~5% Gastrointestinal involvement:
  - ○ Rectum/sigmoid (70%) > appendix > cecum > distal ileum > ascending colon > transverse/descending colon
- Only ~50% incidence of additional endometriotic lesions in such women
- Common symptoms: bloating, crampy abdominal pain, tenesmus, change in bowel habits, ↓ bowel movements, hematochezia, anorexia
- Serosa and muscularis are most often affected, whereas the mucosa is rarely involved (Panganiban 1972); if the endometriotic lesion is ≥1.75 cm, all patients had lymph node involvement (Abrao 2006).
- May be removed laparoscopically if located far enough from the anus and a skilled laparoscopic surgeon is present with the ability to do segmental colonic resection

DIAGNOSIS

Examination

- Localized tenderness of cul-de-sac
- Nodularity of the uterosacral ligaments
- Obliteration of the cul-de-sac
- Fixed retroversion of the uterus
- Ovarian enlargement
- Lateral cervical displacement (resulting from uterosacral scarring) (Propst 1998)

Transvaginal Sonography

- Useful in diagnosis of endometrioma → homogeneous hypoechoic carpet of low-level echoes or *ground-glass* appearance (Kupfer 1992)

Laparoscopy

- Most common sites: ovary, post–cul-de-sac, broad ligament, uterosacral ligaments, rectosigmoid colon, bladder
- Endometriomas involve the *left* ovary more frequently than
  the *right* ovary (Jenkins 1986).
  - Cells regurgitated through the right tube are more exposed
    to the clockwise peritoneal current and may be removed
    by the macrophage disposal system (Rosenheim 1979).
- Women with endometriotic lesions of the *left* hemipelvis
  have a greater risk of disease recurrence and delay of future
  pregnancy compared to those with disease confined to the
  right hemipelvis (Ghezzi 2001).
- Diaphragmatic endometriotic lesion distribution: right-only =
  66%, left-only = 6%, bilateral = 27% (Vercellini 2007); this
  supports the menstrual reflux theory as the cells get stuck on
  the right hemidiaphragm by the falciform ligament.
- Blue-black "powder burn" lesion (older, enclosed implant?)
- Varied appearance: red, white, yellow, clear (active lesions?
  higher vascularity and mitotic activity)
- In women with no visible endometriosis, a biopsy of
  normal-appearing peritoneum shows evidence of endometriosis in 6% of cases (Balasch 1996).
- Deep endometriosis when lesion penetrates through mesothelium (Koninckx 1991)

RECTOVAGINAL ENDOMETRIOSIS
CLASSIFICATION BASED ON LOCATION

- Type I/RV septum nodules (10%): within the RV septum
  between the posterior wall of the vaginal mucosa and the
  anterior wall of the rectal muscularis
- Type II/posterior vaginal fornix nodules (65%): posterior
  fornix (retrocervical) toward the RV septum
- Type III/hourglass-shaped nodules (25%): posterior fornix
  lesions extending cranially to the anterior rectal wall; average size is 3 cm.

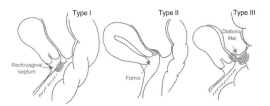

Source: Adapted from Donnez J, Pirard C, Smets M, et al. Surgical managment of
endometriosis. *Best Practice Res Clin Obstet Gynecol* 18(2):329, 2004.

AMERICAN SOCIETY FOR REPRODUCTIVE MEDICINE CLASSIFICATION

- American Society for Reproductive Medicine (ASRM) staging (American Society for Reproductive Medicine 1997):

Patient's Name _____ Date _____

Stage I (Minimal) - 1-5
Stage II (Mild) - 6-15
Stage III (Moderate) - 16-40
Stage IV (Severe) - >40
Total _____

Laparoscopy _____ Laparotomy _____ Photography _____
Recommended Treatment _____
_____

Prognosis _____

	ENDOMETRIOSIS	<1cm	1-3cm	>3cm
PERITONEUM	Superficial	1	2	4
	Deep	2	4	6
OVARY	R Superficial	1	2	4
	Deep	4	16	20
	L Superficial	1	2	4
	Deep	4	16	20

	POSTERIOR CULDESAC OBLITERATION	Partial	Complete
		4	40

	ADHESIONS	<1/3 Enclosure	1/3-2/3 Enclosure	>2/3 Enclosure
OVARY	R Filmy	1	2	4
	Dense	4	8	16
	L Filmy	1	2	4
	Dense	4	8	16
TUBE	R Filmy	1	2	4
	Dense	4*	8*	16
	L Filmy	1	2	4
	Dense	4*	8*	16

*If the fimbriated end of the fallopian tube is completely enclosed, change the point assignment to 16.

Denote appearance of superficial implant types as red [(R), red, red-pink, flamelike, vesicular blobs, clear vesicles], white [(W), opacifications, peritoneal defects, yellow-brown], or black [(B) black, hemosiderin deposits, blue]. Denote percent of total described as R___%,W___% and B___%. Total should equal 100%.

Additional Endometriosis: _____   Associated Pathology: _____
_____   _____
_____   _____

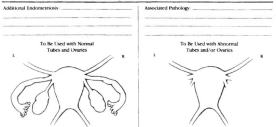

To Be Used with Normal Tubes and Ovaries

To Be Used with Abnormal Tubes and/or Ovaries

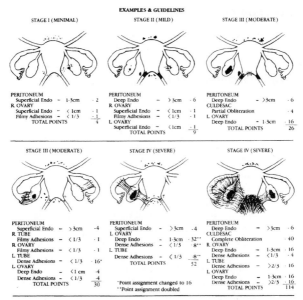

American Society for Reproductive Medicine revised classification of endometriosis. Endo, endometriosis.

Source: Reproduced with permission from Revised American Society for Reproductive Medicine classification of endometriosis: 1996. *Fertil Steril* 67(5):817, 1997.

TREATMENT

1. Expectant management
2. Surgical management
3. Medical treatment
4. Assisted reproductive technology

- Note: In >60% of cases, reappearance of lesions occurs within 1–5 year (10% per year) after hormonal and/or surgical treatment (Regidor 1996).

Expectant Management

- Long-term pregnancy rate: 55–90% for stages I–III with age-related adjustments downward as age advances

Surgical Management

Conservative Surgery

- Excisional and ablative treatments seem to have similar efficacy in treating pain (Wright 2005).
- Regression of disease in 30–40% of women on second-look laparoscopy after initial surgery used to diagnose the disease (Harrison and Barry-Kinsella 2000).
- Uterosacral nerve ablation:
  o Two randomized controlled trials (RCTs) reveal no evidence to support an additional laparoscopic uterine nerve ablation (LUNA) procedure for women undergoing surgical treatment for endometriosis pain (Johnson 2004b; Vercellini 2003a).
- No controlled trials have documented a benefit of preoperative or postoperative medical treatment to ↑ pregnancy rate over surgery alone.
- 30%/2 years recurrence risk after laparoscopic cystectomy (Koga 2006); factors that increase risk of recurrence:
  o prior medical therapy (OR = 2.3)
  o larger (>5 cm) cyst diameter (OR = 1.18)
- In an RCT, laparoscopic cystectomy had a better 24-month pregnancy rate than drainage and coagulation (67% vs. 24%, P <.05) (Beretta 1998).
- 2.4% incidence of ovarian failure following excision of bilateral endometriomas
- Normal ovarian tissue found adjacent to excised endometrioma in ~59% compared with ~5% with other benign cysts (Matsuzaki 2009).
- Laparoscopic excision of endometriomas and ovarian reserve (Somigliana 2003):
  o 32 patients over 46 cycles who had endometriomas removed from one ovary
  o 53% ↓ in number of dominant follicles (IVF cycles) in ovary with prior endometriomas (P <.001):

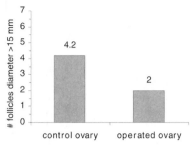

Source: Adapted from Somigliana E, Ragni G, Benedetti F, Borroni R, Vegetti W, Crosignani PG. Does laparoscopic excision of endometriotic ovarian cysts significantly affect ovarian reserve? Insights from IVF cycles. *Hum Reprod.* 18(11):2450–3, 2003.

- Laparoscopic cystectomy for endometrioma (>3 cm) before an IVF cycle does not improve fertility outcomes; likewise, conservative surgical treatment of endometriomas does not impair IVF success rates (Garcia-Velasco 2004).
- Ovarian reserve as judged by antral follicle count may be less impaired by sutured ovaries after cystectomy than in those electrocoagulated for hemostasis (Coric 2011).
- Endometriomas are associated with a reduced responsiveness (mean diameter follicles >15 mm) to gonadotropins (Somilgiana 2006); however, the pregnancy rates seem unaffected (Banaglia 2013).
- IVF outcome is impaired in women having excision of bilateral ovarian endometriomas (4% vs. 17% delivery rate for controls) (Somigliana 2008).
- Removal of unilateral endometriomas prior to IVF compared with no treatment has no significant effect on IVF pregnancy rates (Tsoumpou 2009). See figure that follows.
- The mere presence of an endometrioma is associated with lower AMH values; excision of endometriomas may have a further negative impact on AMH with a **mean decline in AMH by ~1–1.5 ng/mL** (Raffi 2012; Uncu 2013).

Study	Treated endometrioma n/N	Non-treated endometrioma n/N		Weight %	OR 95% CI
Garcia-Velasco 2004	37/147	14/63		53.09	12.18 (0.58, 2.37)
Pabuccu 2004	11/44	8/40		22.75	1.33 (0.58, 2.37)
Wong 2004	17/36	13/38		24.16	1.72 (0.67, 4.39)
Total	65/227	35/141		100.00	1.34 (0.82, 2.20)

n, clinical pregnancy; N, IVF cycle

0.2 0.5 1 2 5

Favors non-treatment   Favors treatment

Source: Adapted from Tsoumpou I, Kyrgiou M, Gelbaya, et al. The effect of surgical treatment for endometrioma on in vitro fertilization outcomes: a systematic review and meta-analysis. *Fertil Steril* 92:75-87. 2009.

- Evidence of enhanced fertility by conservative surgical treatment (minimal-mild endometriosis):):
  - **Endocan (Canadian study) (Marcoux 1997)**
    - → RCT; data collected for 36 weeks; stage I–II (30% stage II); infertility ~2 years

n = 341	Ablation (%)	Diagnostic Laparoscopy Only (%)
Cumulative pregnancy[a]	31.0[b]	18.0
Fecundity[c]	4.7	2.4

[a] >20 weeks' gestation.
[b] $P < .01$.
[c] Rates of 20-week pregnancies per 100 person months (RR, 95% CI=1.7, 1.2-2.6).

- - - 8 women need surgery to achieve one additional pregnancy; however, because we cannot diagnose endometriosis preoperatively, the number may actually double to 16 surgeries for one pregnancy.

    - Of the 29/168 pregnancies in the diagnostic laparoscopy group, 4 underwent fertility treatment that month compared to 0 of the 50/172 pregnancies in the ablation group; suggesting fertility treatment, if anything, led to an overestimation of the effect on the diagnostic laparoscopy group.

    - Clear or pink vesicular lesions (may be *most active*!) not included
  - **Gruppo Italiano (Italian study) (Parazzini 1999)**
    - → RCT; data collected for 12 weeks; stage I–II (60% stage II); unexplained infertility ≥2 years

n = 96	Ablation	Diagnostic Laparoscopy Only
Spontaneous conceptions	24%	29%

○ Marcoux + Gruppo Italiano common odds ratio benefit:

	Common Odds Ratio Benefit
All conceptions	1.7 (95% CI, 1.1–2.6)
>20-week pregnancy	1.6 (95% CI, 1.0–2.7)

CI, confidence interval.

→ NNT = 12 meaning for every 12 women having stage I or II endometriosis there will be 1 additional successful pregnancy if resection is performed compared to no treatment; Therefore, modest efficacy of endometriosis ablation in ↑ pregnancy rate in infertile women with minimal-mild endometriosis

Retrospective observational study on impact of surgery for stage I–II and stage III–IV (Coccia 2008).

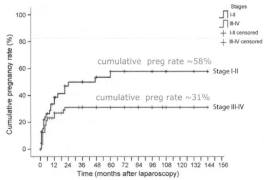

Reproduced with permission from Coccia ME, Rizzello F, Cammilli F, et al. Endometriosis and infertility Surgery and ART: An integrated approach for successful management. *Eur J Obstet Gynecol Reprod Biol.* May;138(1):54-9, 2008.

Definitive Surgery

- Symptoms refractory to medicine/conservative surgery
- Hysterectomy with bilateral salpingo-oophorectomy: 90% rate of success (Lamvu 2011)
- Recurrence rate: 0–5% (same if patient taking estrogen treatment)
- Posthysterectomy + oophorectomy estrogen replacement may start in the postoperative period without ↑ incidence of symptom recurrence (Hickman 1998); addition of a progestin is unnecessary.

Postoperative Adjuvant Drug Therapy

- Six randomized trials:

Regimen	Length of Treatment (months)	n	Results
Danazol vs. medroxy-progesterone acetate vs. placebo	6	51	↓ Pain in treatment groups at 1 year
GnRH-a vs. placebo	3	53	No difference in pain at 1 year[a]
GnRH-a vs. placebo	6	93	↓ Pain at end of treatment but no difference at 1 year[a]
Danazol vs. no treatment	3	77	No difference in pain at 9 months[a]
GnRH-a vs. no treatment	6	210	No difference in pain at 1 year[a]
GnRH-a vs. no treatment	3	89	No difference in pain at 18 months[a]

Dz, danazol; GnRH-a, gonadotropin-releasing hormone agonist.
[a]Low statistical power to detect smaller, though clinically significant, differences.
Source: Adapted from Telimaa S, Ronnberg L, et al. Placebo-controlled comparison of danazol and high-dose medroxyprogesterone acetate in the treatment of endometriosis after conservative surgery. *Gynecol Endocrinol* 1(4):363, 1987; Parazzini F, Fedele L, et al. Postsurgical medical treatment of advanced endometriosis: results of a randomized clinical trial. *Am J Obstet Gynecol* 171(5):1205, 1994; and Hornstein MD, Hemmings R, et al. Use of nafarelin vs. placebo after reductive laparoscopic surgery for endometriosis. *Fertil Steril* 68(5):860, 1997.

Medical Treatment

Progestins

- Results in endometrial decidualization—atrophy and pseu-dodecidualization (Silverberg 1986; Maruo 2001).
- 5 mg/day oral norethindrone acetate
- 20–30 mg/day oral medroxyprogesterone acetate or progestin-only pill
- Levonorgestrel-intrauterine device (lng-IUD, Mirena) delivers 20 µg levonorgestrel/day over 5 years.

Oral Contraceptives

- Continuously; 60–90% effective; 1st-year recurrence =
  17%, 5–10% annual recurrence rate
  - → RCT (cyclic OCs vs. placebo) with radiologically-
    confirmed endometrioma: dysmenorrhea score
    significantly reduced (Harada 2008)
  - → RCT: continuous monophasic OC vs. GnRH agonist
    + norethindrone acetate 5 mg (Guzick 2011)
    - equally effective
- Continuous use of oral contraceptives after surgery for endo-
  metriomas greatly reduces the long-term recurrence rate:

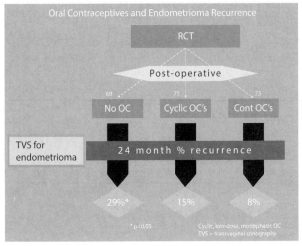

Source: Adapted from Seracchioli R, Mabrouk M, Frascà C et al Long-term cyclic and
continuous oral contraceptive therapy and endometrioma recurrence: a randomized
controlled trial. *Fertil Steril.* Jan;93(1):52-56, 2010.

Gonadotropin Releasing Hormone Agonist

- To avoid flare effect, initiate GnRH-a at
  - Midluteal phase or
  - After 2 weeks of OCs (started on cycle day 1 or 2) over-
    lapping by 1 week
- Side effects: breakthrough bleeding (BTB), vasomotor
  symptoms (2nd month), vaginal dryness, mood altera-
  tion, insomnia, irritability, headache, depression, reversible bone mineral density loss (loss of 5% by dual-energy
  x-ray absorptiometry (DXA) at conclusion of 6 months of
  therapy)

Lupron Depot, 3.75 mg IM q28 days, or
Goserelin, 3.6 mg SC q28 days, or
Nafarelin, 400–800 mg/day intranasally in divided doses

Early-onset BTB

1. Rule out pregnancy.

2. Withdrawal bleed after 1st cycle is common.

3. Confirm adequate suppression ($\downarrow E_2$) if on GnRH-a.

4. Initiate GnRH-a closer to onset of menses.

5. Consider progestin or oral contraceptive pretreatment 2 weeks pre–GnRH-a.

Late-onset BTB

1. Rule out pregnancy.

2. Confirm scheduling.

3. Confirm adequate suppression ($\downarrow E_2$).

4. Rule out atrophic bleeding (treatment: low-dose estrogen replacement therapy)

BTB, breakthrough bleeding; E_2, estradiol; GnRH-a, gonadotropin-releasing hormone agonist.

- 75–90% effective, pain symptoms return within 1 year of treatment with GnRH-a, 20% having recurrent symptoms requiring retreatment (Hornstein 1995)
- Empiric GnRH-agonist is not given to adolescents <16 years old due to concerns on long-term bone density.
- Add-back therapy:
  - Used for vasomotor symptoms and bone preservation.
    → Therapeutic window:

E_2 (pg/mL)	E_2-Dependent Ramification
<80	Lipid metabolism compromised
<60	Vaginal epithelial atrophy
<40	Vasomotor symptoms
<20	Bone density deterioration

E_2, estradiol.
Note: Optimal (E_2) 30–50 pg/mL for endometriosis.
Source: Adapted from Barbieri RL. Hormone treatment of endometriosis: the estrogen threshold hypothesis. *Am J Obstet Gynecol* 166:740, 1992.

- ○ Add-back options
  - → Norethindrone acetate, 5 mg PO/day
  - → Estradiol, 25 μg transdermal patch each week
  - → Conjugated equine estrogen, 0.625 mg/day

Add-Back Therapy for GnRH-a Patients

Author (reference)	Groups	Symptoms	Vaso-motor Symptoms	BMD
Hornstein 1998 (n = 201) 1 year of treatment	a) Placebo	↑	88%	↓
	b) NETAc (5 mg/day)	↓	47%	No change
	c) NETAc (5 mg/day) + CEE (0.625 mg/day)	↓	58%	No change
	d) NETAc (5 mg/day) + CEE (1.25 mg/day	↓	40%	No change

Note: A significantly higher percentage of patients terminated due to lack of symptom relief in group (d) than in group (a).

Freundl 1998 (n = 27) 6 months of treatment	a) Placebo	↓	92%	-6.5
	b) Ethinyl estradiol (20 mg/day) + desogesterel (0.15 mg/day)	↓	57%	-2.0

Note: Dysmenorrhea for both groups but dyspareunia only in group (a); ASRM scoring after treatment not as diminished in group (b) as for group (a) suggesting oral contraceptives may induce more rapid lesion recurrence.

CEE, conjugated equine estrogens; GnRH-a, gonadotropin-releasing hormone agonist; NETAc, norethindrone acetate.

Depo-subQ Provera 104™ (Crosignani 2006; Schlaff 2006)

- Clinical data show that depo-subQ provera 104 is equally as effective for treating pain as GnRH-a with significantly less decline in bone mineral density and lower incidence of hot flashes; 17% incidence of abnormal vaginal bleeding.

Aromatase Inhibitor

- Regimen: letrozole, 2.5 mg/day; norethindrone acetate, 5 mg/day; vitamin D, 800 IU/day; calcium citrate, 1.25 g/day
- In the limited studies to date, aromatase inhibitors combined with add-back treatment (i.e., NETAc 5 mg PO daily) may effectively reduce endometriosis-pain (Ferrero 2011)
- Estradiol levels decrease by 97–99% with doses of 1–5 mg of aromatase inhibitors.
- Possible adverse effects: hot flashes (without add-back), mild headache, joint stiffness, nausea and diarrhea

SUMMARY OF MEDICAL AGENTS USED TO TREAT ENDOMETRIOSIS

Class	Drug	Dosage
Androgen	Danazol[a]	100–400 mg PO twice a day 100 mg per vagina daily
Aromatase inhibitor	Anastrozole[b] Letrozole[b]	1 mg PO daily 2.5 mg PO daily
Estrogen-Progestin combinations	Monophasic estrogen/progestin[a]	Low ethinyl estradiol dose continuously
Gonadotropin-releasing hormone agonist	Goserelin[ab] Leuprolide depot[ab] Nafarelin[ab]	3.6 mg SC monthly (10.8 mg IM every 3 months) 3.75 mg IM monthly (11.75 mg IM every 3 months) 200 mg intranasally twice a day
Gonadotropin-releasing hormone antagonist	Cetrorelix	3 mg SC weekly

(Continues on next page)

(Continued from previous page)

Progestin	Depo-subQ Provera 104[a]	104 mg/0.65 mL SC every 3 months
	Dienogest[c]	2 mg daily
	Etonogestrel-releasing implant	1 for 3 years
	Levonorgestrel-releasing IUS	1 for 5 years
	Medroxyprogesterone acetate	30 mg daily PO for 6 months, followed by 100 mg IM every 2 weeks x 2 months, then 200 mg IM monthly x 4 months
	Norethindrone acetate[a]	5 mg daily

[a] **FDA-approved for endometriosis**

[b] With add-back, i.e., norethindrone acetate 5 mg daily + vitamin D 800 IU daily + Calcium 1.25 gm daily

[c] Dienogest is a 19-nortestosterone derivative that is approved in the European Union for treatment of endometriosis. It is not available in the USA as a separate drug. It is only available in the oral contraceptive Natazia (estradiol valerate/dienogest), which is a newer four-phasic pack that contains dienogest.

Assisted Reproductive Technologies

- Fertility: No role for drug therapy (OC, progestins) in the treatment of infertility associated with endometriosis
- Superovulation in women with endometriosis:

Regimen	n	Cycle Fecundity Rate (%)	
		Treatment Group	*Expectant Group*
Clomiphene citrate, IUI	67	9.5	3.3
Human menopausal gonadotropin, human chorionic gonadotropin, IUI	49	15.0	4.5

(Continues on next page)

(Continued from previous page)

Follicle-stimulating hormone, IUI	103	11[a]	2[a]

IUI, intrauterine insemination.
[a]Live birth rate (%).
Source: Adapted from Deaton JL, Gibson M, et al. A randomized, controlled trial of clomiphene citrate and intrauterine insemination in couples with unexplained infertility or surgically corrected endometriosis. *Fertil Steril* 54(6):1083, 1990; Fedele L, Bianchi S, et al. Superovulation with human menopausal gonadotropins in the treatment of infertility associated with minimal or mild endometriosis: a controlled randomized study. *Fertil Steril* 58(1):28, 1992; and Tummon IS, Asher LJ, et al. Randomized controlled trial of superovulation and insemination for infertility associated with minimal or mild endometriosis. *Fertil Steril* 68(1):8, 1997.

- IVF outcome: endometriosis only vs. tubal factor only, meta-analysis:

Regimen	Pregnancy Rate		
	Stage I–II	*Stage II–IV*	*Control Group*
In vitro fertilization	21.1%	13.8[a]	27.7

[a]Odds ratio, 0.46 (0.28, 0.74).
Source: Adapted from Barnhart K, Dunsmoor-Su R, et al. Effect of endometriosis on in vitro fertilization. *Fertil Steril* 77(6):1148, 2002.

- GnRH-a pretreatment before IVF: prospective, randomized trial:

Regimen	n	Cycle Pregnancy Rate (%)
No GnRH-a	26	55
GnRH-a × 3 months	25	80[a]

GnRH-a, gonadotropin-releasing hormone agonist.
[a]$P <.05$; NNT = 4.
Source: Adapted from Surrey ES, Silverberg KM, et al. Effect of prolonged gonadotropin-releasing hormone agonist therapy on the outcome of in vitro fertilization–embryo transfer in patients with endometriosis. *Fertil Steril* 78(4):699, 2002.

- 3 RCT utilizing 3–6 months of GnRH agonist prior to IVF in women with stage II–IV endometriosis led to a fourfold increase in clinical pregnancy rates (Sallam 2006)

Treatment Algorithms

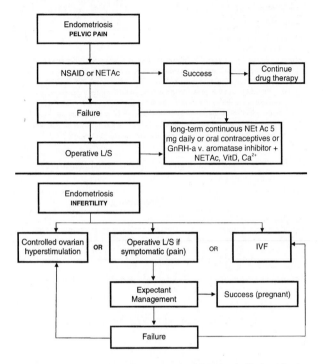

GNRH-a, gonadotropin-releasing hormone agonist; IVF, in vitro fertilization; L/S, laparoscopy; NETAc, norethindrone acetate; NSAID, nonsteroidal anti-inflammatory drug; OC, oral contraceptive; VitD, vitamin D.

17
Fibroids

PREVALENCE

- Cumulative incidence of fibroids by age 50 of 70–80%
  (Baird 2003)
- 70–80% cumulative incidence of fibroids at 50 yo.
- Prevalence of uterine myomas in the 1st trimester of pregnancy (prospective cohort study) (Laughlin 2009):
  - **18% in African-American women**
  - **10% in Hispanic women**
  - **8% in white women**

CLASSIFICATION

Submucosal

- Fibroid distorts the uterine cavity.

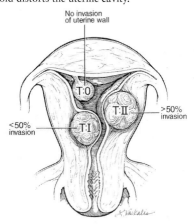

Source: Reproduced with permission from Cohen L, Valle R. Role of vaginal sonography and hysterosonography in the endoscopic treatment of uterine myomas. *Fertil Steril* 73(2):197–204, 2000.

Intramural

- <50% protrudes into the serosal surface.
- >50% of the myoma is within the myometrium.

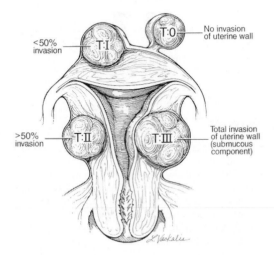

Source: Reproduced with permission from Cohen L, Valle R. Role of vaginal sonography and hysterosonography in the endoscopic treatment of uterine myomas. *Fertil Steril* 73(2):197–204, 2000.

Subserosal

- >50% protrudes out of the serosal surface (sessile or pedunculated).

FIBROIDS AND BLEEDING

- Most common symptom is menorrhagia or hypermenorrhea.
- Obstructive effect on uterine vasculature may lead to endometrial venule extasia → proximal congestion in the myometrium/endometrium → hypermenorrhea.
- ↑ Size of uterine cavity (sometimes appreciated on hystero-salpingogram) leads to greater surface area for endometrial sloughing.

FIBROIDS AND PAIN *(Lippman 2003)*

- ↑ Severity of dyspareunia and noncyclic pelvic pain with the presence of fibroids
- Dysmenorrhea not more common in those with fibroids vs. those without fibroids
- Fibroids in the fundus may be associated with more severe dyspareunia and pelvic pain.

FIBROIDS AND INFERTILITY

- Sole factor for infertility in <10% of infertility cases (Wallach and Vu 1995)
- Submucosal is most likely to cause infertility, then intramural, then subserosal (Farhi 1995).
- Prospective study of small (≤5 cm) intramural fibroids on the cumulative outcome of up to 3 attempts of IVF/ICSI: (Khalaf 2006)
  - ↓ 40% pregnancy rate with each cycle.
  - ↓ 45% cumulative ongoing pregnancy rate.
  - ↓ 49% cumulative live birth rate
  - However, it is still unclear if this negative impact can be ameliorated by a myomectomy.
- Submucosal mechanism of infertility:
  - Dysfunctional uterine contractility (Vollenhoven 1990)
  - Focal endometrial vascular disturbance
  - Endometrial inflammation; endometritis
  - Secretion of vasoactive substances
  - Enhanced androgen environment (Buttram and Reiter 1981)
- Patients are advised to wait 4–6 months after myomectomy before attempting to conceive.
- Uterine artery embolization is not recommended in patients considering future fertility.

FIBROIDS AND REPRODUCTIVE OUTCOME

- 80% of fibroids remain the same size or diminish during pregnancy (Lev-Toaff 1987).
- Complications: miscarriage, ectopic, preterm labor (15–20%), abdominal pain, abruption, intrauterine growth restriction (10%), obstructed labor, postpartum hemorrhage, malpresentation (20%) (Phelan 1995)

- Five retrospective cohort studies:

	Pregnancy Rate (%)	Spontaneous Abortion (%)[a]
Submucosal	9	40
Intramural	37	33
Subserosal	16	33
Control	29	20

[a]Small numbers.
Source: Adapted from Bajekal N, Li TC. Fibroids, infertility, and pregnancy wastage. *Hum Reprod Update* 6:614, 2000.

Reproductive Outcome

	CPR-RR	Spontaneous Abortion Rate
Submucosal	**0.36** (CI 0.18–0.74)	**1.68** (CI 1.37–2.05)
Intramural	**0.71** (CI 0.44–1.15)	**2.38** (CI 1.11–5.12)

CPR-RR, clinical pregnancy rate-relative risk.

Bold signifies P<0.05 (Source: Adapted from Pritts EA, Parker WH, Olive DL. Fibroids and infertility: an updated systematic review of the evidence. *Fertil Steril.* Apr;91(4):1215–23, 2009.)

- Review of 27 studies: No conclusive evidence on whether number, size, or location of fibroids before myomectomy influenced postoperative pregnancy (Vercellini 1998).
- Markers of endometrial receptivity (HOXA10, HOXA11, LIF and BTEB1 proteins) were significantly decreased in adjacent and surface endometrium of uteri from the women with **submucosal myomas** (Rackow 2008).
- Using an oocyte donation model, the presence of intramural leiomyomas without cavity distortion, regardless of size and number, had **no detrimental effect on ongoing pregnancy rates** or implantation genes within the endometrium (Horcajadas 2008).

SUBMUCOSAL FIBROIDS

- RCT of hysteroscopic myomectomy for submucousal fibroids (Shokeir 2010):

	Pregnant
Hysteroscopy-diagnostic	29/103 **(28.2%)**
Hysteroscopy with resection of fibroid	64/101 **(63.4%)**

RR=2.1 (95% CI 1.5-2.9), **NNT=3**

Note: **There was no difference in fertility rate for those with type II myomas.**

Source: Modified from Shokeir T, El-Shafei M, Yousef H, Allam AF, Sadek E. Submucous myomas and their implications in the pregnancy rates of patients with otherwise unexplained primary infertility undergoing hysteroscopic myomectomy: a randomized matched control study. *Fertil Steril.* 94(2):724-9, 2010.

- The majority of women who conceive do so within the first year after a myomectomy.
- Many of the studies demonstrating a higher pregnancy rate after myomectomy are nonrandomized and suffer from an inherent selection bias. There is no prospective data addressing myomectomy outcomes for women with subserosal and/or intramural fibroids without intracavitary involvement. If there is no cavity distortion, then there is no information (Surrey 2001).

AROMATASE INHIBITOR *(Parsanezhad 2010)*

- Aromatase inhibitors (letrozole 2.5 mg daily for 3 months) have been shows to reduce the size of uterine myomas more effectively than after use of a GnRH agonist.
- Further study will deterimine if hypoestrogenic side effects and follicular recruitment can be minimized while on aromatase inhibitors

PREOPERATIVE GONADOTROPIN-RELEASING HORMONE AGONIST

Background

- Greater potency and longer half-life (t½) than native GnRH
- Analogs: decapeptide with substitutions at positions 6 and 10
- Initially stimulates gonadotropin release—lasts 1–2 weeks
- Fibroid growth stimulated by estrogen and progesterone

- Down-regulation with GnRH-a induces a state of hypoestrogenism (<30 pg/mL) and anovulation.
- Long-term treatment with GnRH-a is limited due to side effects (bone mineral density loss and hot flashes)
- Myoma volume ↓ 30% using GnRH-a (leuprolide) in a double-blind, placebo-controlled study (Schlaff 1989).
- Randomized, placebo-controlled study did not find that GnRH-a preoperative treatment led to ↓ size of small myomas, rendering them undetectable at surgery and early recurrence (Friedman 1992).
- Fibroids regrow after discontinuing GnRH-a
- Therefore, GnRH-a used mainly in preoperative setting for definitive therapy (hysterectomy) or conservative therapy (myomectomy).
- Prospective, RCT found no benefit from preoperative GnRH-agonist treatment prior to hysteroscopic resection of submucosal fibroids (Mavrelos 2010)

Outcomes of Gonadotropin-Releasing Hormone Agonist–Treated Groups vs. Nontreated

Preoperative Gonadotropin-Releasing Hormone Agonist Treatment × 3–4 Months

	Weighted Mean Difference	95% Confidence Interval
↑ Hematocrit	3.1%	1.8 to 4.5
↓ Uterine volume	−159 mL	−169 to −149
↓ Gestational size	−2.2 weeks	−2.3 to −1.9
↓ Fibroid volume	−12 cc	−18.3 to −6.6
Pelvic symptom score	−2.1	−2.4 to −1.9

Source: Data from Lethaby A, Vollenhoven B, Sowter M. Efficacy of pre-operative gonadotropin hormone releasing analogues for women with uterine fibroids undergoing hysterectomy or myomectomy: a systematic review. *BJOG* 109:1097, 2002.

Intraoperative Outcomes

	Myomectomy	**Hysterectomy**
Blood loss	ND	↓ 58 mL (–76 to –40)
Duration of surgery	ND	↓ 5.2 minutes (–8.6 to –1.8)
Hospital stay	ND	ND
Rate of blood transfusions	ND	ND
Proportion of vertical skin incisions	0.11 (0.1–0.8)	0.4 (0.2–0.6)

ND, no difference.
Source: Data from Lethaby A, Vollenhoven B, Sowter M. Efficacy of pre-operative gonadotropin hormone releasing analogues for women with uterine fibroids undergoing hysterectomy or myomectomy: a systematic review. *BJOG* 109:1097, 2002.

Postoperative Outcomes

	Myomectomy	**Hysterectomy**
Postoperative complications	ND	↑ 0.6% (0.4–0.9)
Postoperative hematocrit	ND	↑ 1.8% (1.1–2.4)
Fibroid recurrence[a]	4.0[b] (1.1–14.7)	Not applicable

ND, no difference.

[a]Only two published trials.

[b]May not see small fibroids at the time of surgery in pretreated women.
Source: Data from Lethaby A, Vollenhoven B, Sowter M. Efficacy of pre-operative gonadotropin hormone releasing analogues for women with uterine fibroids undergoing hysterectomy or myomectomy: a systematic review. *BJOG* 109:1097, 2002.

Interventions to Reduce Blood Loss During Myomectomy

- Misoprostol (200–400 mg vaginally), intramyometrial injection of vasopressin (20 U in 50 cc NS) and tourniquets; more research is needed as studies to date have been underpowered studies to date (Kongnyuy 2007).

Laparoscopic Myomectomy: Outcomes of Gonadotropin-Releasing Hormone Agonist–Treated Groups vs. Nontreated

Preoperative Gonadotropin Releasing Hormone Agonist Treatment × 2 Months

	Value	P Value
Blood loss	↓ 60.3 mL	<.01
Duration of surgery		
Fibroids with high echogenicity	↓ 24.4 minutes	<.05
Fibroids with low echogenicity	↑ 13.4 minutes	<.05

Source: Adapted from Zullo F, Pellicano M, et al. A prospective randomized study to evaluate leuprolide acetate treatment before laparoscopic myomectomy: efficacy and ultrasonographic predictors. *Am J Obstet Gynecol* 178(1 Pt 1):108, 1998.

Recurrence after Myomectomy *(Parker 2007; Hanafi 2005; Brahma 2006)*

- Risks for recurrence (Hanafi 2005):
  - multiple leiomyomata
  - > 10 week sized uterus
  - high BMI
  - weight gain
  - insulin resistance, diabetes

Overall 10 year recurrence after myomectomy

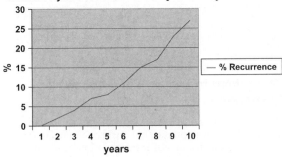

Source: Reproduced with permission from Parker WH. Uterine myomas: management. *Fertil Steril.* Aug;88(2):255–71, 2007.

18
Polycystic Ovary Syndrome

- ~8% of reproductive-aged women have polycystic ovary syndrome (PCOS)
- Genetics:

Affected 1st-Degree Relative	Risk of Polycystic Ovary Syndrome (%)
Mother	35
Sister	40

Source: Adapted from Kahsar-Miller MD, Nixon C, Boots LR, et al. Prevalence of polycystic ovary syndrome (PCOS) in first-degree relatives of patients with PCOS. *Fertil Steril* 75(1):53, 2001.

- Mothers of women with PCOS have elevated low-density lipoprotein/androgen levels as well as markers of insulin resistance (IR) consistent with a heritable trait (Sam 2006).
- PCOS patients frequently develop regular menstrual cycles when aging (Elting 2000), possibly resulting from ↓ size of the follicle cohort? Or from ↓ inhibin?
- **Theory of etiology:** *enhanced serine phosphorylation unification theory* → ↑ CYP17 activity in the ovary (hyperandrogenism) and ↓ insulin receptor activity peripherally (insulin resistance [IR]) (Dunaif 1995) lead to the endocrine dysfunction of PCOS.

CLINICAL SIGNS AND SYMPTOMS

Menstrual Dysfunction

- Onset at menarche: oligo/amenorrhea

Infertility

- Ovulatory dysfunction

Obesity

- Obesity occurs in 35–65% of women with PCOS (>80% are obese before puberty).
- Androgens converted to E_1 in peripheral fat and can contribute to endometrial hyperplasia.
- Fat contributes to insulin resistance.

Hirsutism

- Gradual onset over months to years; onset usually with puberty
- Dark, coarse hairs in androgen-dependent locations
- Associated with hyperandrogenemia (classic PCOS) and idiopathic increased end organ sensitivity
- *Ferriman-Gallwey* scores (see Appendix B in this chapter) are used to quantify degree of hirsutism and grade responses to treatments (Ferriman and Gallwey 1961); on a day-to-day clinical basis, most endocrinologists rely on patient perceptions and frequency of waxing or electrolysis.

Variable Other Signs and Symptoms

- **Acne:** no known correlation between the severity of acne and plasma free T (Slayden and Azziz 1997)
- **Acanthosis nigricans:** usually seen with significant insulin resistance; called the *h*yperandrogenism, *i*nsulin *r*esistance–*a*canthosis *n*igricans (**HAIR-AN**) syndrome:
  o Dermal hyperkeratosis and papillomatosis presenting as a brown or gray, velvety, occasionally verrucous, hyperpigmented area over the neck, vulva (most common), axillae, groin, umbilicus, and submammary areas
- **Insulin Resistance** (~30%) or overt non–insulin-dependent diabetes mellitus (NIDDM) (~8%) (Dunaif 1997)
- Skin tags
- **Polycystic-appearing ovaries** (PCAOs) not necessarily a prerequisite for diagnosis (see criteria in the following text); present in 30% of population:

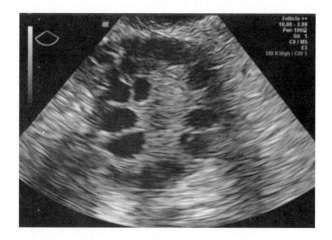

CLINICAL EVALUATION OF POLYCYSTIC OVARY SYNDROME/HIRSUTISM

- Revised 2003 Rotterdam European Society for Human Reproduction and Embryology (ESHRE)/American Society for Reproductive Medicine (ASRM)–sponsored PCOS consensus on diagnostic criteria for PCOS (**two out of three**) (Rotterdam ESHRE/ASRM-Sponsored PCOS Consensus Workshop Group 2004):

1. Oligo- and/or anovulation

2. Clinical and/or biochemical (total testosterone >70 ng/dL (2.4 nmol/L); androstenedione >245 ng/dL (8.6 nmol/L); DHEA-S >248 µg/dL (6.7 µmol/L)) signs of hyperandrogenism

3. Polycystic ovaries (≥12 follicles [2–9 mm diameter]) or increased ovarian volume (>10 cm³) in either ovary.

Exclusion of other etiologies (e.g., nonclassic congenital adrenal hyperplasia [NCAH], hyperprolactinemia, Cushing's syndrome, and androgen-secreting tumors)

- NIH panel recommendation identifying the specific patient phenotype (Source: NIH Evidence-based Methodology Workshop on Polycystic Ovary Syndrome, Dec 2012)
  o androgen excess + ovulatory dysfunction
  o androgen excess + polycystic ovarian morphology
  o ovulatory dysfunction + polycystic ovarian morphology
  o androgen excess + ovulatory dysfunction + polycystic ovarian morphology

- In most cases, the diagnosis can be made on history and physical examination (H&P) alone; ~10% incidence

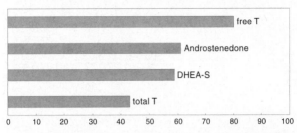

Frequency of elevation of each of the androgens in 138 women with polycystic ovary syndrome (Wild 1983), listed as a percentage. DHEA-S, dehydroepiandrosterone sulfate; T, testosterone. (Source: Adapted from Wild RA, Umstot ES, Andersen RN, et al. Androgen parameters and their correlation with body weight in one hundred thirty-eight women thought to have hyperandrogenism. *Am J Obstet Gynecol* 146[6]:602, 1983.)

Diagnostic Studies *(Phipps 2001)*

Testosterone

- Unbound (free) T (uT), total T
- Most testosterone assays have poor sensitivity and accuracy in the female ranges, even for women with PCOS.
- Circulating levels vary by: menstrual phase, time of day, food intake.
- Total T upper limit = 200 ng/dL (6.9 nmol/L); free T upper limit = 2.2 pg/mL (7.6 pmol/L)
- Rule out ovarian androgen-producing tumor if T levels >200 ng/dL (6.9 nmol/L).
- % Free T of total T:
  - Normal men: 3%
  - Normal women: 1%
  - Hirsute women: 2% (ovary is major source of ↑ T and A_4)
  - A single androgen level may not be representative of the average because the secretion is pulsatile; a single serum T level may differ by 38% from the 24-hr mean.
- Measure free T by (a) equilibrium dialysis or (b) ammonium sulfate precipitation.
  - Androgens return to basal level ~8 weeks following discontinuation of oral contraceptives (Sanchez 2007)

Estradiol and Follicle-Stimulating Hormone

- May be helpful to exclude hypogonadotropic hypogonadism (↓ E_2, ↓ FSH) and premature ovarian failure (POF) (↓ E_2, ↑ FSH).

Dehydroepiandrosterone Sulfate

- Upper limit = 430 μg/dL (11.7 μmol/L)
- Rule out adrenal androgen-producing tumor if >700 μg/dL (19 μmol/L).
- Note: may not be of benefit if T is normal, as all androgen-producing adrenal tumors will present with increased testosterone (personal communication, Leon Speroff, MD)

17-Hydroxyprogesterone (in Follicular Phase, 8:00 a.m.) + Progesterone

- 17-OHP upper limit = 200 ng/dL (6 nmol/L)
- Rule out nonclassic 21-hydroxylase deficiency.
- P_4 is drawn to be sure that the patient is not in the luteal phase when 17-OHP is naturally elevated; want P_4 <3 ng/mL (104 pmol/L)

24-Hour Urinary Cortisol

- Cortisol usually <50 μg/24 hr (<135 nmol/24 hr); Cushing's diagnosed if the urinary cortisol is greater than 3 times the upper limit of normal
- Consider additional testing for Cushing's syndrome if patient is hypertensive.

Prolactin

- Upper limit = 30 ng/mL
- Rule out hyperprolactinemia as cause of ovulatory dysfunction.
- Also check thyroid-stimulating hormone (TSH) to rule out hyperprolactinemia from hypothyroidism.

Thyroid-Stimulating Hormone

- Rule out thyroid disease as cause of ovulatory dysfunction.

Glucose Tolerance Testing

- Insulin resistance is present in both lean and obese PCOS
- Screening ought to be done every 2 years for those with normal values and every year if insulin resistant.
- Hemoglobin A1c:
  - 5.7–6.4% = insulin resistance
  - ≥ 6.5% = diabetes (confirm with repeat test)

	Fasting Plasma Glucose (mg/dL)	**2-hr Plasma Glucose (mg/dL)**
Normal	≤99	≤139
Impaired	100–125	140–199
Type II diabetes mellitus	≥126	≥200

Source: Adapted from American Diabetes Association Diagnosis and classification of diabetes mellitus. *Diabetes Care* 33 (Suppl1):S62-S69, 2010.

- Incidence of IR or NIDDM in women with PCOS (Legro 1999):
  - IR: 31.1%
  - Type II DM: 7.5%

Lipid Profile

- Cholesterol, high-density lipoprotein (HDL), low-density lipoprotein (LDL), triglycerides (Orio 2004)

Adrenocorticotropic Hormone Stimulation Test

- For those with moderately elevated 17-OHP (200–400 ng/dL), in setting of normal P_4 (<3ng/mL), in whom NCAH is suspected (see page 190 on Nonclassic Congenital Adrenal Hyperplasia)

Pelvic Ultrasound

- For PCAO (polycystic-appearing ovaries) and endometrial thickness
- **PCAO** in ~30% of all reproductive-aged women
  - May occur from a variety of causes (Givens 1984)
  - Ovarian volume may be proportional to the level of circulating insulin (Pache 1993)
- **Endometrium:** Incidence of endometrial abnormalities in 56 obese women with PCOS (Cheung 2001):
  - Hyperplasia: 36%
  - Atypia: 9%
    - → Progression to carcinoma (Kurman 1985):
      - 2% of untreated hyperplasia without atypia
      - 23% untreated hyperplasia with atypia
  - Evidence for ↑ risk of endometrial carcinoma in PCOS is incomplete and contradictory; it may apply only to the subgroup who are obese (BMI >27) (Hardiman 2003)

RULE OUT OTHER DIAGNOSES

Virilizing Ovarian or Adrenal Tumor

- *Rapid* onset and *progressive* course of virilizing symptoms
- *Severe* hirsutism: male pattern balding, clitoromegaly, weight gain
- Total T >200 ng/dL (6.9 nmol/L) or DHEA-S >700 µg/dL (19 µmol/L)
  - Positive predictive value of a repeat total T >250 ng/dL → 9%; negative predictive value of 100% (Waggoner 1999)

		Presence of Tumor		
		Yes	**No**	
T>250 ng/dL { 1/11	**Y**	1	10	1/11
467/467	**N**	0	467	467/467
		Sensitivity	**Specificiy**	

  - Computed tomography (CT) of pelvis and adrenals with contrast if tumor suspected (may require selective venous catheterization of ovarian/adrenal veins)
  - Most common virilizing ovarian tumor: *arrhenoblastoma*
  - Adrenal tumor: suspect if DHEA-S >700 µg/dL (19 µmol/L)
    → Diagnosis: Dexamethasone, 0.5 mg PO q6 hr × 2 days
      - Measure DHEA-S and 17-OHP, before and after steroid course
        ❖ If no decrease to normal → virilizing adrenal tumor (Cushing's syndrome), although some tumors may suppress DHEA-S.
        ❖ If levels decrease → NCAH vs. PCOS; need to check 17-OHP

Cushing's Syndrome

- If patient is hypertensive, assess 24-hr free urinary cortisol

Idiopathic Hirsutism

- Clinical hyperandrogenism with normal androgen levels and regular ovulatory cycles
  - Women with PCOS have greater 5α-reductase activity than healthy women (Fassnacht 2003).
  - The enzyme responsible for the degradation of dihydrotestosterone (DHT) (3α-hydroxysteroid dehydrogenase, type III) may be deficient in some hirsute women (Steiner 2004).

Nonclassic Congenital Adrenal Hyperplasia

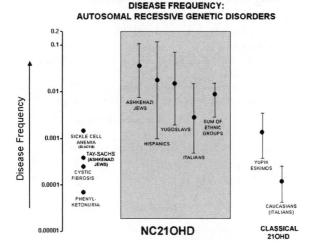

Source: Reproduced with permission from New MI. Nonclassical 21-Hydroxylase *Deficiency J Clin Endo Metab* 91:4205–4214, 2006.

Ethnic Group	n	Disease Frequency	Carrier Frequency
Ashkenazi Jews	56	1:27	1:3
Hispanics	9	1:40	1:4
Slavics[1]	8	1:50	1:5
Italians	12	1:300	1:10
Heterogeneous population of New York City	249	1:100	1:6

[1] From Croatia.
Source: Reproduced with permission from New MI. Nonclassical 21-hydroxylase deficiency. *J Clin Endo Metab* 91:4205–4214, 2006.

- 17-OHP and P_4 to discriminate between PCOS and NCAH:
  - a.m. follicular phase, due to circadian variability
- The presenting signs of NCAH in children include premature pubarche, cystic acne, accelerated growth and advanced bone age. Patients are tall children but short adults (New 2006).

17-Hydroxyprogesterone (17-OHP) (ng/dL)	Diagnosis
<200	Polycystic ovary syndrome
200–400	Cortrosyn stimulation test[a]
>400	Nonclassic congenital adrenal hyperplasia

[a]Cortrosyn stimulation test: Measure 17-OHP at t = 60 after 0.25 mg IV adrenocorticotropic hormone administration (see list below).

t = 60 17-Hydroxyprogesterone (ng/dL):

>1,500 = NCAH

>1,000 = Likely NCAH

<1,000 = Polycystic ovary syndrome

- **21-Hydroxylase deficiency** (gene: *CYP21A2*) (20–50% enzyme activity) is an autosomal-recessive trait with variable genotype-phenotype patterns. More than 40 CYP21A2 mutations have been found in association with NCAH due to 21-hydroxylase deficiency.
  - Incidence: 1/1,000
  - Treatment: 5.0–7.5 mg prednisone in two divided doses
    → May restore ovulation but relatively ineffective for existing hirsutism; monitor for iatrogenic Cushing's syndrome (rapid weight gain, hypertension, pigmented striae, and osteopenia).
    → Treatment efficacy is considered a target 17-OHP between 1 and 10 ng/mL measured at the nadir of steroid blood levels.

TREATMENT DURING PREGNANCY:

Mother Is a Carrier and Had a Previous Child with CAH

- If she becomes pregnant with the same partner, the fetus has a 1-in-4 chance of having CAH
- Consider IVF with PGD to look for CAH
- Dexamethasone (not inactivated by placental enzymes and thus provides more effective suppression of fetal adrenals) if PGD is not performed and the gender and CAH status of the current fetus is unknown (Lo 1999). The goal here is

to suppress endogenous androgen production by the fetal adrenal and thus prevent virilization.

- o Dexamethasone 20 μg/kg in divided oral doses t.i.d. (it is unclear why such a high dose is needed)
- o Since maternal estriol (E_3) is derived from the placental metabolism of fetal adrenal androgens, serum E_3 levels can be used to monitor glucocorticoid therapy: **Aim for E_3 between 0.2–10 nmol/L**
- Nevertheless, ~15% of female fetuses who receive glucocorticoid treatment will still have some virilization
- Since genitalia begin virilization just 6 weeks after conception, to be effective, corticosteroid treatment (see below for dosage recommendations) must be started before 9 weeks, although this is controversial. Informed consent is suggested—see "Rationale for withholding glucocorticoid replacement." Steroids are continued until genetic diagnosis from chorionic villous biopsy or cell-free circulating DNA at 10-12 weeks. If the results show a CAH-affected female fetus, dexamethasone is continued in order to diminish fetal virilization from high maternal androgen exposure.

In a Mother with CAH or NCAH

- Screen the father for CAH/NCAH
- Start glucocorticoid replacement before 9 weeks of gestation using prednisolone or hydrocortisone to lower maternal androgens and avoid virilization of female fetus; prednisolone or hydrocortisone is inactivated by placental enzymes and hence do not suppress fetal adrenal androgens, but they do reduce maternal androgen production. If a male karyotype is determined, corticosteroids can be discontinued.
- o Prednisolone 7 mg/day, range from 4 to 10 mg/day
- o Hydrocortisone 30 mg/day, range from 15 to 40 mg/day
- Aggressive suppression of maternal androgens in pregnancy is **probably not warranted** since the placenta can effectively aromatize maternal androgens. However, if the aromatase enzyme is saturated by extremely high androgen levels, then theoretically, virilization of a female fetus could occur. This is extremely rare with maternal CAH (Oglivie 2006).

Rationale for Withholding Glucocorticoid Replacement

- Adverse effects to the mother: weight gain, edema, striae, signs of Cushing syndrome
- Adverse effects to the fetus:
  - glucocorticoids are increasingly recognized as having potent genomic imprinting effects in utero with the following potential adverse effects to the fetus: postnatal failure to thrive, psychomotor developmental delay, neuropsychological dysfunctions, increased risk of orofacial clefts
- Clinical Practice Guidelines statement for CAH due to 21-hyroxylase deficiency published in 2010 by the Endocrine Society: "We recommend that prenatal therapy continue to be regarded as experimental" (qtd. in Speiser 2010).
- Conundrum treating all at risk for only 1 in 8 affected female fetus (Miller 2013):
  - Since only 1 in 4 will be affected, and only half of the affected fetuses will be females (those most benefiting from treatment) then treatment would be directed toward only 1 in 8 fetuses. Put another way, one would be exposing 7 of 8 fetuses (4 of 4 males and 3 of 4 females) to high dose dexamethasone to treat the one affected female.

- o Maternal blood testing for fetal Y-chromosomal DNA
  can determine fetal sex and thus improve the probability

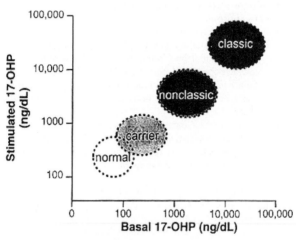

Nomogram for comparing 17-hydroxyprogesterone (17-OHP) ratio before and after administration of 0.25-mg IV cosyntropin (carriers = heterozygotes). (Source: Reproduced with permission from White PC, Speiser PW. Congenital adrenal hyperplasia due to 21-hydroxylase deficiency. *Endocr Rev* 21[3]:2454, 2000.)

of treating an affected female fetus from 1 in 8 to 1 in 4.
- o Diagnosis with ACTH stimulation test (0 and 60 min) (Lutfallah 2002):
- • 3β-Hydroxysteroid dehydrogenase deficiency (gene: *HSDB2*): less common and no consensus on this diagnosis

PATHOPHYSIOLOGY OF POLYCYSTIC OVARY SYNDROME

Endocrine Dysfunction

Hypersecretion/Elevation of Luteinizing Hormone

- • ↑ Pulse amplitude and frequency, ↑ luteinizing hormone (LH) bioactivity (abnormal LH secretion is secondary to ovarian dysfunction):
  - o Lack of negative feedback (↓ progesterone [P_4])?

- ○ Programming of the hypothalamic-pituitary axis by androgens?
- ○ ↓ Sex hormone–binding globulin (SHBG) from hyper-insulinemia and hyperandrogenemia leads to ↑ free estradiol levels, lowering follicle-stimulating hormone (FSH) relative to LH.
  - → Insulin is the most potent inhibitor of SHBG (Nestler 1991).

Hyperinsulinemia

- Hyperinsulinemia leads to ↓ SHBG, ↓ IGF-binding protein (IGFBP)-I and ↑ free androgens.
- Total serum IGF-I levels are normal in PCOS, but ↓ IGFBP-I concentrations can lead to ↑ **free IGF-I**.
- IGF-I and -II → ↑ LH stimulation of androgens in theca cells.
- Insulin may also ↑ androgen production directly or may ↑ LH secretion from the pituitary (Dorn 2004).
- **Waist-hip ratio** >0.85 (central obesity) is significantly related to insulin sensitivity, but body mass index (BMI) is not.

Androgen Excess

- Ovarian production: ↑ LH results in theca hyperplasia (theca cell dysfunction), resulting in ↑ testosterone (T), androstenedione (A_4), dehydroepiandrosterone (DHEA), 17-hydroxyprogesterone (17-OHP), and estrone (E_1). Ovarian estradiol (E_2) production is unchanged.
- Adrenal is a secondary source of elevated serum androgens. Nonclassic adrenal hyperplasia (NCAH)—a genetic defect in either the 21-hydroxylase (*CYP21B*) or the 3β-hydroxysteroid dehydrogenase (3bHSD) genes—results in elevated levels of primarily adrenal androgens (i.e., DHEA-sulfate [DHEA-S]).
- ↓ SHBG leads to ↑ free androgen and estrogen (↓ SHBG from elevated insulin, hyperandrogenemia, hyperprolactinemia).
- 30% of patients with PCOS show mild hyperprolactinemia (Isik 1997).

Prevalence of Different Androgen Excess Disorders in 950 Women Referred Because of Clinical Hyperandrogenism Organ Dysfunction

	Number of Patients	% of Total Number of Patients
Classic PCOS	538	56.6
Ovulatory PCOS	147	15.5
Idiopathic hyperandrogenism	150	15.8
Idiopathic hirsutism	72	7.6
NCAH	41	4.3
Androgen-secreting tumors	2	0.2

Source: Reproduced with permission from Carmina E, Rosato F, Janni A et al. Extensive clinical experience: relative prevalence of different androgen excess disorders in 950 women referred because of clinical hyperandrogenism. *J Clin Endo Metab.* 91(1):2–6, 2006.

Potential Long-Term Consequences of Polycystic Ovary Syndrome

Definite or Very Likely Consequences of Polycystic Ovary Syndrome	Possible Consequences of Polycystic Ovary Syndrome
Insulin resistance; type II diabetes mellitus (greater than weight-matched controls)	Hypertension
	Dyslipidemia
Coronary heart disease	Ovarian cancer (conflicting data)
Endometrial hyperplasia/atypia	Spontaneous abortion (may not be greater than for subfertility population)
Gestational diabetes	
Sleep apnea (even when controlled for body mass index)	
Depression	

- Hyperlipidemia (Mahabeer 1990; Orio 2004) may increase levels of plasminogen activator inhibitor (PAI; major inhibitor of fibrinolysis); PAI is an independent risk factor for atherosclerosis.

- ↑ Left ventricular mass index noted in asymptomatic women with PCOS compared with controls (Orio 2004).
- Studies showing no clear association between PCOS and cardiovascular events may be biased due to PCOS study patients having had wedge resection (Pierpoint 1998; Wild 2000).
- Type II diabetes mellitus (DM): 3–7× ↑ incidence in PCOS patients

TREATMENT
Goals

- Prevent endometrial hyperplasia/cancer
- Restore normal menstruation; resolution of anovulation/infertility
- Improve hirsutism and acne

Weight Reduction

- As little as 5–7% of body weight reduction can reduce hyperandrogenism, improve insulin sensitivity, and restore spontaneous ovulation and fertility in 75% of women with PCOS (Kiddy 1992).
  - Low-calorie diet (1,000–1,500 kcal/day)
  - Waist-hip ratio >0.85 at greater risk for morbidity
  - Metformin may promote weight loss.

Oral Contraceptives

- 1st line of drug treatment (use at least 30 μg of ethinylestradiol and avoid norgetrel and levonorgestrel)
- Method of action: ↑ SHBG, suppression of LH, inhibition of 5α-reductase and androgen receptor binding
- Greatest efficacy against acne (hirsutism usually requires the addition of antiandrogens)
- Avoid levonorgestrel-containing oral contraceptives (OCs), due to the androgenic properties of the progestin (e.g., Alesse, Levlen, Nordette, Triphasil).
- OCs ↓ LH but not to normal levels (Polson 1988).
- Gonadotropin-releasing hormone (GnRH) agonist plus add-back no better than OCs alone (Carr 1995).

Progestins

- Give progestins q month or q 2–3 months to prevent endometrial hyperplasia.

Antiandrogens

- Antiandrogens are effective in the treatment of hirsutism after 6–9 months; however, cessation of antiandrogen therapy is followed by recurrence (Yucelten 1999).
  - **Spironolactone** (Aldactone, 100–200 mg/day) plus OCs (Lobo 1985; Young 1987); *Contraception is mandatory* with the use of spironolactone, as incomplete virilization of a male fetus may occur. Wait ≥2 months after discontinuance of spironolactone before beginning attempts at conception.
    - → Aldosterone antagonist, K+-sparing diuretic:
      - Inhibits steroidogenic enzymes and binds the DHT receptor at the hair follicle
      - Can cause irregular uterine bleeding
      - 25-mg tablets are generic and inexpensive
  - **Finasteride** (Proscar, 5 mg/day), type II 5α-reductase inhibitor; shows signs of being an excellent and safe antiandrogen
    - → ↓ Circulating DHT levels; not effective topically (Price 2000); not approved by the U.S. Food and Drug Administration (FDA) for this purpose
    - → Low dose (2.5 mg) every 3 days is as effective as continuous administration in ↓ hirsutism (Tartagni 2004).
    - → *Contraception is mandatory* (Ciotta 1995; Wong 1995; Fruzzetti 1999) because its use during the late first trimester may ↑ risk of hypospadias and other genital abnormalities in male fetuses.
  - **Cyproterone acetate (Androcur)**, not approved in the United States (used extensively in Europe [Diane 35] and Israel for hirsutism)
    - → Androgen receptor antagonist, decreases 5α-reductase activity, impairs androgen synthesis
    - → Reports of liver tumors in beagles have kept this effective drug from the U.S. market.
  - **Eflornithine** (Vaniqa, 13.9% topical cream b.i.d.)
    - → Irreversibly inhibits ornithine decarboxylase (ODC) to inhibit follicle polyamine synthesis necessary for hair growth
    - → Effect seen over 4–8 weeks; *reversible* if medicine is stopped
    - → <1% systemic absorption; skin irritation may occur
    - → Category C drug

Hair Removal Systems

- Systemic treatment of hyperandrogenism and hirsutism should be combined with hair removal (shaving, waxing, depilatories [short-acting], or electrolysis or laser [long-acting]) for maximum effect on existing hair.

Electrolysis

- Electric current (through needle in hair follicle) destroys hair follicle.
- Blend most effective: galvanic electrolysis and thermolysis
- Expensive, painful, and time-consuming but can be permanent
- Scarring if not done correctly

Laser-Assisted Hair Removal

- Thermal injury targeted to follicular melanin ("selective photothermolysis") destroys hair follicle (Hobbs 2000).
- Works best for those with light skin and dark hair, although newer lasers are better at light hair.
- May cause pigment changes: hypo- or hyperpigmentation
- Requires multiple (4–6) treatments; effect may be improved by waxing before procedure.
- Avoid in patients who form keloids or hypertrophic scars or who are on retinoids.
- For dark skin, choose longer wavelength: Nd:YAG and Diode; avoid long-pulsed Ruby (Lanigan 2003).
- Types of Lasers
  - **Nd:YAG:** 1064 nm, Q-switched or long-pulsed, temporary hair loss, uses carbon solution massaged into hair follicles
  - **Ruby:** 694 nm, long-pulsed, long-term reduction in hirsutism, pigment changes can occur
  - **Alexandrite:** 755 nm, long-pulsed, may have fewer pigment changes, long-term reduction
  - **Diode:** 800 nm, long-term hair loss, fewer pigment changes, works less well on fine hair

Insulin Sensitizing Drugs

Metformin (Glucophage)

- Biguanide oral hypoglycemic agent
- Inhibits hepatic glucose production; increases peripheral tissue insulin sensitivity; ↓ LH, free T, and PAI-I
  - Avoid metformin if: creatinine >1.4 mg/dL (124 μmol/L); liver function tests (LFTs) are elevated → ↑ risk of lactic

acidosis; severe congestive heart failure; history of alcohol abuse

○ Metformin may cause dizziness and/or gastrointestinal (GI) discomfort (10–25% of patients) and should not be taken with IV contrast dye (e.g., hysterosalpingogram [HSG])

○ Metformin XR regimen (no consensus regarding optimal dose [Nestler 2001]):

○ Stop after 1st trimester, although preliminary studies suggest no teratogenicity.

500 mg — 1 week → 1000 mg metformin XR QHS

Source: Fulghesu AM, Romualdi D, Di Florio C, et al. Is there a dose-response relationship of metformin treatment in patients with polycystic ovary syndrome? Results from a multicentric study. *Hum Reprod.* Oct;27(10):3057–66, 2012.

CMRMN Study (Legro 2007)

• 6-month randomized trial comparing clomiphene, metformin, or both for PCOS.

• Live birth rate was 22.5% in clomiphene group, 7.2% in metformin group, and 26.8% in the combination group (p <0.001 for metformin vs. either other group).

• Rate of multiple pregnancy was 6% (clomiphene), 0% (metformin), and 3.1% (combination-therapy group).

• No significant difference in first TM loss although metformin was discontinued with a positive pregnancy test (not adequately powered).

• No placebo-only group.

• Placebo-controlled randomized trial: metformin vs. placebo (Morin-Papunen 2012)

○ Metformin significantly increases the live birth rate with an NNT of 7.6

• Metformin and the incidence of preeclampsia and perinatal mortality—single study with unsubstantiated results (Hellmuth 2000).

○ Metformin vs. insulin-treated: 32% vs. 10% incidence of preeclampsia (p <.001)

○ Metformin vs. insulin- or sulfonylurea-treated: 11.6% vs. 1.3% incidence of perinatal mortality (p <.02)

• In a randomized, controlled trial, metformin reduced the incidence of diabetes in persons at high risk ($\downarrow$ 31% over 3 years; number needed to treat = 14) (Jakubowicz 2002).

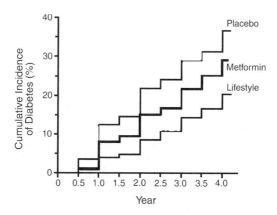

Reproduced with permission from Knowler WC, Barrett-Connor E, Fowler SE, et al. Reduction in the incidence of type 2 diabetes with lifestyle intervention or metformin. *N Engl J Med.* 2002;346(6):393.

TREATMENT OF ANOVULATION AND INFERTILITY

- In a couple in whom the woman is diagnosed with PCOS the prevalence of additional infertility factors are as follows (McGovern 2007):
  - 10% Oligospermia
  - 4% Nonpatency of tubes
  - 1% Hyperprolactinemia
  - 1% Uncontrolled thyroid disease

- **Weight loss** (5%): Guzick (1994) compared weight loss to no weight loss in obese, hyperandrogenic, anovulatory women. Women in the treatment group displayed ↑ SHBG, ↓ free T, and ↓ fasting insulin levels. Four of six spontaneously ovulated. As little as a 7% ↓ in body weight significantly improves hyperandrogenism (Kiddy 1992). 5–10% ↓ in body weight is enough to restore ovulation in 55–100% within 6 months (Kiddy 1992).
- **Metformin:** See page 199
- **CC or aromatase inhibitors:** treatment of choice
  - If nonresponsive, a higher dose of CC or AI may be initiated without inducing menses = "stair-step" protocol (Hurst 2009)

- o 10-day letrozole protocol (2.5 mg cycle days 1–10) may be more effective than a standard 5-day protocol (Badawy 2009)
- o Ovulatory rates of ~80%
- o Pregnancy rates of 60–70% within the first 6 months
- **Gonadotropins:** PCOS patients are highly susceptible to hyperstimulation; start with low doses.
- **Glucocorticoids**
  - o Steroid treatment appears to be related to the suppression of excessive androgen levels (Steinberger 1979).
  - o Three randomized trials revealed ↑ pregnancy rates (40–75% vs. 4–35%) in CC-resistant women (Daly 1984; Elnashar 2006; Parsanezhad 2002).
  - o Response seen for those with or without elevated DHEA-S levels.
  - o One protocol is to utilize **2 mg dexamethasone from cycle days 5 through 14** in conjunction with ovulation induction medicine (Parsanezhad 2002).
- **Laparoscopic ovarian cautery/drilling:**
  - o Restores spontaneous ovulation in ~50% of CC-resistant hyperandrogenic women (Gjønnæss 1984; Daniell and Miller 1989; Abdel Gadir 1990; Gjønnæss 1998; Lazovic 1998; Vegetti 1998).
  - o Consider the balance between reducing androgen levels and potential negative effects:
    - → Postoperative adhesion formation
    - → General endotracheal anesthesia
    - → Iatrogenic diminished ovarian reserve
  - o Spontaneous abortion (SAB) rate may be lower for ovarian cautery compared with medical induction of ovulation (Abdel Gadir 1992).
  - o Predictors of success:
    - → Good responders:
      - ■ Women with hyperinsulinemia respond better to ovarian drilling than do those with normoinsulinemia with respect to lowered glucose and insulin values (Saleh 2001).
      - ■ LH >10 IU/L (Amer 2004)
      - ■ Lean PCOS women (<25 kg/m² BMI) (Baghdadi 2012)
    - → Poor responders (Amer 2004):
      - ■ BMI ≥35 kg/m²
      - ■ Total T ≥4.5 nmol/L or 130 ng/dL
      - ■ Duration of infertility >3 years

- In women with PCOS, the pregnancy rate at 12 and 18 months after drilling is 55% and 70%, respectively (Felemban 2000).
- 18-20 years after ovarian cauterization in anovulatory PCOS women, 74% were still ovulating (Gjønnaess 1998)
- Randomized, controlled trial for CC-resistant women with PCOS: ovarian cauterization or recombinant FSH:

Technique	Pregnancies (%)	Live Births (%)
r-hFSH	67	60
Ovarian cauterization	34	34
Ovarian cauterization → anovulatory women given CC	29	29
Ovarian cauterization → anovulatory women given r-hFSH after failed CC	65	52

CC, clomiphene citrate (Clomid); r-hFSH, recombinant human follicle-stimulating hormone.
Source: Adapted from Bayram N, Van Wely M, et al. Using an electrocautery strategy or recombinant follicle stimulating hormone to induce ovulation in polycystic ovary syndrome: randomised controlled trial. *BMJ* 328(7433):192, 2004.

COCHRANE LIBRARY REVIEW CONCLUDING STATEMENT CONCERNING OVARIAN DRILLING

There is a lack of controlled data, and relatively few RCTs of this surgical technique have been carried out. With such a small number of patients studied in a controlled way and underpowered studies, conclusions about the effectiveness of laparoscopic treatment of the polycystic ovarian syndrome remain uncertain. Although observational data show that it is likely that ovarian drilling has a beneficial effect on ovulation and pregnancy rates for anovulatory PCOS patients wishing to conceive, more data on the short- and long-term safety of the procedure are required.

TREATMENT SUMMARY

	Dose/ Technique	Mechanism of Action	Side Effects
Spironolac-tone	100–200 mg b.i.d.	Aldosterone antagonist Competitive AR blockage 5α-Reductase and CYP17 inhibitor Inhibits androgen synthesis	AUB, head-aches, mastal-gia, ambiguous genitalia in male offspring
Finasteride	5 mg q.d.	Azasteroid 5α-Reductase inhibitor	Ambiguous genitalia in male offspring
Metformin XR	1,500 mg q.d.	Biguanide oral hypoglycemic Reduces ovarian cytochrome p450c17α; ↑ sex hormone–binding globulin	Gastrointestinal: nausea, vomit-ing, flatulence, diarrhea
Ovarian drilling	5–8/ovary (electrocauteri-zation) (Gjøn-næss 1998) 25–40/ovary (laser) (Daniell and Miller 1989)	Alteration of the intraovarian steroid environ-ment and, in turn, the feedback to the hypothalamic pituitary axis May last >18 years (Gjønnæss 1998)	Adhesion formation; risk of premature ovarian failure

APPENDIX A

Ferriman-Gallwey Scores

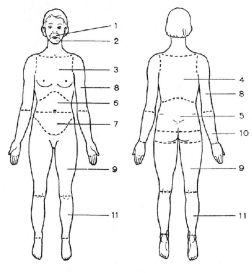

Site	Grade	Definition
Upper lip	1	Few hairs at outer margin
	2	Small moustache at outer margin
	3	Moustache extends halfway from outer margin
	4	Moustache extending to midline
Chin	1	Few scattered hairs
	2	Scattered hairs with small concentrations
	3, 4	Complete cover, light and heavy
Chest	1	Circumareolar hairs
	2	With midline hair in addition
	3	Fusion of these areas, with ¾ cover
	4	Complete cover
Upper back	1	Few scattered hairs
	2	Rather more, still scattered
	3, 4	Complete cover, light and heavy

(Continues on next page)

(Continued from previous page)

Lower back	1	Sacral tuft of hair
	2	With some lateral extension
	3	¾ Cover
	4	Complete cover
Upper abdomen	1	Few midline hairs
	2	Rather more, still midline
	3, 4	Half and full cover
Lower abdomen	1	Full midline hairs
	2	Midline streak of hair
	3	Midline band of hair
	4	Inverted V-shaped growth
Arm	1	Sparse growth affecting ≤¼ limb surface
	2	More than this; cover still incomplete
	3, 4	Complete cover, light and heavy
Forearm	1, 2, 3, 4	Complete cover of dorsal surface; two grades of light and two grades of heavy growth
Thigh	1, 2, 3, 4	As for arm
Leg	1, 2, 3, 4	As for arm
Total Score:	____	

Source: Reproduced with permission from Ferriman D, Gallwey JD. Clinical assessment of body hair growth in women. *J Clin Endocrinol Metab* 21:1440, 1961.

APPENDIX B

Steroid Hormone Synthesis

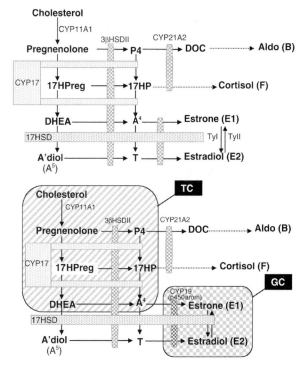

A_4, androstenedione; A'diol, androstenediol; Aldo (B), aldosterone; DHEA, dehydro-epiandrosterone; DOC; 17HP, 17OH-progesterone; GC, granulosa cell; HSD, hydroxysteroid dehydrogenase; 17-HPreg, 17OH-pregnenolone; P_4, progesterone; T, testosterone; TC, theca cell; TyI, type I; TyII, type II.

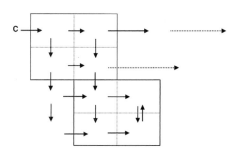

Steroid biosynthesis worksheet.

19
Female Subfertility

BASIC INFERTILITY

Fast Facts

- 12% of all couples suffer from infertility.
  - Monthly pregnancy rate (PR) in couples with unexplained subfertility after 18 months' duration → 1.5–3.0%
  - Cumulative PRs for couples with unexplained subfertility 1 year and 3 years after the first visit are 13% and 40%, respectively.
- Approximately 50% of healthy women become clinically pregnant during the first two cycles, and between 80% and 90% during the first 6 months (Gnoth 2003; Wang 2003).

DEFINITIONS

- **Subfertility:** failure to conceive after 1 year of unprotected intercourse (Gnoth 2005)
- **Fecundability:** conception rate; usually *per month*
  - Normal → 20%
  - 38-year-old with 3-year history of infertility → 2%
- **Fecundity:** birth rate per 1 month

ETIOLOGY

Cause of Infertility	%
Female factors (single)	
Tubal Factor	40%
Ovulatory dysfunction	40%
Unexplained infertility	10%
Unusual problems	10%
Male Factor in 35% of infertile couples	

Source: Adapted from Fritz MA, Speroff L. Infertility. In *Clinical Gynecologic Endocrinology and Infertility*. 8th ed. Philadelphia: Lippincott Williams & Wilkins, 2011.

MATERNAL AGE

- Fertility decreases with maternal age.

Age	Subfertile (%)
≤30 years old	25
30–35 years old	33
35–40 years old	50
>40 years old	>90

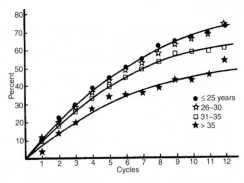

Effect of age on the cumulative pregnancy rate in a donor insemination program. The younger age groups (<31 years) were significantly different from the older groups. (Source: Reproduced with permission from Schwartz D, Mayaux MJ. Female fecundity as a function of age: results of artificial insemination in 2193 nulliparous women with azoospermic husbands. Federation CECOS. *N Engl J Med* 306:404, 1982.)

EVALUATION OF THE FEMALE

Family History

- Endometriosis
- Recurrent spontaneous abortions
- Premature ovarian failure/early menopause

Past Medical History

- Infections, sexually transmitted infections, pelvic inflammatory disease (PID)
- Postpartum or postabortion infections
- Appendicitis (ruptured?)

Surgery

- Ovarian cysts
- Appendectomy
- Tubal surgery (i.e., ectopic, hydrosalpinx, tubal ligation)

Menstrual History

- Length of cycles: normal = 24–35 days
- Flow: Hypermenorrhea suggests fibroids or anovulation.
- Cramps: Ovulation is often associated with some dysmenorrhea.

Coital History

- Dyspareunia suggests salpingitis or endometriosis.
- Sperm survive in vaginal secretions up to 1.5 days and in cervical mucus up to 4 days after coitus (Settlage 1973)
- Frequency is important:
  - More than q.o.d. may cause a ↓ count
  - Infrequent coitus ↓ fecundity
  - Must antecede ovulation (see figure on page 216)

Physical Examination

- Body hair distribution, thyromegaly, breast development, galactorrhea, clitoromegaly, male escutcheon, adnexal mass, uterosacral nodularity
- Vagina: Amenorrheic women with **polycystic ovary syndrome (PCOS)** are well estrogenized, whereas **hypothalamic amenorrhea** is associated with vaginal atrophy

Imaging

- Transvaginal ultrasound
  - uterine appearance
  - ovarian morphology and antral follicle count
  - endometrium reaches a plateau in growth at ~cycle day 9 (Bromer 2009):

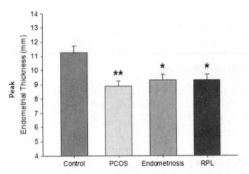

Source: Reproduced with permission from Bromer JG, Aldad TS, et al. Defining the proliferative phase endometrial defect. *Fertil Steril* 91(1):698–704, 2009.
Asterisks refer to the difference from the control group. *P<0.05, **P<0.01.

- Hysterosalpingogram (HSG) or Saline Infusion Sonography (SIS)
  - perform CD 6–12
  - Consider prophylactic antibiotics in high-risk patients:
    - → Azithromycin 1 g PO qhs night before HSG/SIS
    - → Doxycycline 100 mg PO b.i.d. night before and day of HSG/SIS

Laboratory Testing

- PRL: normal <20 mg/mL; if magnetic resonance imaging reveals an adenoma, check insulin-like growth factor-I for growth hormone tumor (acromegaly), 25% of which will produce PRL as well
- TSH > 2.5mIU/mL: treat with 50 µg levothyroxine daily (see Chapter 29)
- Hirsutism laboratory tests: **free testosterone** (a.m. follicular phase), **total testosterone, dehydroepiandrosterone sulfate, 17-hydroxyprogesterone, P_4** (if unsure of time of cycle), HbA1c (diabetes if ≥ or equal to 6.5), **24-hr urinary cortisol** is patient hypertensive
- Ovarian reserve testing AMH or day 2–5 FSH
  - Variability does not affect the prognostic category (Scott 1990).
    - → Variability in different months is just as bad (Buyalos 1998)
  - Basal FSH screening retains its predictive value in women with one ovary (Khalifa 1992).
  - Values >15 mIU/mL are associated with lower live birth rates

Reproductive Physiology of Oviduct *(Lyons 2006)*

- Progressive ↓ in the proportion of ciliated cells from fimbria (>50%) to the isthmus (<35%)
- High serum progesterone leads to atrophy and deciliation
- The strokes of cilia are synchronized and oriented toward the uterine cavity at the time of ovulation
- Post-ovulation, the oocyte takes ~8 hours to reach the ampullary-isthmic junction (site of fertilization); the embryo remains in the tube a further 72 hours
- Following intrauterine insemination it takes ~30 seconds for sperm to reach the oviduct (Schmiedehausen 2003)
- Sperm populate the oviduct within 5 minutes of coitus; there's a constant level of sperm in the oviduct from 15 to 45 minutes following deposition of sperm in the proximal vagina (Settlage 1973).
- The tubal epithelium is the likely site for sperm storage

- o Density of sperm: isthmus > ampulla
- Smoking >20 cigarettes/day leads to ~fourfold risk of ectopic gestation
- Both *Neisseria gonorrhoeae* and *Clamydia trahchomatis* destroy tubal cells

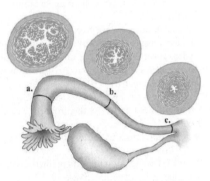

Illustration of the human fallopian tube, showing the longitudinal folds in cross-section at the (a) infundibulum, (b) ampulla and (c) isthmus. (Source: Reproduced with permission from Lyons RA, Saridogan E, et al. The reproductive significance of human fallopian tube cilia. *Hum Reprod Update* 12(4):363–372, 2006.)

Evaluation of Specific Functions

- Timing of diagnostic tests

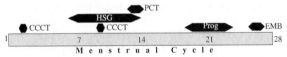

CCCT, clomiphene citrate challenge test; EMB, endometrial biopsy (historical purposes only); HSG, hysterosalpingogram; PCT, postcoital test (historical purposes only); Prog, progesterone.

- *Chlamydia trachomatis* titers if subfertile <1 year (controversial):
  - o ≥1:256 immunoglobulin G serum antibody titers → treat with doxycycline (both partners)
  - o Associated with tubal occlusion, odds ratio (OR), 2.4 (confidence interval [CI], 1.7–3.2) (comparing fertile control subjects to infertile control subjects) (Hubacher 2001)
- Ovulation
  - o Basal body temperature (BBT) chart: normal → biphasic, 12- to 14-day luteal phase; not helpful for timing of coitus

- o Luteinizing hormone (LH) stimulates resumption of meiosis (germinal vesicle [GV] $\longrightarrow$ meiosis II [MII])
- o **LH urine detection kits**
  - → The rise in **serum** LH begins ~36 hours before ovulation
  - → The LH surge appears in **urine** 12 hours after it appears in serum
  - → Therefore, **a positive urine LH kit occurs ~24 hours (95% CI, 14-26 hours) before ovulation (Miller and Soules 1996)**
  - → Note: ovulation occurs ~36 hours after human chorionic gonadotropin (hCG) administration
  - → Despite a positive LH surge by OPK, 7% of women may actually be anovulatory (McGovern 2004)
- o What is the best way to time the IUI?

Type of Study (Using Clomiphene Citrate [Clomid])	No Difference in Pregnancy Rate
Retrospective (Awonuga and Govindbhai 1999)	LH-timed hCG-timed hCG-boost (after positive LH)
Randomized, cross-over (Zreik 1999)	LH-timed hCG-timed

hCG, human chorionic gonadotropin; LH, luteinizing hormone.

- o Key points on **ovulation predictor kits** (from Fertility Plus Web site: http://www.fertilityplus.org/faq/opk.html):
  1. Best time to test → 2 p.m.; anytime between noon and 8 p.m. is fine; first morning urine is not recommended because most women experience a surge in the morning, but it can take 4 hours to show up in the urine.
  2. Clomiphene citrate (CC; Clomid) can cause a false-positive result if tested too soon; should wait at least 3 days (3–7 regimen → start on day 10; 5–9 regimen → start on day 12) after finishing the CC.
  3. Most kits do not show a full positive result until ≥25–40 mIU, but many will show a faint line with LH >10 mIU.
  4. The BBT thermal shift occurs **after ovulation** in response to $\uparrow$ progesterone (P_4) production; positive kits allow timing **before ovulation.**
  5. False-negative results can occur if peak LH concentrations are <40 IU/l, and this may occur in up to 35% of ovulatory cycles (Arici 1994).

   6.   False negative OPKs occur in up to 25% of cycles
        and false positives occur in up to 4%.
- **Fertility monitors** assess LH, estrogen, and P_4 levels.
- Serum P_4: mid-luteal (8 days post-LH surge)
  → 3–5 ng/mL → ovulatory
  → ≥10 ng/mL → adequate P_4 production
- Nearly all pregnancies can be attributed to IC during a
  6-day period ending on the day of ovulation (Wilcox 1995).

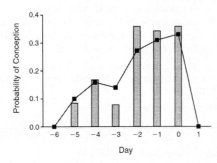

"0" denotes the day of ovulation. (Source: Reproduced with permission from
Wilcox AJ, et al. Timing of sexual intercourse in relation to ovulation. Effects on the
probability of conception, survival of the pregnancy, and sex of the baby. *N Engl J Med*
333:1517–1521, 1995.)

- Cervical mucus: postcoital test (no longer performed, no
  correlation found)
  - Postcoital (Simms-Huhner) test performed preovulatory
    once LH kit is positive; 2–18 hours postcoital
    → Normal: **1 motility sperm/3-of-5 hpf**; copious mucus;
      Spinnbarkeit, 8–10 cm; acellular
    → Poor validity, lack of standard methodology, and
      unknown reproducibility (Griffith and Grimes 1990)
    → No significant effect on PR (Oei and Helmerhorst 1998)
    → Could be useful if male partner needs an incentive to
      obtain a semen analysis because of prior refusal

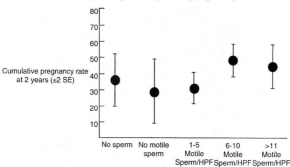

Postcoital testing fail to predict pregnancy

Cumulative pregnancy rates by number of sperm per high-power field (HPF) on postcoital test. (Source: Reproduced with permission from Griffith CS, Grimes DA. The validity of the postcoital test. *Am J Obstet Gynecol* 162:615, 1990.)

TREATMENT

Abnormal Semen Analysis

- See Chapter 20, Male Subfertility.

Ovulatory Dysfunction

- Treat endocrine abnormalities: Bromocriptine; thyroid replacement; progesterone supplementation
- Induce ovulation: CC, letrozole, recombinant human FSH, hCG
  - If a basal ovarian cyst is present (> or equal to 10 mm) there is a lower rate of ovulation upon CC therapy (81% vs. 98%) (Csokmay 2006).
- βhCG 8–11 days after injection of 10,000 mIU/mL should be <50 mIU/mL (Liu 1988)
- After injection of HCG a rise in serum hCG between days 10-12 and a subsequent assay would be indicative of pregnancy (Damewood 1989)
- Using a Danish population of 54,362 women with infertility problems, **no strong association was found between the use of fertility drugs and ovarian cancer**; caveat: many of these women have not yet reached the peak age for ovarian cancer (Jensen 2009). Another, case control study in 1,900 women found no increased risk of ovarian tumors with a history of infertility or use of infertility drugs (Asante 2013).
- The pooled odds ratio for pregnancy (Van Rumste 2008):
  - 1 vs. 2 follicles = 1.6

- - 1 vs. 3 follicles = 2
  - 1 vs. 4 follicles = 2
- The risk of multiple gestations after 2, 3 and 4 follicles increased by 6, 14 and 10% (Van Rumste 2008)
- Clomiphene citrate
  - Weak estrogen that functions as anti-estrogen
  - Requires intact hypothalamic-pituitary-ovarian axis
  - Follow follicular size with ultrasound and increase CC by 50 mg until follicular recruitment obtained
  - Consider IUI especially in couple with unexplained infertility
  - Available as ~3 to 2 ratio of two triphenylethylene derivative geometric isomers: enclomiphene (62% inactive isomer) and **zuclomiphene** (38% active isomer)
  - Half-life = 5 days
  - Risk of twins 10%
  - Body weight and hyperandrogenemia are the predominant predictors for **ovulation** after CC, whereas age and cycle history dictate **pregnancy** chances in **ovulatory women** (Imani 1998; Imani 1999).
  - CC may inhibit E_2-induced endometrial epithelial cell proliferation by inhibiting the recruitment of steroid receptor coactivator-1 (SRC-1) and estrogen receptor α (Amita 2010)
  - Ovulation rate by dose: 50 mg (52%), 100 mg (22%), 150 mg (12%), 200 mg (7%), 250 mg (5%) (Gysler 1982)
  - Baseline pregnancy rates of **1–2%** in patients with **unexplained infertility** may be enhanced to **2–4%** per cycle with CC (Hughes 2000).
  - ⅔ of patients who conceived reach this endpoint within the 1st three ovulatory CC treatment cycles

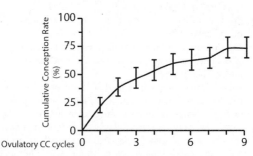

CC, clomiphene citrate. (Source: Reproduced with permission from Imani B, et al. Predictors of chances to conceive in ovulatory patients during clomiphene citrate induction of ovulation in normogonadotropic oligoamenorrheic infertility. *J Clin Endocrinol Metab* 84:1617–1622, 1999.)

- Rare visual changes (palinopsia = prolonged afterimages or shimmering of the peripheral field) that may be irreversible (Purvin 1995)
- Letrozole (Femara® or generic): When used in conjunction with FSH, letrozole reduces FSH dose; PR often equivalent to FSH-only (Mitwally and Casper 2003)
  - Letrozole's terminal elimination half-life is approximately 2 days
  - Letrozole use for ovulation induction is off-label
  - Compared to clomiphenecitrate there was no difference in rate of congenital malformations (Zulaudi 2006, Badawy 2008)
  - Letrozole, 5–7.5 mg/day, days 3–7, and FSH injection (50–150 IU/day starting on day 7 until the day of hCG [10,000 IU])
  - Hybrid cycles denote utilizing both letrozole and FSH in an effort to limit cost as well as maintain efficacy and perhaps diminish high order multiples (Ryan 2005)
  - Clinical studies:
    → Prospective: 324 treatment cycles
    → Prospective trial: unexplained infertility or mild male factor

Method (+ Intrauterine Insemination)	Clinical Pregnancy Rate (%)[a]
FSH	21.4
FSH + CC	11.1
Letrozole + FSH	22.2

CC, clomiphene citrate; FSH, follicle-stimulating hormone.
[a]$P < .05$.
Source: Adapted from Mitwally MF, Casper RF. Aromatase inhibition reduces gonadotropin dose required for controlled ovarian stimulation in women with unexplained infertility. *Hum Reprod* 18(8):1588, 2003.

Drug	Half-Life (Days)	Pregnancy Category
Clomiphene citrate (Clomid)	5	X
Aromatase inhibitor (Femara)	2	X

Cycle Characteristics Using Letrozole as a Single Agent for 5 Days of Ovulation Induction

	Letrozole Dose (mg)		P-value
	5	7.5	
No. of follicles ≥18 mm	**1.4**	**3.4**	<0.05
Cycle day	**11.6**	**9.6**	<0.05
Endometrial thickness (mm)	8.2	10.2	<0.05

Source: Adapted from Badawy A, Metwally M, Fawzy M. Randomized controlled trial of three doses of letrozole for ovulation induction in patients with unexplained infertility. *Reprod Biomed Online.* May;14(5):559–62, 2007.

Gonadotropins (FSH or FSH/Luteinizing Hormone [LH] Combinations)

- Candidates
  - Hypothalamic-pituitary failure
  - Hypothalamic-pituitary dysfunction
    - → PCOS or other anovulatory menstrual disorders
  - Unexplaned infertility or endometriosis
- Informed consent essential
  - Risk of multiple gestation (~20%)
  - Risk of ovarian hyperstimulation depends on stimulation
- Exogenous FSH does not seem to increase the risk of fetal aneuploidy (Massie 2011)
- LH trigger between 9 p.m. and 12 a.m. with IUI ~36 hours thereafter; there is a suppressive effect of FSH treatment on endogenous LH secretion—mechanism unknown (Messinis 1987)
- Luteal phase support: RCT in patients using FSH/IUI randomized to Crinone 8% gel (QD) vs. no support: live birth rate/cycle 17.4% vs. 9.3%, respectively (P<0.05) (Erdem 2009).
- **Glucocorticoids**
  - Glucocorticoid treatment (dexamethasone 0.5 mg/day) can suppress androgen levels in some cases (Steinberger 1979).
  - Two randomized trials revealed ↑ pregnancy rates (40–75% vs. 5–35%) in CC-resistant women (Daly 1984; Parsanezhad 2002).
  - Reserved for PCOS patients with DHEAS high-normal or above

Tubal Disease

- Hydrosalpinx
- Remove or clip hydrosalpinx
  - Meta-analysis: hydrosalpinx ↓ PR by 50% and ↑ spontaneous abortion ×2 (Camus 1999)

Mechanism of Adverse Effect (Strandell and Lindhard 2002)

↓ Nutrients in hydrosalpinx fluid

Toxic effect of fluid on embryos (Sachdev 1997) and/or sperm (Ng 2000)

↓ Endometrial: $\alpha_v\beta_3$, LIF, HOXA10 (Meyer 1997)

Embryo wash-out effect from fluid

↑ Endometrial peristalsis due to hydrosalpinx fluid

↓Endometrial and subendometrial blood flow (Ng 2006)

↑Endometrial inflamatory cells (Copperman 2006)

- Ligation of the hydrosalpinx or salpingectomy restores normal PR (Johnson 2002; Strandell 2001a Kontoravdis 2006)
- Number needed to treat calculation: Seven to eight women would need to have a salpingectomy before IVF to gain one additional live birth (Johnson 2002). A cost-effectiveness analysis of salpingectomy prior to IVF proved this to be a reasonable intervention (Strandell 2005).
- Salpingectomy if hydrosalpinx seen on ultrasound:
  - → Salpingectomy restores endometrial HOXA10 expression (Daftary GS 2007)
  - → No compromise of ovarian stimulation (Strandell 2001b)
  - → RCT (192 patients; outcome = birth rate after first embryo transfer):

	Birth Rate (%)[a]
Salpingectomy	28.6
No intervention	16.3

[a]$P < .05$.

Source: Adapted from Strandell A, Lindhard A, et al. Hydrosalpinx and IVF outcome: a prospective, randomized multicentre trial in Scandinavia on salpingectomy prior to IVF. *Hum Reprod* 14:2762–2769, 1999.

- RCT for ultrasound-guided hydrosalpinx aspiration during IVF resulted in greater clinical pregnancy rates than for controls (31.3% vs. 17.6%). Small numbers however and fluid likely to reaccumulate post aspiration. Utilize i.v. Unasyn 1.5 gm intra-operatively and then Azithromycin 500 mg × 3 days following procedure (Hammadieh 2008)
- Extended doxycycline therapy may be an effective option when surgery is not feasible (Hurst 2001)

Tubal Reversal

- Tubal length (≥4 cm) after reanastomosis is most important; duration of sterilization not important; laparoscopic tubal anastomosis has a 50% PR at 6 months (Bissonnette 1999)
  - Consider female age and presence of male factor when counseling
- Pregnancy success rates after microsurgical tubal reversal: clip > ring > coagulation = Pomeroy (Gordts 2009)

Uterine Abnormalities

- Hysteroscopic resection of adhesions, septum, submucosal leiomyoma, polyp
- Non-cavity-distorting fibroids do not seem to affect IVF pregnancy rates (Klatsky 2007).
- Type O and I submucosal fibroids ought to be resected (see page 175) (Shokeir 2010).
- Polyps (Lee 2010)
  - Prevalence in reproductive-aged women = 1.7%
  - Polyps may regress spontaneously (DeWaay 2002)
  - Endomerial micropolyps are associated with endometrial inflammation (Cicinelli 2005)
  - Mechanism for subfertility:
    - → Overexpression of endometrial aromatase (Pal 2008)
- Prospective study on the frequency of uterine polyps (Shokeir 2004):
  - ~16% in infertile eumenorrheic (n=35/244)
  - ~3% in fertile eumenorrheic (n=1/31)
- Office hysteroscopy prior to IVF found polyps in 32% of 1,000 women (Hinckley 2004).
- In eumenorrheic, infertile women with a normal ultrasound the incidence of uterine polyps with hysteroscopy was 6% (n=41/678) (Fatemi 2010).

- RCT of polypectomy vs. no polypectomy (Peréz-Medina 2005) (also see page 456):
  - Spontaneous pregnancy rate of 29% for polypectomy group vs. 3% in the control group
  - Clinical pregnancy rate of 63% in the polypectomy group compared with 28% in the control group with subsequent FSH/IUI; NNT=3.
  - No difference with respect to size of polyps

Endometriosis

- Medical therapy: suppressive not curative
- See Endometriosis chapter

Unexplained Infertility

- Ultrasound monitoring to time IUI has no significant effect on success rate in patients with unexplained infertility though reasons to perform a sono include: (Lewis 2006)
  - Difficulties with OPKs
  - Patient preference
  - Assess response in order to plan future cycles appropriately
- Success rates for various treatments
  - Retrospective analysis of 45 reports (Guzick 1998)

Method	Pregnancy Rate (%)
Intercourse	4
IUI	4
CC	5.6
CC + IUI°	**8**
FSH	7.7
FSH + IUI°	**17**
In vitro fertilization°	**21**

CC, clomiphene citrate; FSH, follicle-stimulating hormone; IUI, intrauterine insemination.
Note: No randomized control trial: CC vs. CC/IUI; CC vs. FSH.
°Statistically significant difference.
Source: Adapted from Guzick DS, et al. Efficacy of treatment for unexplained infertility. *Fertil Steril* 70:207, 1998.

- IUI vs. FSH/IUI (randomized) (Guzick 1999)

Method	Pregnancy Rate (%)	LB/Couple (%)	LB/Cycle (%)
IUI	18	13	4
Follicle-stimulating hormone/IUI[a]	**33**	**22**	**8**

IUI, intrauterine insemination; LB, live birth.
[a]Statistically significant difference.
Source: Adapted from Guzick DA, et al. Efficacy of superovulation and intrauterine insemination in the treatment of infertility. National Cooperative Reproductive Medicine Network. *N Engl J Med* 340:177, 1999.

- Treatment of infertility usually does not make the difference between conceiving and not conceiving; the difference lies in conceiving sooner rather than later. The risks of the "sooner" option in terms of multiple pregnancy, ovarian hyperstimulation syndrome, emotional stress, and financial costs may be unacceptably high (te Velde and Cohlen 1999).

MULTIPLE PREGNANCY RISKS

- Incidence of cerebral palsy in multiple pregnancies

0.15%	Singletons (general prevalence)
1.5%	Twins
8%	Triplets
43%	Quadruplets

Source: Adapted from Yokohama Y, Shimizu T, et al. Prevalence of cerebral palsy in twins, triplets and quadruplets. *Int J Epidemiol* 24(5):943, 1995.

INTERPREGNANCY INTERVAL

- An infant born between 20 and 60 months after the delivery of a previous child had the lowest risk of low birth-weight, preterm, and/or small size for gestational age (Conde-Aqudelo 2006)

APPENDIX A

Non–Assisted Reproductive Technology Treatment Outcomes

Diagnostic Group	Treatment (unit)	Live Birth Rate (%)
Amenorrhea	None (3 years)	6
	Clomid (cycle)	19
	Gonadotropins (cycle)	21
Oligomenorrhea	None (3 years)	46
	Clomid (cycle)	9
	Gonadotropins (cycle)	21
	Metformin + Clomid (cycle)	11
	Ovarian cauterization (1 year)	38
Hyperprolactinemia	None (3 years)	30
	Bromocriptine (1 year)	31
Tubal obstruction	None (3 years)	5
	Tubal surgery (1 year)	18
Other tubal disease	None (3 years)	22
	Tubal surgery (1 year)	28
	Gonadotropins + IUI (cycle)	8
Endometriosis, I–II	None (3 years)	25
	Laparoscopic ablation (1 year)	18
	CC + IUI (cycle)	5
	Gonadotropins + IUI (cycle)	8
Endometriosis, III–IV	None (3 years)	10
	Surgery (1 year)	30
	Gonadotropins+ IUI (cycle)	8
Azoospermia	None (3 years)	5
	Therapeutic donor insemination (cycle)	13
Oligospermia	None (3 years)	32
	IUI (cycle)	5
	Gonadotropins + IUI (cycle)	5
Unexplained infertility	None (3 years)	36
	CC + IUI (cycle)	5
	Gonadotropins + IUI (cycle)	8

CC, clomiphene citrate; Gns, gonadotropins; IUI, intrauterine insemination.
Source: Adapted from Collins JA, Van Steirteghem A. Overall prognosis with current treatment of infertility. *Hum Reprod Update* 10:309–316, 2004.

APPENDIX B

Odds of Pregnancy

Baseline Chance of Pregnancy	Three Attempts
5%	14%
8%	22%
10%	27%
12%	32%
15%	39%
20%	49%
25%	58%
30%	66%
35%	73%
40%	78%
45%	83%
50%	88%

Equation: $1-((1 - \% \text{ chance of conceiving})^3)$, wherein $1 - \%$ chance of conceiving is the probability of not getting pregnant in a month. One then calculates this probability of not getting pregnant the first month x the probability of not getting pregnant the following month, times the probability of not getting pregnant in the third month. This does not account for diminishing returns, which are increasingly important with improving effectiveness of therapy.

APPENDIX C

Probability for Natural Conception by Age and Month of Trying

	Month				
	1	2	3	6	12
<25 yo	50%	40%	30%	20%	4%
25-34 yo	40%	30%	20%	10%	2%
35-40 yo	30%	20%	10%	5%	1%

Source: Adapted from Gnoth C, Godehardt D, Godehardt E, et al. Time to pregnancy: results of the German prospective study and impact on the management of infertility. Hum Reprod Sep;18(9):1959–66, 2003.

APPENDIX D

Summary of Options

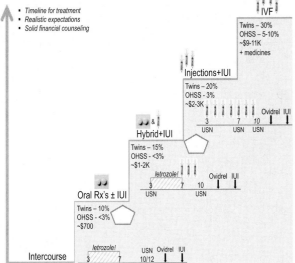

- Timeline for treatment
- Realistic expectations
- Solid financial counseling

IVF
Twins – 30%
OHSS – 5-10%
~$9-11K
+ medicines

Injections+IUI
Twins – 20%
OHSS - 3%
~$2-3K

3   7   10   Ovidrel IUI
USN   USN   USN

Hybrid+IUI
Twins – 15%
OHSS - <3%
~$1-2K

letrozole!
3   7   10   Ovidrel IUI
USN   USN

Oral Rx's ± IUI
Twins – 10%
OHSS - <3%
~$700

letrozole!
3   7   USN   Ovidrel IUI
       10/12

Intercourse

Oral Rx's = Clomiphene citrate, letrozole
Hybrid = oral drugs + gonadotropin injections
IUI = intrauterine insemination
IVF = in vitro fertilization
OHSS = ovarian hyperstimulation syndrome
USN = ultrasound

APPENDIX E

Success Rates Using Superovulation Based on Age and Diagnosis

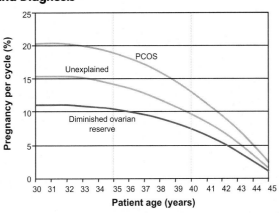

20
Male Subfertility

- A male factor is solely responsible in approximately 20% of subfertile couples and contributory in another 30–40%. (Thonneau 1991)
- A history of male fertility is not an accurate predictor of a normal semen analysis (Lucidi 2005).
- Causes of male factor subfertility can be divided into four main categories:
  - Idiopathic (40–50%)
  - Testicular (30–40%)
  - Posttesticular (10–20%)
  - Pretesticular (1–2%)

EVALUATION OF THE MALE PATIENT

- Evaluation of the male should be done before one year of unsuccessful attempts at conception if 1) there are known male infertility risk factors, 2) female infertility risk factors including female age ≥35), 3) the couple questions the male's fertility potential (AUA best practice statement 2010).
- At a minimum, evaluation should include reproductive history and two semen analyses.

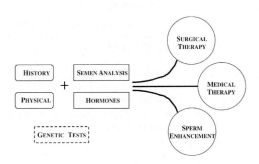

- Goals are to identify:
  - Potentially correctable conditions
  - Irreversible conditions that are amenable to assisted reproductive technologies (ARTs) using the sperm of the male partner
  - Irreversible conditions that are not amenable to ART, and for which adoption or donor insemination is an option.
  - Life- or health-threatening conditions that may underlie the subfertility and require medical attention
    → Men with male factor infertility were 2.8 times more likely to develop testicular cancer than other men (Walsh 2009)
  - Genetic abnormalities that may affect the health of offspring if ART is used

Semen Analysis

- Men make ~1200 sperm/heartbeat.
- Collect × 2 if first one is abnormal (one test is not enough). Patient must be abstinent for 2–3 days before collection of semen; optimal duration of abstinence may be as short as 1 day (Levitas 2005).

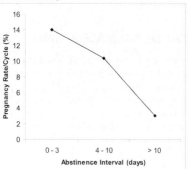

Source: Reproduced with permission from Jurema MW, Vieira AD, Bankowski B, et al. Effect of ejaculatory abstinence period on the pregnancy rate after intrauterine insemination. *Fertil Steril.* Sep;84(3):678–81, 2005.

- Collect by masturbation or by intercourse using special semen collection condoms that do not contain substances detrimental to sperm; do not use lubricants with masturbation when collecting.
- Collect at home or in the laboratory; should be kept at room temperature during transport and examined within 1 hour of collection
- Parameters can vary widely over time, even among fertile men, and exhibit seasonal variation; also, each lab may have different semen reference limits

Parameter	Reference Value (5th %ile)	50th %ile	Possible Pathologies
Volume	1.5mL	3.7	Low: ejaculatory dysfunction, hypogonadism, poor collection technique
Concentration	>15 million/mL	73	Azoospermia or oligospermia: varicocele, genetic, cryptorchidism, endocrinopathy, drugs, infections, toxins or radiation, obstruction, idiopathic
Total motile count	≥10 million	≥165	10–20 would warrant IUI therapy
Motility	>40%	61%	Asthenospermia: prolonged abstinence, antisperm antibodies, partial obstruction, infection, sperm structural defects, idiopathic
Normal morphology	>4% normal	15%	Teratospermia: varicocele, genetic, cryptorchidism, drugs, infections, toxins or radiation, idiopathic

Source: Adapted from Cooper TG, Noonan E, von Eckardstein S, et al. World Health Organization reference values for human semen characteristics. *Hum Reprod Update.* May–Jun;16(3):231–45, 2010.

Total Motile Count (see pages 250–251)

- Total motile count (TMC) before processing (× million = volume × concentration × % motility):
  o 10–20 million: intrauterine insemination (IUI) helpful
  o 5–10 million: in vitro fertilization (IVF)
  o <5 million: intracytoplasmic sperm injection (ICSI)

Morphology

- If abnormal (<1% normal Kruger) → urology consultation (Kruger 1987)
  o 4–14% intermediate rates of fertilization (Guzick 2001)

- ○ **Sperm morphology and IUI:** meta-analysis (Van Waart 2001)

Morphology	Other	Recommendation
>4%	Irrespective	IUI
≤4%	IMC >1 million Motility >50% ≥2 follicles	4 IUI cycles
≤4%	IMC <1 million Motility <50%	Intracytoplasmic sperm injection/in vitro fertilization

IMC, inseminating motile count; IUI, intrauterine insemination.

Source: Adapted from Van Waart J, Kruger TF, Lombard CJ, et al. Predictive value of normal sperm morphology in intrauterine insemination (IUI): a structured literature review. *Hum Reprod Update* 7(5):495, 2001.

- If sperm morphology ≤1%, intracytoplasmic sperm injection is recommended.

Motility

- <40% problematic (longer abstinence may result in higher density and lower motility)

Antisperm Antibodies

- sperMAR ≥20% necessitates obtaining immunobead testing wherein head-binding antibodies are worse than tail, and >50% head-binding antibodies are worrisome (Clarke 1985).
- Pregnancy rates are lower when >50% of sperm are antibody-bound (Ayvaliotis 1985).
- ICSI can circumvent adverse effects of antisperm antibodies (ASAs).
- Screen for ASA when there is isolated asthenospermia with normal sperm concentration, sperm agglutination, or an abnormal postcoital test
- ASAs found on the surface of sperm by direct testing are more significant than ASAs found in the serum or seminal plasma by indirect testing.
- ASA testing is not needed if sperm are to be used for ICSI.

Round Cells

- Leukocytes and immature germ cells appear similar and are properly termed *round cells*.
- When >5 million/mL or >10/high power field (high power field = 40× magnification), must differentiate using cytologic staining and immunohistochemical techniques.

- Mild prostatitis, epididymitis?
- Leukocytospermia is defined as >1 million WBCs/mL (WHO); should be followed up with a semen culture.
- No strong evidence for treatment regimens of leukocytospermia, however; typical practice patterns include antibiotic + NSAID (i.e., doxycycline 100 mg b.i.d. or ciprofloxacin 500 mg b.i.d. × 14–21 days + ibuprofen 600 mg t.i.d. × 7 days)

Postejaculatory Urinalysis

- Clearly beneficial in those patients with failure to have emission with ejaculation.
- Perform in patients with volumes <1 mL, unless patient has bilateral vasal agenesis, clinical signs of hypogonadism, collection problems, or short abstinence interval: All offer an explanation.
- Centrifuge for 10 minutes at a minimum of 300 g and inspect at 400× magnification.
- Significant numbers of sperm found in urine of patients with low volume oligospermia suggests retrograde ejaculation although "significant numbers" has not been defined.

Specialized Clinical Tests on Semen and Sperm

- Not required for diagnosis
- May be useful in a small number of patients for identifying a male factor contributing to unexplained infertility or for selecting therapy such as ART.

Sperm DNA Fragmentation Testing

- Assays: Low sensitivity, high specificity
- More frequent DNA fragmentation in those with recurrent pregnancy loss compared to those undergoing IVF or therapeutic donor insemination (Carrell 2003).
- Routine use of DNA integrity testing in the evaluation of an infertile couple remains questionable; its effect on embryo development is still unclear (ASRM Committee Opinion 2011), insufficient evidence to warrant routine use of this test (AUA Best Practice Statement).
- Weak evidence that varicocelectomy or treatment of a semen infection may reduce sperm DNA fragmentation
- At present, results of sperm DNA integrity testing do not predict pregnancy rates achieved with IUI, IVF or ICSI.
- Treatments to improve DNA integrity have not been shown to have clinical value as of yet.

- Varicocelectomy can decrease sperm DNA fragmentation (35.2% to 30.2% based on Smit 2010) but since other sperm parameters also improved it is not certain if this alone is clinically significant.

Sperm Viability Tests

- Recommended to rule out necrospermia when motility is <5–10%.
- Assessed by mixing fresh semen with a supravital dye, such as eosin or trypan blue, or by the use of the hypoosmotic swelling (HOS) test
- Determine whether nonmotile sperm are viable by identifying which sperm have intact cell membranes.
- Nonmotile but viable sperm, as determined by the HOS test, may be used successfully for ICSI.

Sperm Penetration Assay

- Removal of the zona pellucida from hamster oocytes allows human sperm to fuse with hamster ova (hamster egg penetration assay [HEPA]).
- Number of penetrations per egg by the sperm of the test subject is compared to that observed using sperm from a known fertile individual.
- Evaluates capacitation, the acrosome reaction, fusion with the oocyte, and ability to penetrate membrane
- Results are sensitive to culture conditions and difficult to standardize.
- Not widely available, costly, time-consuming
- Sperm function can also be evaluated using human zona pellucida–binding tests; not often used

Computer-Assisted Sperm Analysis (Davis 1993)

- Computer-assisted sperm analysis requires sophisticated instruments to generate digitized video images for quantitative assessment of sperm motion characteristics: Kinematics may be more specific.
- May be important factors in determining sperm fertility potential.

Acrosome Reaction

- This testing is primarily used for research testing.
- Acrosome reaction: fusion of acrosome and plasma membrane → release of acrosomal enzymes and exposure of sperm head

- Infertile men have increased prevalence of spontaneous acrosome loss and decreased acrosome reactivity assessed by fluorescein-labeled pea or peanut agglutinins and specific monoclonal antibodies in response to challenge by calcium ionophore.
- Not necessary for routine evaluation because uncommon problem

Biochemical Tests

- Measurements of sperm creatine kinase and reactive oxygen species (ROS) (Aitken 1989)
  - May detect a probable cause for low fertilization rates or failed IVF
  - Sperm creatine phosphokinase enzyme is involved in generation, transport, and use of energy within the sperm.
  - ROS interfere with sperm function by peroxidation of sperm lipid membranes and creation of toxic fatty acid peroxides.
  - Studies have yielded conflicting results.

History

Medical History

- Childhood illnesses and developmental history, including testicular descent, pubertal development, loss of body hair or decreased shaving frequency, school performance
  - Systemic illness: diabetes, cancer, upper respiratory diseases, infection
  - Surgical history: mumps orchitis, cryptorchidism, herniorrhaphy, trauma, torsion, retroperitoneal/prostate surgery, vasectomy, bladder neck/prostate surgery
  - Medication use: nitrofurantoin, cimetidine, sulfasalazine, spironolactone, α-blockers; testosterone replacement therapy
- History of radiation or chemotherapy

Fertility History

- Duration of subfertility and prior fertility; previous infertility treatments

Sexual History

- Sexually transmitted infections; coital frequency and timing; erectile function; lubricants

Family History

- Cryptorchidism, midline defects (Kallmann syndrome), hypospadias, primary ciliary dyskinesia (immotile cilia syndrome), infertility, cystic fibrosis

Social and Occupational History

- Gonadal toxin exposure:
  - More than mild ethanol use, cocaine and other recreational drugs, anabolic steroids
  - Exposure to ionizing radiation, chronic heat exposure → ↓ count and motility
  - Aniline dyes, pesticides, heavy metals (lead)
  - Tobacco → ↓ motility
  - Marijuana → ↓ count, motility, testosterone, and acrosome reaction (Whan 2006); cannabinoid-binding sites found on human sperm (Rossato 2005)

Physical Examination

Penis Examination

- Including the location of the urethral meatus

Palpation of the Testes and Measurement of Their Size

- Normal testicular size: 4 × 3 cm or 20 mL in volume (Charney 1960)
- Examine for testicular mass, small soft testes suggest testicular failure.

Presence and Consistency of Both the Vas Deferens and Epididymis

- Epididymides should be palpated for fullness or suspicion of obstruction.
- Diagnosis of congenital bilateral absence of the vas deferens is made by physical examination alone and does not require scrotal sonography or exploration.

Presence of a Varicocele

- Incidence:
  - 11%: Normal semen analysis
  - 25%: Abnormal semen analysis
  - 35%: Infertile men with primary infertility
  - Up to 80%: Men with secondary infertility
  - 53%: Sons of fathers with a varicocele
- The mechanism of injury to sperm is uncertain:
  - Impaired blood drainage from testis leading to ↑ stromal temperature, hypoxia, ↑ testicular pressure, and reflux of adrenal metabolites
- Associated with ↓ testosterone (statistically significant but not necessarily clinically significant); ↓ total sperm count, morphology, and motility
  - No consistent semen analysis pattern distinguishes men with a varicocele.
- Repair improves testosterone deficit, although change may not be clinically significant. Repair will decrease sperm DNA fragmentation as well as increase total motile sperm count (Smit 2010).
- Randomized, controlled trial analyzing utility of varicocelectomy over observation in infertile men with palpable varicoceles (grades 1–3) and impaired semen quality: (Abdel-Meguid 2011)
  - Spontaneous pregnancy achieved in 14% of control arm vs. 33% surgical arm
  - The mean of all semen parameters improved significantly during follow up vs baseline in the surgical arm compared to the control arm
  - Odds ratio of 3.04 (95% CI, 1.33–6.95)
  - Number needed to treat –5.26 patients
- Outcome after subclinical (detected by ultrasound, not clinical examination) varicocelectomy is significantly less beneficial than after repair of clinical varicocele (Jarow 1996); subclinical varicoceles found by ultrasound but not by palpation should not be repaired (Yamamoto 1996).

Criteria to Repair Varicoceles (All Should Be Met):

1) Varicocele is palpable
2) Couple has known infertility
3) Female partner has normal fertility or potentially treatable cause of infertility
4) Man has abnormal semen parameters or sperm function tests

- Azoospermic patients have shown return of sperm to the ejaculate but will typically still require ART to conceive (Abdulmaaboud 1998; Segenreich 1998; Perimenis 2001).
- Larger series report a 30–50% spontaneous pregnancy rate after varicoclectomy with an average time of 8 months from treatment to pregnancy (Pryor 1987).

Secondary Sexual Characteristics

- Body habitus, hair distribution, and breast development
  - Men with Klinefelter's syndrome (47,XXY) are classically tall and eunuchoid, with gynecomastia and small testes.

Digital Rectal Examination

- Defines size and symmetry of the prostate and may reveal the presence of midline cysts or dilated seminal vesicles suggesting ejaculatory duct obstruction.

Hormones

- Hypogonadism is found in:
  - 45% of men with non-obstructive azoospermia
  - 43% of men with oligospermia
  - 35% men with with normal semen parameters (Sussman 2008).
- Evaluation of the pituitary-gonadal axis (1.7% incidence of abnormalities); evaluate if <10 million/mL sperm concentration, impaired sexual function, or other clinical findings suggestive of a specific endocrinopathy.
  - Testosterone: ↓ if prolactinoma or hypogonadotropism
    → If low, obtain a repeat measurement of total and free testosterone.
  - FSH: ↑ in germ cell aplasia
  - Hyperprolactinemia: can result in ↓ libido and problems with impotence
  - Thyroid-stimulating hormone (TSH): leads to hyperprolactinemia

Clinical Condition	Follicle-Stimulating Hormone	Luteinizing Hormone	Testosterone	Prolactin
Normal spermatogenesis	Normal	Normal	Normal	Normal
Hypogonadotropic hypogonadism	Low	Low	Low	Normal
Abnormal spermatogenesis[a]	High/normal	Normal	Normal	Normal
Complete testicular failure/hypergonadotropic hypogonadism	High	High	Normal/low	Normal
Prolactin-secreting pituitary tumor	Normal/low	Normal/low	Low	High

[a]Many men with abnormal spermatogenesis have a normal serum follicle-stimulating hormone, but a marked elevation of serum follicle-stimulating hormone is clearly indicative of an abnormality in spermatogenesis.

Urologic Evaluation

- *Transrectal ultrasonography* indicated in azoospermic patients with palpable vasa and low ejaculate volumes to determine if ejaculatory duct obstruction is present.
  - Findings of dilated seminal vesicles, dilated ejaculatory ducts, and/or midline prostatic cystic structures are suggestive of complete or partial ejaculatory duct obstruction.
  - Normal seminal vesicles are <1.5 cm in AP diameter (AUA Best Practice Statement)
  - Complete ejaculatory duct obstruction: low-volume, fructose-negative, acidic, azoospermic ejaculates
  - Partial ejaculatory duct obstruction: low volume, oligoasthenospermia, and poor forward progression
  - Transscrotal ultrasonography may be useful to clarify ambiguous findings on examination or in patients in whom a testicular mass is suspected.
  - May identify nonpalpable varicoceles, but these have not been shown to be clinically significant and should not be repaired.

GENETICS OF MALE SUBFERTILITY

Male Fertility Genetics in a Nutshell

Up to 15% of men with azoospermia have a genetic abnormality on karyotype, Y-chromosome microdeletion or in cystic fibrosis transmembrane conductance regulator (CFTR) gene.

239

1. Karyotype
   a. Severe OATS (oligoasthenoteratozoospermia)
   b. Azoospermia and severe oligospermia (<5 million/mL)
   c. Counsel men for possible health implications, pregnancy loss, birth defects and transmission
2. Y-chromosome microdeletion (AZF)
   a. Deletion present in 13% of men with non-obstructive azoospermia
   b. Check prior to microdissection TESE
   c. Successful sperm retrieval has never been reported in men with AZFa or AZFb deletions
   d. Sperm retrieval is possible for ICSI in men with AZFc deletions
   e. Couple should be counseled on inheritance of subfertility to male offspring if man has AZFc deletion
3. CF testing
   a. Men with obstructive azoospermia due to CBAVD likely have a CFTR abnormality
   b. Almost all males with clinical CF have CBAVD
   c. Female partners of men with CBAVD or CFTR abnormalities should undergo testing to rule her out as a carrier if they plan to use his sperm to conceive
   d. CFTR testing should include, at minimum, a panel of common point mutations and 5T allele (See Chapter 33)

Cystic Fibrosis Gene Mutations

- Strong association between congenital bilateral absence of vas deferens (CBAVD) and mutations of the cystic fibrosis (CF) transmembrane regulator gene on chromosome 7.
  - CBAVD is associated with mutations within the CF gene in 70–80% of men.
  - CBAVD in 1% of infertile males
- Besides CF gene mutations, a second genetic etiology involves abnormal differentiation of the mesonephric ducts.
- One of the more common diagnoses in patients with obstructive azoospermia
- Seminal volume low (<1 cc), pH <7.0
- Important to test patient's partner before performing IVF/ICSI with his sperm, because of the risk that his partner may be a CF carrier.

Chromosomal Abnormalities Resulting in Impaired Testicular Function

- Prevalence of karyotypic abnormalities in infertile men: 7%
- Infertile men have an eight- to tenfold higher prevalence of chromosomal anomalies than fertile men.
- Frequency is inversely proportional to sperm count.
  - 10–15% in azoospermic men
  - 5% in severe oligospermic men (<5 million/mL)
  - <1% in normospermic men
- Klinefelter's syndrome (47,XXY or 46,XY/47,XXY) accounts for ⅔ of the chromosomal abnormalities observed in subfertile men.
  - these men may undergo testicular sperm extraction and ICSI as most sperm from Klinefelter's syndrome patients have a normal 23,X or Y complement
- Structural abnormalities of the autosomal chromosomes, such as inversions and translocations, are also observed at a higher frequency in infertile men than in the general population.
- Couple is at increased risk for miscarriages and children with chromosomal and congenital defects when the male has gross karyotypic abnormalities.
- Karyotyping should be offered to men who have nonobstructive azoospermia (NOA) or severe oligospermia (<5 million/mL) before IVF with ICSI.
- Genetic counseling should be provided whenever a genetic abnormality is detected.

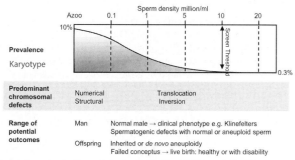

Source: Reproduced with permission from McLachlan RI, O'Bryan MK. Clinical Review: State of the art for genetic testing of infertile men. *J Clin Endocrinol Metab.* Mar;95(3):1013–1024. 2010.

Y Chromosome Microdeletions Associated with Isolated Spermatogenic Impairment

- Y-chromosome analysis should be offered to men who have NOA or severe oligospermia (<5 million/mL) before ICSI.
- Found in approximately 10–15% of men with azoospermia or 5% if severe oligospermia (<5 million/mL)
- Too small to be detected by standard karyotyping but can be found by using polymerase chain reaction
- The intervening large segment of the Y chromosome, known as the *male specific Y*, contains many genes involved in spermatogenesis.
- Regions prone to microdeletion: *AZFa*, *AZFb*, and *AZFc* (most common).

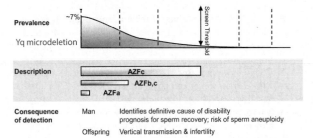

Source: Reproduced with permission from McLachlan RI, O'Bryan MK. Clinical Review: State of the art for genetic testing of infertile men. *J Clin Endocrinol Metab.* Mar;95(3):1013-24. 2010.

- Microdeletion in *AZFc* region in 1 in 4,000 men; most common molecular cause of NOA
  - Approximately 70% of men with an *AZFc* microdeletion possess sperm recoverable by testicular sperm aspiration.
  - 13% of men with NOA possess *AZFc* microdeletion.

- ○ Approximately 5% of men with severe oligospermia, <5 million/mL, possess *AZFc* microdeletion.

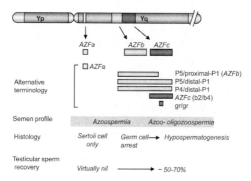

Source: Reproduced with permission from McLachlan RI, O'Bryan MK. Clinical Review: State of the art for genetic testing of infertile men. *J Clin Endocrinol Metab.* Mar;95(3):1013–1024. 2010.

CAUSES OF MALE SUBFERTILITY (Turek 2004)

- Four main areas:
  1. Pretesticular (hypothalamic/pituitary disease) (1–2%)
  2. Testicular (primary hypogonadism) (30–40%)
  3. Posttesticular (disorders of sperm transport) (10–20%)
  4. Idiopathic (40–50%)

Hypothalamic Disease

Gonadotropin Deficiency (Kallmann Syndrome)

- Rare (1 in 50,000 persons) disturbance of neuron migration from the olfactory placode during development
- Two most common clinical deficits: anosmia and absence of GnRH
- Other signs and symptoms:
  - ○ Facial asymmetry, color blindness, renal anomalies, microphallus, cryptorchidism, and, the hallmark of the syndrome, → delay in pubertal development
- Low testosterone, low luteinizing hormone (LH), and low FSH levels
- Sperm production can be promoted by exogenous FSH and LH

Isolated Luteinizing Hormone Deficiency ("Fertile Eunuch")

- Rare; due to partial gonadotropin deficiency
- Enough LH is produced to stimulate intratesticular testosterone production and spermatogenesis, but

insufficient testosterone to promote virilization. Eunuchoid body proportions, variable virilization, and often gynecomastia.

- Normal testis size, but the ejaculate contains reduced numbers of sperm.
- FSH levels are normal, but serum LH and testosterone levels are low-normal.

Isolated Follicle-Stimulating Hormone Deficiency

- Extremely rare; insufficient FSH
- FSH levels are uniformly low and do not respond to stimulation with GnRH. Sperm counts range from azoospermia to severely low numbers (oligospermia).

Congenital Hypogonadotropic Syndromes

- Prader-Willi syndrome (1 in 20,000 persons): genetic obesity, cognitive impairment, small hands and feet, and hypogonadism
- Caused by a deficiency of hypothalamic GnRH
- Single-gene deletion associated with this condition is found on chromosome 15.
- Spermatogenesis can be induced with exogenous FSH and LH.
- Bardet-Biedl syndrome: rare, autosomal recessive, results from GnRH deficiency (cognitive impairment, retinitis pigmentosa, polydactyly, and hypogonadism)
- The hypogonadism can be treated with FSH and LH.

Pituitary Disease

Pituitary Insufficiency

- Tumors, infiltrative processes, operation, radiation

Hyperprolactinemia

- Systemic diseases and medications should be ruled out.
- PRL-secreting pituitary adenoma is the most common etiology
- Elevated PRL usually results in decreased FSH, LH, and testosterone levels and causes infertility.
- Associated symptoms include loss of libido, impotence, galactorrhea, and gynecomastia.
- Signs and symptoms of other pituitary hormone derangements (adrenocorticotropic hormone, TSH) should also be investigated.

Testicular (Primary Hypogonadism) Effects

- Effects of primary hypogonadism are, at present, largely irreversible.
- Etiology
  - **Chromosomal** (Klinefelter's syndrome [47,XXY], 46,XX sex reversal, 47,XYY syndrome)
  - **Noonan's syndrome** (male Turner syndrome): 75% have cryptorchidism.
  - **Myotonic dystrophy:** testis atrophy; fertility has been reported.
    - → Testis biopsies show seminiferous tubule damage in 75% of cases.
- **Vanishing testis syndrome** (bilateral anorchia): rare, occurring in 1 in 20,000 males
- **Sertoli-cell only syndrome** (germ cell aplasia) –25% micro-TESE retrieval rate
- **Y chromosome microdeletions** (see page 242)
- **Gonadotoxins (radiation, drugs)**
  - Ketoconazole, spironolactone, and alcohol inhibit testosterone synthesis; cimetidine is an androgen antagonist.
  - Marijuana, heroin, and methadone are associated with lower testosterone.
  - Pesticides are likely to have estrogen-like activity.
- **Systemic disease** (renal failure, liver failure, sickle cell anemia)
- **Defective androgen activity**
  - 5α-Reductase deficiency
    - → Normal development of the testes and wolffian duct structures (internal genitalia) but ambiguous external genitalia
  - Androgen receptor deficiency: X-linked
- **Testis injury (orchitis, torsion, trauma)**
- **Cryptorchidism**
- **Varicocele** (see page 237)
  - Objectives of repair:
    - → Relieve pain
    - → Improve semen parameters
    - → Improve pregnancy rates in couples with male factor infertility associated with varicocele

Posttesticular Causes of Infertility

Reproductive Tract Obstruction

Congenital Blockages

- Congenital absence of the vas deferens
- **Young syndrome:** triad of chronic sinusitis, bronchiectasis, and obstructive azoospermia. The obstruction is in the epididymis.
- Idiopathic epididymal obstruction
- Polycystic kidney disease: usually secondary to obstructing cysts in the epididymis or seminal vesicles
- Ejaculatory duct obstruction: Transurethral resection of an obstruction results in increased semen volume in approximately ⅔ of affected men and returns sperm to the ejaculate in approximately ½ of azoospermic men.

Acquired Blockages

- **Vasectomy:** 5% of men have the vasectomy reversed, most commonly because of remarriage.
  - ○ Overall pregnancy rate: 50%
  - ○ Choice may also depend on presence of female factors.
  - ○ Pregnancy rate decreases as the time passes since the vasectomy
- **Groin surgery** can result in inguinal vas deferens obstruction in 1% of cases.
- **Infection** *may* involve the epididymis, with scarring and obstruction.

Vasectomy Reversal Depending on Time since Vasectomy

Years since Vasectomy	Pregnancy Rate (%)
2	77
5	49
10	43
15	30

Source: Adapted from Belker AM, Thomas AJ, Jr., et al. Results of 1,469 microsurgical vasectomy reversals by the Vasovasostomy Study Group. *J Urol* 145(3):505, 1991.

Functional Blockages

- **Sympathetic nerve injury:** In men with spinal cord injuries, demyelinating neuropathies, or diabetes, and in those who have had retroperitoneal lymph node dissections, ejaculation can be achieved with vibratory stimulation, and in those who do not respond, electroejaculation.
- If the total motile count is >4 million, it is reasonable to perform electroejaculation/IUI if no anesthesia (high cost) is necessary. If

anesthesia costs are incurred or total motile count is <4 million, then proceeding to IVF/ICSI is warranted (Ohl 2001).
- **Pharmacologic:** Antihypertensives, antipsychotics, antidepressants

Disorders of Sperm Function or Motility

- **Immotile cilia syndromes:** Kartagener syndrome is a subset of this disorder (1 in 40,000 males) that presents with the triad of chronic sinusitis, bronchiectasis, and situs inversus. Most immotile cilia cases are diagnosed in childhood with respiratory and sinus difficulties.
- **Maturation defects:** seen in vasectomy-induced blockage
- **Immunologic infertility:** Autoimmune infertility has been implicated as a cause of infertility in 10% of infertile couples.
- **Infection**
- **Age-related effects:** Several studies show that semen volume and sperm motility may decrease continuously between 22 and 80 years of age (Eskenazi 2003).

Disorders of Coitus

- **Impotence**
- **Hypospadias** can cause inappropriate placement of the seminal coagulum too distant from the cervix.
- Timing and frequency: Appropriate frequency is every 2 days, within the periovulatory period.
- Avoid lubricants if at all possible (see Appendix B).

Exogenous Hormones

- Testosterone replacement therapy for hypogonadism resulting in decreased pituitary gonadotropin production and decreased intratesticular testosterone and decreased spermatogenesis
- Anabolic steroid use, same effect as testosterone replacement

Other Endocrinopathies as Etiologies for Infertility

- Androgen excess, hyperprolactinemia, estrogen excess
- Obesity resulting in aromatization of testosterone to estradiol
- Testicular malignancies: destruction of spermatogenic tissue, alter intratesticular blood flow, increase intratesticular temperatures, and paracrine effects
- Congenital adrenal hyperplasia, 21-hydroxylase deficiency is the most common deficiency, abnormally high production of adrenal androgen resulting in suppression of gonadotropins

- Hormonally active adrenocortical tumors or Leydig cell tumors of the testis

TREATMENT

Abnormal Semen Analysis

Antibiotics

- Culture for urethritis; empiric therapy for epididymitis, prostatitis

Surgery

- Varicocele repair: ↑ sperm parameters and clinical pregnancy rates

Intrauterine Insemination

Total Motile Count (Million)	Live Birth Rate (%)*
<10	**1.4**
>10	**6.8**

*This includes natural-IUI, clomiphene-IUI, gonadotropins-IUI.

Source: Adapted from Van Voorhis BJ, Barnett M, Sparks AE, et al. Effect of the total motile sperm count on the efficacy and cost-effectiveness of intrauterine insemination and in vitro fertilization. *Fertil Steril* 75(4):661, 2001.

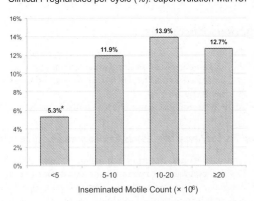

Clinical Pregnancies per cycle (%): superovulation with IUI

Inseminated Motile Count (× 10⁶)

*P<0.02

Source: Adapted from Khalil MR, Rasmussen RE, Erb K, Laursen SB, Rex S, Westergaard LG. Homologous intrauterine insemination. An evaluation of prognostic factors based on a review of 2,473 cases. *Acta Obstet Gynecol Scand* 80:74, 2001.

- Timing of IUI (Rahman 2011)
  - Pregnancy rate/cycle ~15% for 36 hours post-hCG vs. ~9% for 24 hours
- Sperm washing allows for removal of seminal plasma to avoid prostaglandin-induced contractions; also, washing of sperm is associated with much lower rates of pelvic infection.
- No difference in pregnancy rate with double inseminations compared with single (Ghanem 2011)
- Ultrasound-guided IUI offers no added benefit than blind insemination (Ramon 2009)
- IUI is superior to intracervical inseminations (RCT with frozen, donor sperm) (Patton 1992)

Therapeutic Donor Insemination

- Frozen to prevent human immunodeficiency virus transmission

In Vitro Fertilization with Intracytoplasmic Sperm Injection

- Indications: morphology ≤1%; motility <10%; TMC <5 million
- No correlation between chromosomal anomalies and ICSI in cases of normal semen analysis
- Risk of a birth defects: (Davies 2012)
  - **5.7% for a spontaneous birth in fertile population**
  - 8.7% for a spontaneous birth in infertile population
  - 7.1% for a fresh or frozen embryo transfer following IVF
  - **10.7% for a fresh embryo transfer following IVF/ICSI**
  - 6.6% for a frozen embryo transfer following IVF/ICSI
- Testicular or epididymal (frozen are equivalent to fresh) can be used for ICSI
- See page 276 for further information on risk of birth defects with IVF and IVF/ICSI; there seems to be a higher percentage of sex chromosome abnormalities following IVF/ICSI when compared to the general population (Bonduelle 1998).

Aberration	General Public (%)	ICSI (%)
Autosomal	0.020 (2 in 1,000)	0.83 (8 in 1,000)
Sex chromosomal	0.25 (1 in 400)	0.83 (1 in 125)
Structural de novo (i.e., nonbalanced)	0.07	0.36

Source: Adapted from Bonduelle M, Aytoz A, et al. Incidence of chromosomal aberrations in children born after assisted reproduction through intracytoplasmic sperm injection. *Hum Reprod* 13(4):781, 1998.

Hormonal Therapy

- Indications: Low testosterone/high estradiol, non-obstructive azoospermia (NOA) or idiopathic oligospermia.
- Use of aromatase inhibitor, clomiphene citrate, hCG and human menopausal gonadotropins can result in sperm in an ejaculate for ~65% of those with **idiopathic oligospermia** and **11% for NOA**. If still azoospermic they may have a greater likelihood of sperm acquisition from testicular sperm extraction (Hussein 2005; Hussein 2013).

APPENDIX A

Approach to Diagnosis of Male Subfertility

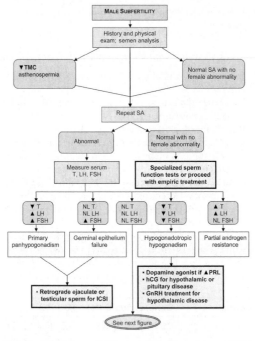

FSH, follicle-stimulating hormone; GnRH, gonadotropin-releasing hormone; hCG, human chorionic gonadotropin; ICSI, intracytoplasmic sperm injection; LH, luteinizing hormone; NL, normal; PRL, prolactin; SA, semen analysis; T, testosterone; TMC, total motile count. (Adapted with permission from: Swerdloff RS, Wang C. Evaluation of male infertility. In: UpToDate, Inc. For more information visit www.uptodate.com.)

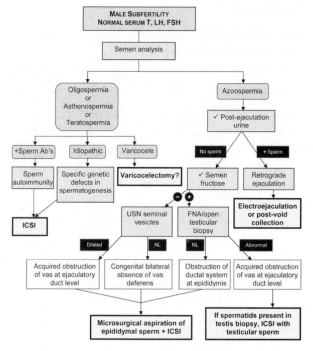

Ab's, antibodies; FNA, fine-needle aspiration; FSH, follicle-stimulating hormone; ICSI, intracytoplasmic sperm injection; LH, luteinizing hormone; NL, normal; T, testosterone; USN, ultrasound. (Adapted with permission from: Swerdloff RS, Wang C. Evaluation of male infertility. In: UpToDate, Inc. For more information visit www .uptodate.com.)

APPENDIX B

Sperm Retrieval Techniques for Nonobstructive and Obstructive Azoospermia

	Technique	Advantages	Disadvantages	Comments
PERCUTANEOUS	TFNA (fine needle aspiration of testis	Simple; Minimally invasive (22 gauge needle)	Very low sperm yield; Lower % motile sperm than in epididymis	No demonstrated benefit over PercBiopsy
	PercBiopsy (percutatneous testis bipsy)	Simple; minimally invasive (14 gauge needle); improved sperm yield over TFNA	Large needle—w/o apparent inc risk of cx over TFNA	Preferred percutaneous approach to sperm retrieval
	PESA (percutaneous epididymal aspiration)	Higher potential sperm yield; larger %motile sperm than in testis	Not always successful; sperm retrieved often of poor quality (motility) with macrophage contamination; difficult after multiple operations; risk to testicular blood supply	Variable success—requires avail of back-up technique without distinct advantages
OPEN	TESE (testicular sperm extraction/open biopsy	Reliable yield of sperm	Invasive procedure w/o sperm quality seen for MESA; may transiently affect testicular function	Unnecessarily invasive for obstructed patients
	MESA (microsurgical epididymal sperm aspiration)	Yields high numbers of motile sperm usable for multiple IVF cycles with good reliability (>99%); low complication rate	Invasive procedure with longer recovery than percutaneous approaches; Requires microsurgical skills	Preferred approach for couples who may undergo multiple IVF cycles
	Micro TESE (microsurgical testicular sperm extraction)	Excellent technique for non-obstructive azoospermia; low complication rate	Invasive; requires microsurgical skills	Not indicated for obstructive azoospermia

Source: Reproduced with permission from Schlegel PN. Causes of azoospermia and their management. *Reprod Fertil Dev*, 16(5):561–72, 2004.

- Timing of sperm retrieval procedure
  - In obstructive azoospermen men as well as non-obstructive azoospermic (NOA) men, success rates for cryopreserved testicular or epididymal sperm are similar to those for fresh samples as long as adequate sperm are available. In fact, the frozen sperm may have better outcomes (Kalsi 2011)
  - In NOA with successful retrievals with microTESE, quantities of sperm obtained are sometimes inadequate for cryopreservation.
  - Sperm retrieval for obstructive azoospermia can usually be done on the day of egg collection via PESA
  - Consider scheduling sperm retrieval for NOA (micro-TESE) on the day of egg collection due to (a) low number of retrieved sperm and (b) only 50% chance of retrieving viable sperm
- Isolated diagnostic testicular biopsy is rarely, if ever, indicated anymore due to microdissection testicular sperm extraction (microTESE) (Kalsi 2012; Ramasamy 2007;

Schoor 2002). High FSH is not a contraindication for micro-TESE (Ramasamy 2009).

○ Counsel couple about use of donor sperm or oocyte cryopreservation as part of back-up strategy in case of failure to obtain any sperm

APPENDIX C

Lubricants and Sperm

Vaginal Lubricants: Effect on Sperm

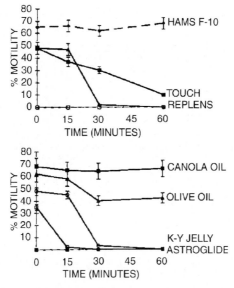

Motility determined by computer-assisted semen analysis of various sperm-lubricant treatments at 1, 15, 30, and 60 minutes. Control media (Hams F-10) shown in the top graph had minimal effect on sperm motility. A spermicidal agent with nonoxynol 9 had immediate and prolonged inhibitory effects on sperm motility (shown as a *dashed line* at the bottom of each graph). (Source: Reproduced with permission from Kutteh WH, Chao CH, et al. Vaginal lubricants for the infertile couple: effect on sperm activity. *Int J Fertil Menopausal Stud* 41[4]:400, 1996.)

• Pre-Seed™ does not cause a decrease in sperm motility or chromatin integrity.

APPENDIX D

Algorithm for Genetic Tests in Azoospermia or Severly Oligozoopermia

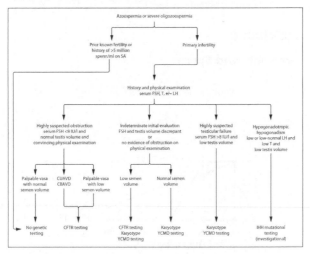

Source: Reproduced with permission from Stahl PJ, Schlegel PN. Genetic evaluation of the azoospermic or severely oligozoospermic male. *Curr Opin Obstet Gynecol.* Aug;24(4):221–228, 2012.

21

Diminished Ovarian Reserve

DEFINITION

- *Diminished ovarian reserve* (DOR) refers to the condition of having a low number of normal oocytes (Scott 1995).

BACKGROUND

- ↑ Age is associated with ↓ fecundity (ability to get pregnant), ↓ live birth rate, ↑ early follicular phase follicular-stimulating hormone (FSH) levels, ↓ anti-müllerian hormone (AMH), ↑ miscarriage rates, and ↑ in vitro fertilization (IVF) cancellation rates due to poor stimulation (Pearlstone 1992; Pellestor 2003; Stein 1985).
- For ~95% of women by the age of 30 years only 12% of their maximum pre-birth non-growing follicles population is present whereas for those at age 40 years only 3% of these follicles remain (Wallace 2010)

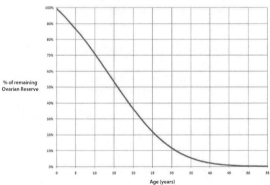

Source: Reproduced with permission from Wallace WH, Kelsey TW. Human ovarian reserve from conception to the menopause. *PLoS One*. Jan 27;5(1):e8772, 2010.

- Despite age, some young, normally cycling women do not become pregnant with repetitive cycles of IVF, experience frequent miscarriage, or do not respond well to exogenous gonadotropins.
- From 1969 to 1994, the number of women older than 30 years having their first child ↑ from 4.1% to 21.2% (Heck 1997)
- Donor insemination recipients' 1-year pregnancy rate (Schwartz and Mayaux 1982):
  - <31 years old = 74%
  - 31–35 years old = 62%
  - **>35 years old = 54%**

IMPLICATIONS

- Fragile X carrier screening (FMRI premutation) should be considered in women with diminished ovarian reserve (ACOG Committee Opinion No. 469, October 2010).
- Women with low ovarian reserve have ↓ fecundity with stimulated IVF cycles.
- The combination of an abnormal ovarian reserve test AND a poor ovarian response in the 1st IVF cycle predicts a very low response in subsequent cycles (Klinkert 2004).
- This **does not mean** that they do not ovulate, that they will not respond to gonadotropins or oral ovulation induction, or that there are **no** good eggs remaining within the ovary.
- It **does** mean, however, that **there are no means by which to selectively stimulate the good eggs to ovulate and recruitment of additional follicles is unlikely.**
- Before embarking on aggressive surgery or infertility treatment to enhance fertility, it is a good idea for some patients to undergo ovarian reserve testing.
- There is no significant decline in ovarian response in patients undergoing up to 3 repetitive IVF cycles (Luk 2010).
- Natural cycle IVF may be a reasonable alternative (Schimberni 2009).
- Adjuvant therapy that may improve success rates with IVF for those with diminished ovarian reserve: Coenzyme Q10, dehydroepiandrosterone, growth hormone, microdose GnRH agonist flare protocol, transdermal testosterone, vitamin D (Bosdou 2012; Duffy 2010; Kahraman 2009; Rudick 2012; Turi 2010; Urman 2012).
- DOR testing has been found to correlate with embryonic aneuploidy (Katz-Jaffe 2013):

	Normal Reserve	DOR	P
Aneuploid blastocysts	51.7%	66%	0.048
All aneuploid blastocysts	14.3%	35.1%	<0.001

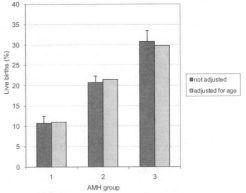

Live birth rate per started cycle, without (mean values +/- SEM, black) and with age adjustment (gray). Group 1: antimullerian hormone (AMH) <0.84 ng/mL (25th percentile); group 2: AMH 0.84–2.94 ng/mL; group 3: AMH >2.94 ng/mL (75th percentile). N = 1230 in vitro fertilization-intracytoplasmic sperm injection treatment cycles.

Source: Reproduced with permission from Brodin T, Hadziosmanovic N, Berglund L, et al. Antimüllerian hormone levels are strongly associated with live birth rates after assisted reproduction. *J Clin Endocrinol Metab.* Mar;98(3):1107–14, 2013.

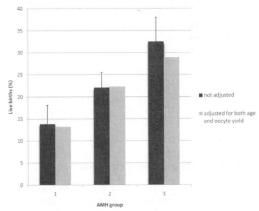

Live birth rate per ovum pickup. This finding suggests that AMH, independent of age, to some extent may reflect the qualitative aspect of ovarian reserve.

Source: Reproduced with permission from Brodin T, Hadziosmanovic N, Berglund L, et al. Antimüllerian hormone levels are strongly associated with live birth rates after assisted reproduction. *J Clin Endocrinol Metab.* Mar;98(3):1107–14, 2013.

HORMONAL TESTS

Caveats

- Different assays may report varying hormone levels from the same serum samples. It is important to calibrate the assay to that in the original studies (Sharara 1998).
- Studies have equal validity in women who have just one ovary (Khalifa 1992); although data from the National Health and Nutrition Examination Survey suggest that FSH levels were increased in women with one ovary removed (Backer 1999).
- A normal FSH or AMH does not improve a woman's age-related ↓ fecundity (Sharara 1998)

Hypothetical representations of ovarian reserve impact on IVF cycles. The spheres may represent oocyte yields and quality parameters based on age and AMH levels. Abnl = abnormal; darkened spheres = poor quality oocytes (Brodin 2013; Katz-Jaffe 2013)

Case scenarios

→ 40 yo with AMH >4:
  - Same # eggs as a 20 yo with AMH >2?
    - Possible but likely fewer viable oocytes
→ 20 yo with AMH <0.05:
  - Likely not as much a hit on quality as for a 40 yo with AMH <0.05 but a hit nonetheless (seen in the aneuploidy study)

HORMONES

Day 3 Follicle-Stimulating Hormone

- FSH on day 3 of <10 IU/L is normal. Levels between 10 IU/L and 14 IU/L are a gray zone with decreasing fertility as levels rise. FSH >14 IU/L results in a <1% chance of a live birth per cycle (Levi 2001)
- Most centers consider CD 3 FSH > 13 IU/L as worrisome and ≥20 IU/L as abnormal.
- If a single CD 3 FSH is ≥20 IU/L, the pregnancy rate per initiated cycle is 5% (Martin 1996).

- Variability does not affect the prognostic category (Buyalos 1998; Scott 1990; Abdalla 2006).
- Valid to test basal FSH on CD 2–5 (Hansen 1996)
  - Nocturnal pulses begin 4 weeks postpartum (Liu 1983)
- Basal FSH screening may not be of value in the general subfertility population with ovulatory menstrual cycles (Van Montfrans 2000).
- Threshold values of D3 FSH (Scott 2007):

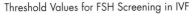

Threshold Values for FSH Screening in IVF

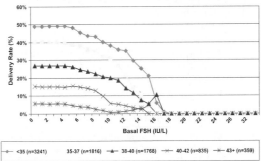

Source: Reproduced with permission from Scott RT Jr., Elkind-Hirsch KE, Styne-Gross A, et al. The predictive value for in vitro fertility delivery rates is greatly impacted by the method used to select the threshold between normal and elevated basal follicle-stimulating hormone. *Fertil Steril.* Apr;89(4):868–878, 2008.

Day 3 Estradiol

- Levels typically nadir at CD 3 (Sharara 1998).
- Elevated E_2 levels on CD 3 indicate advanced follicular phase; this is due to a premature rise in FSH in the luteal phase and reflects DOR (Sharara 1998).
- Inappropriately high E_2 can suppress FSH back into the normal range by CD 3, and therefore may mask DOR.
- E_2 >80 pg/mL have higher cancellation rates with IVF (Smotrich 1995).
- CD 3 E_2 <20 pg/mL or ≥80 pg/mL have an ↑ risk for canceled IVF cycles, but these levels do not seem to predict pregnancy outcome nor correlate with ovarian response in those patients not canceled (Frattarelli 2000).

Anti-Müllerian Hormone (AMH)

- AMH is produced by granulosa cells of all follicles beyond the primordial follicle stage but not yet entered selection for dominance (Weenan 2004)

- AMH seems to be influenced by combined contraception (oral contraceptives, transdermal patches and vaginal rings) with signficant decreases in serum AMH levels after 9 weeks of continuous use (~50% decline from baseline values) (Kallio 2013)
- Measuring AMH on day 7 of the pill-free interval seem to reflect accurate levels (Van den Berg 2010)
- <1.26 mg/mL was predictive of reduced ovarian reserve (IVF) ≤4 oocytes retrieved (Gnoth 2008)
- Measuring AMH at the onset of FSH stimulation for IVF cycles was predictive of pregnancy rates per initiated cycle (P<0.0001): (Blazar 2011)
  - ≤1 ng/mL – 23.4%
  - >3 ng/mL – 60.3%
- Treatment success in patients with poor ovarian reserve (Brodin 2013; Gordon 2013; La Marca 2011; Polyzos 2012)
- There is reason to believe AMH may be a more useful measure of diminished ovarian reserve than FSH (Toner 2013).

Clinical usefulness of AMH values

AMH (ng/mL)	Clinical situation	Implications for management
Low (<0.5)	Impending onset of menopause	Counseling; consider possible options of HRT, DEXA
	Impending POF	Above, plus option for donated eggs
	Impending cancer treatment	Fertility preservation
	Test for ovarian reserve	Realistic expectations
		Option of aggressive OI, DHEA, CoQ10, vitamin D
Midrange (1.0–3.5)	Ovarian reserve testing	Guide dose selection for OI/IVF
		Consideration of fertility preservation if having treatment for cancer or for social reasons
		Provide insight into options for exclusive vs. split egg donors (i.e., the higher the AMH, the more likely to split donor)
Elevated (>3.5)	PCO or PCO-like ovaries	Consider possible option of metformin
	Increased risk for OHSS	Gentle stimulation protocols; consider GnRH agonist trigger; consideration of transferring fewer goodquality embryos

Source: Reproduced with permission from Toner JP, Seifer DB. But isn't antimüllerian hormone still better than follicle-stimulating hormone? *Fertil Steril.* 99(7):1825-30, 2013.

Approximate Live Birth Rates with Low AMH

AGE	% LB FSH/IUI	% LB per IVF[a] cycle		% LB per NC IVF[b] cycle	
		Cycle start	Embryo transfer	Cycle start	Embryo transfer
<35	8%	12%	15%	14%	30%
35–40	6%	10%	13%	10%	28%
>40	2%	5%	10%	5%	15%

[a] AMH < 0.4 (La Marca 2011); AMH <0.84 (Brodin 2013)
[b] AMH < 0.5 (Gordon JD, personal communication)
FSH/IUI, follicle stimulation hormone/intrauterine insemination; IVF, in vitro fertilization; LB = live birth; NC IVF, natural cycle in vitro fertilization
(Brodin 2013; La Marca 2011; Polyzos 2012)

Comparison of ovarian reserve markers FSH and AMH

Feature	FSH	AMH
Site of secretion	Anterior pituitary	Granulosa of pre- and small antral follicles
Temporal change indicating ovarian aging	Latest	Earliest
Timing requirement	Cycle day 2–4 only	Any cycle day
Need for concomitant assay	E_2	None
Cycle to cycle variability	High	Low
Sensitivity for low response	Moderate	Moderate
Sensitivity for high response (risk of OHSS)	None	High
Specificity for low response	High	High
Specificity for high response	None	High
Age-specific values	Limited	Extensive information
Methodology	Automated (1 h)	ELISA (6 h)

Source: Reproduced with permission from Toner JP, Seifer DB. But isn't antimüllerian hormone still better than follicle-stimulating hormone? *Fertil Steril.* 99(7):1825-30, 2013.

Antral Follicle Count (AFC)

- Antral follicles 2–10 mm in diameter should be measured on days 2–4 of the menstrual cycle.
- AFC are a reproducible measure of remaining follicle pool and are directly correlated with likelihood of pregnancy after assisted reproductive technology treatments and inversely correlated with cancellation rates. No antral follicle count, however, can be used as an absolute predictor of pregnancy or cancellation during ART treatments. An antral follicle count of <4 is associated with a high (41–69%) cancellation rate. There is a negative linear correlation between antral follicle counts and gonadotropin dose required to achieve response (Change 1998; Frattarelli 2000, Frattarelli 2003).
- Antral follicle numbers ↓ with advancing chronologic age. The rate of this decline is biphasic, with mean yearly decline of 4.8% in women <37 years of age and increasing to a mean of 11.7% thereafter (Scheffer 1999).

POOR OVARIAN RESPONSE (POR) DEFINITION

- Bologna criteria to define POR (consensus statement from ESHRE) 2-out-of-3 of the following:

---

1. Advanced maternal age (≥40 years old) or any other risk factor for POR
2. Previous POR (≤3 oocytes with a conventional stimulation protocol or <4 oocytes collected
3. Abnormal ovarian reserve test (eg, AFC <5–7 follicles or AMH <0.5–1.1 ng/mL)

- POR if 2 episodes of POR after maximal stimulation even in the absence of advanced maternal age or abnormal reserve testing
- If only #1 and 3 above is obtained this is more appropriately termed as "expected POR."

Source: Modified from Ferraretti AP, La Marca A, Fauser BC, Tarlatzis B, Nargund G, Gianaroli L. ESHRE working group on Poor Ovarian Response Definition. ESHRE consensus on the definition of 'poor response' to ovarian stimulation for in vitro fertilization: the Bologna criteria. *Hum Reprod.* 26(7):1616-24, 2011.

22

Assisted Reproductive Technologies

FAST FACTS

- Assisted Reproductive Technologies (ART) by definition are any fertility treatments in which **both egg and sperm** are handled. Accordingly, ART procedures involve the surgical removal of eggs, known as *egg retrieval.*
- In vitro fertilization (IVF) is the most common ART procedure; IVF has been used in the United States since 1980, and data are collected by the Centers for Disease Control and Prevention and published annually (http://www.cdc .gov/art/ARTReports.htm).

DEFINITIONS

- *In vitro Fertilization* (**IVF**): ovulation induction, oocyte retrieval, and fertilization of the oocytes in the laboratory; embryos are then cultured for 3–5 days with subsequent transfer transcervically under abdominal ultrasound guidance into the uterine cavity.
- **Gamete intrafallopian transfer (GIFT)**: ovarian stimulation and egg retrieval along with laparoscopically guided transfer of a mixture of unfertilized eggs and sperm into the fallopian tubes
- **Zygote intrafallopian transfer (ZIFT)**: ovarian stimulation and egg retrieval followed by fertilization of the eggs in the laboratory and laparoscopic transfer of the day 1 fertilized eggs (*zygotes*) into the fallopian tubes
- **Donor egg IVF:** used for patients with poor egg numbers or egg quality; involves stimulation of an egg donor with typical superovulation followed by standard egg retrieval; eggs are then fertilized by the sperm of the infertile woman's

partner, and embryos are transferred to the infertile woman in a standard IVF-like process.

- **Intracytoplasmic sperm injection (ICSI):** developed in the early 1990s to help couples with severe male factor infertility; one sperm is injected directly into each mature egg, typically resulting in a 50–70% fertilization rate.

EVALUATION BEFORE ASSISTED REPRODUCTIVE TECHNOLOGIES

Ovarian Reserve (see Chapter 21, Diminished Ovarian Reserve)

- Ovarian reserve testing determines the number and possibly quality of eggs present before infertility treatment:

Day 3 FSH	FSH on day 3 of <10 IU/L is normal. Levels between 10 and 14 IU/L are a gray zone with decreasing fertility as levels rise. FSH >14 IU/L results in a <1% chance of a live birth per cycle (Levi 2001). Higher levels suggest early follicular recruitment, which results in a poor prognosis.
Anti-müllerian hormone	AMH decreases steadily with increasing age; <0.4 ng/mL associated with significantly reduced fecundity per initiated cycle; likely not affected by day of cycle
Antral Follicle Count	AFC <6 predicts ovarian response but doesn't predict pregnancy rate

FSH, follicle-stimulating hormone.

Evaluation of Tubal Status

- Patients with a hydrosalpinx on ultrasonography (Camus 1999):
  - 50% ↓ pregnancy rate
  - Twofold ↑ miscarriage rate
- Mechanism of adverse effect (Strandell and Lindhard 2002):

Mechanism of Adverse Effect (Strandell and Lindhard 2002)
↓ Nutrients in hydrosalpinx fluid
Toxic effect of fluid on embryos (Sachdev 1997) and/or sperm (Ng 2000)
↓ Endometrial $\alpha_v\beta_3$, LIF, HOXA10 (Meyer 1997)
Embryo wash-out effect from fluid
↑ Endometrial peristalsis due to hydrosalpinx fluid
↓ Endometrial and subendometrial blood flow (Ng 2006)
↑ Endometrial inflamatory cells (Copperman 2006)

- o Ligation of the hydrosalpinx or salpingectomy restores normal pregnancy rate (Strandell 2001a; Johnson 2002; Kontoravdis 2006).
- o RCT for ultrasound-guided hydrosalpinx aspiration during IVF resulted in greater clinical pregnancy rates than for controls (31.3% vs. 17.6%). Small numbers however. Utilize Unasyn 1.5 gm intra-operatively and then azithromycin 500 mg x 3 days following procedure

Evaluation of the Uterine Cavity

- Significantly lower clinical pregnancy rates with IVF if uterine cavity abnormalities are present (8.3% vs. 37.5%) (Shamma 1992).
- Evaluation techniques: sonohysterogram, hysterosalpingogram, hysteroscopy
- Prevalence of unsuspected intrauterine defects ranges from 11–45% (Fatemi 2010)

Uterine mapping (Trial Transfer; Mock Transfer)

- Uterine mapping is performed before ovulation induction with the same type of catheter used for embryo transfer to help ensure atraumatic transfer of the embryos into the uterine cavity.
- Performed before superovulation: under transabdominal sonography with similar catheter as used for ET.
- For severe cervical stenosis one can try placing a Malecot catheter (Yanushpolsky 2000) or laminaria (Glatstein 1997).

Evaluation of Male Factor Infertility

- Semen analysis: Basic semen analysis should include volume of ejaculate, concentration, motility, and morphology using the Kruger strict criteria.

SUPEROVULATION INDUCTION MEDICINES

- Fresh cycle IVF pregnancy rates relative to patient age tend to peak after 10 mature eggs are retrieved. Gonadotropin-releasing hormone agonists (GnRH-a) or antagonists are used to prevent a woman from ovulating on her own before egg retrieval (40% incidence without such medicines).
- Steady state serum FSH concentration with use of exogenous FSH: 9 mIU/mL per 150 IU FSH (Noorhasan 2008)

Gonadotropin-Releasing Hormone Agonists

- Agonists bind to and stimulate the pituitary GnRH receptor (GnRH-R) and have a long half-life. They ultimately down-regulate the GnRH-R, thereby decreasing follicle-stimulating hormone (FSH) and luteinizing hormone (LH) secretion. This eliminates the possibility of an LH surge with continued GnRH-agonist administration. The first injection is usually administered in the luteal phase of a natural cycle to help prevent cysts from forming.

Advantages

- More eggs retrieved
- Elimination of LH surge
- ↑ Cohort synchronization
- Improved pregnancy rates
- Not FDA approved for fertility but GnRH-a are commonly used as an off-label indication

Disadvantages

- ↑ Cost
- ↑ Gonadotropin medication requirement
- Possible administration during an early conception

Gonadotropin-Releasing Hormone Antagonists

- Synthetic GnRH molecule that has antagonist properties on the GnRH-R. Immediately binds to and blocks GnRH binding to the receptor. GnRH antagonist is usually initiated on day 6 of stimulation or once a 14 mm follicle is present.

Advantages

- Immediate onset of action
- ↓ Number of injections

Disadvantages

- ↑ Cost
- ↑ Gonadotropin medication requirement
- Possible reduction in implantation rates

Gonadotropin Preparations

Trade Name, Manufacturer	Source
FSH/LH-containing preparations	
Menopur, Ferring	Urine of menopausal women
Repronex, Ferring	Urine of menopausal women
FSH-containing preparations	
Bravelle, Ferring	Urine of menopausal women
Follistim AQ, Merck & Co.	Recombinant, Chinese hamster ovary cells
Gonal-F, EMD Serono	Recombinant, Chinese hamster ovary cells

FSH, follicle-stimulating hormone; LH, luteinizing hormone.

Human Chorionic Gonadotropin Preparations

Trade Name, Manufacturer	Source	Formulations
Novarel, Ferring	Urine of pregnant females	10,000 IU IM
Ovidrel, EMD Serono	Recombinant, Chinese hamster ovary cells	250 µg SC
Pregnyl, Merck & Co.	Urine of pregnant women	10,000 IU IM

Gonadotropin-Releasing Hormone Agonist/Antagonist Preparations

Trade Name, Manufacturer	Formulations
Cetrotide, EMD Serono (antagonist)	250 µg/1 mL SC
Ganirelex, Merck & Co. (antagonist)	250 µg/0.5 mL SC
Leuprolide (agonist)	1 mg/0.2 mL = 20 U SC
Synarel, Pfizer (agonist)	2 mg/mL intranasal
Zoladex, AstraZeneca (agonist)	3.6 mg SC

STIMULATION PROTOCOLS AND DOSES

- Estimating the patient's responsiveness to the fertility agents:
  - Age, body mass index, day 3 FSH, AMH, antral follicle count, response to prior ovarian stimulation

Oral Contraceptive–Gonadotropin-Releasing Hormone Agonist Stimulation Protocol

- Oral contraceptives (OCs) can help with scheduling of IVF cycles and may help synchronize the ovary and result in a better cohort size. OCs typically increase the amount of medications required during stimulation and may decrease the number of eggs in older women.

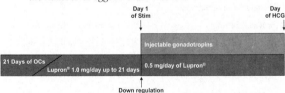

Oral contraceptive (OC)/gonadotropin-stimulating hormone agonist stimulation (Stim). hCG, human chorionic gonadotropin.

1. Start OCs between days 1 and 3 of menstrual cycle. Typically administer for 15–21 days.
2. Start GnRH-a 3–5 days before the completion of the OCs. This overlap of OCs and GnRH-a helps to prevent ovarian cyst formation.
3. Spontaneous menses expected 10–12 days after the 1st day of GnRH-a.
4. Start ovarian stimulation and continue GnRH-a. Stimulation can be with FSH, human menopausal gonadotropin (HMG), or a combination of FSH and HMG.
5. Serial ultrasounds and E_2 levels monitor follicular development; E_2 should ↑ by ~50% each day of stimulation.

6. Once several follicles reach 18–22 mm, administer hCG, typically 5,000–10,000 U SC or IM.
7. Check serum hCG day after hCG injection to verify.
8. Oocyte retrieval is 36 hours after hCG.

Luteal Gonadotropin-Releasing Hormone Agonist Stimulation Protocol

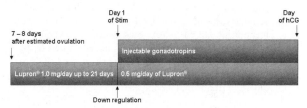

Gonadotropin-releasing hormone agonist stimulation (Stim). hCG, human chorionic gonadotropin.

1. Start GnRH-a on day 21 of menstrual cycle. The luteal start is typically confirmed by a serum progesterone level >5 ng/mL. The luteal start of GnRH-a helps to prevent ovarian cyst formation.
2. Spontaneous menses expected 10–12 days after the 1st day of GnRH-a.
3. Start ovarian stimulation and continue Lupron at lower dose. Stimulation can be with FSH, HMG, or a combination of FSH and HMG.
4. Serial ultrasounds and E_2 levels monitor follicular development; E_2 should $\uparrow$ by ~50% each day of stimulation.
5. Once several follicles reach 18–22 mm, administer hCG, typically 10,000 U SC or IM.
6. Check serum hCG day after hCG injection to verify.
7. Oocyte retrieval 36 hours after hCG

Microdose Gonadotropin-Releasing Hormone Agonist Flare Stimulation Protocol

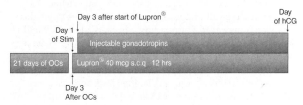

Microdose gonadotropin-releasing hormone agonist flare stimulation (Stim). hCG, human chorionic gonadotropin; OCs, oral contraceptives.

1. Start of OCs between days 1 and 3 of menstrual cycle and administer for 21 days. (Note: Many programs do not use OCs at all for this protocol.)
2. Start Lupron, 40 μg SC q12 hours, 3 days after the end of the OC course (i.e., day 24).
3. Start ovarian stimulation with FSH, HMG, or a combination of FSH and HMG 3 days after the start of Lupron (i.e., day 27) and continue Lupron. (Note: Many programs start the gonadotropins on the same day as the microdose Lupron.)
4. Serial ultrasounds and E_2 levels monitor follicular development; E_2 should ↑ by ~50% each day of stimulation.
5. Once several follicles reach 18–22 mm, administer hCG, typically 5,000–10,000 units SC or IM.
6. Check serum hCG day after hCG injection to verify.
7. Oocyte retrieval is 36 hours after hCG

ORAL CONTRACEPTIVE–GONADOTROPIN-RELEASING HORMONE ANTAGONIST STIMULATION PROTOCOL

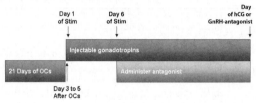

Gonadotropin-releasing hormone antagonist stimulation (Stim). hCG, human chorionic gonadotropin; OCs, oral contraceptives.

1. Start of OCs between days 1 and 3 of menstrual cycle. Typically, administer for 15–21 days.
2. Start ovarian stimulation 3–5 days after discontinuing OCs. Stimulation can be with FSH, HMG, or a combination of FSH and HMG.
3. Serial ultrasounds and E_2 levels to monitor follicular development; E_2 should rise ~50% per day
4. On stimulation day 6, start GnRH antagonist. Administration of the GnRH antagonist can lower endogenous E_2 levels. Typically, no further decrease in gonadotropin dose is recommended. Rather, most clinicians add back FSH/LH drugs at time of antagonist start. Could use GnRH agonist trigger to decrease incidence of OHSS (see Chapter 24).
5. Once several follicles 18–22 mm, administer hCG, typically 5,000–10,000 U SC or IM or 4 mg SC leuprolide (some programs repeat dose in 12 hours).
6. To ensure an adequate response to the trigger, check hCG for the hCG trigger or serum LH and P_4 if

GnRH-agonist utilized (adequate if LH ≥15 mIU/mL and P_4 ≥3 ng/mL).
7. Oocyte retrieval is 36 hours after hCG or GnRH-a.

Natural Cycle IVF

1. Baseline ultrasound between cycle days 2 and 4 of menstrual cycle
2. Monitoring ultrasound on cycle day 7 and serial ultrasounds and E2 levels thereafter
3. When E_2 > 125 pg/mL and follicle >15.5 mm, administer hCG 10,000 U IM.
4. Oocyte retrieval is 36 hours later; aspirate follicle and flush until oocyte is obtained.
   ○ Benefits to natural cycle IVF:
      → Lower costs
      → Elimination of OHSS
      → Single embryo transfer
      → Obviates ethical concerns of patients regarding frozen embryos

Oocyte Retrieval

- Typically performed 36 hours after hCG
- Performed under IV sedation using a 5-MHz vaginal transducer with associated needle guide. A 17-gauge, 35-cm aspiration needle is inserted transvaginally into multiple preovulatory follicles with sequential aspiration (low-grade suction <100 mm Hg) of oocytes. The aspirate is then given to the embryologist for evaluation.
- Complications can include intraabdominal bleeding and infection, typically occurring in <1% of IVF cases.

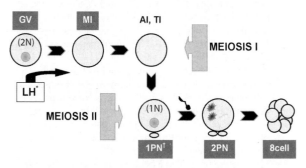

*Arrested at prophase I until luteinizing hormone (LH) surge. †Arrested at metaphase II until fertilization. AI, anaphase I; GV, germinal vesicle; MI, metaphase I; N, nuclei; PN, pronuclei; TI, telophase I.

EMBRYOLOGY PRIMER

- Retrieved eggs are identified in the follicular aspirate. Once they are identified, they are removed from the aspirate and placed in culture dishes.
- Standard IVF insemination is performed by culturing the identified eggs for approximately 16 hours with ≥50,000 sperm/mL. The next morning, the eggs are identified and evaluated for fertilization. The first sign of fertilization is two pronuclei within the cytoplasm.
- ICSI is performed in cases of severe male factor infertility, failed fertilization in a previous cycle, or severe antisperm antibody levels. After identification of the eggs in the follicular aspirate, the eggs are then placed into culture dishes. The cumulus cell complex surrounding the eggs is then removed in a process called *stripping*. Once the eggs are stripped, they are evaluated for maturity. Only metaphase 2 (MII) eggs can be fertilized. All MII eggs are then inseminated by taking one motile, morphologically normal–appearing sperm and injecting it into each mature egg.
- Fertilization rate with standard insemination is approximately 70%. With ICSI fertilization, rates range from 50–70%.
- Embryos are then cultured, typically for 3–5 days, in incubators maintained at body temperature and media specific for human embryo culture. Embryos are typically evaluated on day 3 for their cell number and overall morphology.
- It is possible for embryo transfer to be performed on day 3. However, in most centers, patients with a large number of embryos of high cell count and grade are placed into extended embryo culture for 2 additional days, referred to as the *blastocyst stage*.
- No evidence of a beneficial effect of **preimplantation genetic screening** (PGS) as of 2013 but PGS can decrease pregnancy loss rate by discarding abnormal embryos prior to embryo transfer; some evidence that PGS can lower the live birth rate for women of advanced maternal age (Mastenbroek 2011)
- Blastocyst trophectoderm biopsy with real-time polymerase chain reaction-based comprehensive chromosome screening (CCS) and fresh embryo transfer increases IVF delivery rates (Forman 2013a; Scott 2013a; Scott 2013b; Scott 2013c; Tref 2013); using CCS results in single euploid blastocyst pregnancy rates on par with transferring two untested blastocysts (Forman 2013b).
- Selective use of assisted hatching may be considered for certain patients: ≥2 failed IVF cycles, poor embryo quality and women ≥38 years old (ASRM 2008).

- Small sample sizes have precluded definitive conclusions on live birth rates from assisted hatching (van Wely 2011)

PERCENT FERTILIZATION BASED ON FOLLICLE SIZE AT TIME OF RETRIEVAL *(Rosen 2008)*

	Follicle size (mm)				
	> 18	16–18	13–15	10–12	< 10
IVF	66.8	59.9	47.5	31.3	27.1
IVF-ICSI	66.0	56.1	48.7	35.0	36.5

- Extended embryo culture to the blastocyst stage may help to identify embryos with a better prognosis for pregnancy.
- Blastocyst embryo transfer seems to increase the risk of monozygotic twins compared to day 2–3 embryo transfers (Behr et al. 2000).

POSTRETRIEVAL HORMONAL MANAGEMENT

- Due to the use of GnRH-a and antagonist and the removal of granulosa lutein cells at the time of retrieval, supplemental progesterone is administered IM or vaginally. There is a positive benefit of progesterone support for IVF favoring synthetic progesterone over micronized. There is no difference in the route of administration (van der Linden 2011). This is typically continued until 9–12 weeks of pregnancy.
- Some centers also replace E_2, which is normally concomitantly secreted by the corpus luteum.

EMBRYO TRANSFER

- On either day 3 or day 5, the embryos are transferred transcervically into the uterine cavity with transabdominal guidance.
- The number of embryos transferred is ultimately based on the patient's age, prior IVF history, egg quality, embryo quality, and the IVF center's success rates. Typically, patients <35 years old have one-to-two embryo(s) transferred, whereas those >35 years old have two-to-three embryos transferred.
- ASRM practice committee guidelines on number of embryos transferred:

RECOMMENDED LIMITS ON THE NUMBERS OF EMBRYOS TO TRANSFER

	Cleavage Stage Embryos[a]			
Prognosis	*Age<35*	*Age 35–37*	*Age 38–40*	*Age >40*
Favorable[b]	1–2	2	3	5
All others	2	3	4	5
	Blastocysts[a]			
Favorable[b]	1	2	2	3
All others	2	2	3	3

[a]See text for more complete explanations. Justification for transferring more than the recommended number of embryos should be clearly documented in the patient's medical record.

[b]Favorable = first cycle of *in vitro* fertilization, good embryo quality, excess embryos available for cryopreservation, or previous successful *in vitro* fertilization cycle.

Source Adapted from Practice Committee of American Society for Reproductive Medicine; Practice Committee of Society for Assisted Reproductive Technology. Criteria for number of embryos to transfer: a committee opinion. *Fertil Steril.* Jan;99(1):44–46, 2013.

- Embryo transfer is typically performed under ultrasound guidance. A full bladder helps provide acoustic window and decreases the anterior bend of the cervix in patients with an anteverted uterus. While a Cochrane review (Brown 2010) concludes that there is a benefit in favor of ultrasound guidance, a large RCT has been conducted that **did not** demonstrate a difference in outcomes (Drakeley 2008).
  - Embryo transfer in the mid to lower midportion of the uterus may be optimal in order to avoid the lower cavity where implantation is compromised and avoid upper cavity transfers with associated trauma and contractions (Mains 2010).
  - Following the injection of the embryo(s) one should (a) keep pressure on the syringe plunger until withdrawal of the catheter and (b) slowly withdraw the catheter in order to avoid negative pressure.
- Emerging studies suggest elective cryopreservation may ultimately have better success rates than fresh embryo transfers as well as fewer low birth weight singletons after frozen transfers compared to fresh (Imudia 2013; Kalra 2011; Maheshwari 2013; Pinborg 2013).

RISKS OF IN VITRO FERTILIZATION

- **High-order gestations:** Multiple pregnancies ultimately depend on the number of embryos transferred. Transferring two high-quality embryos in patients <35 years of age: twins → 20–40%, and triplets → 1–3%.

- **Ectopic pregnancy:** The uterus at the time of embryo transfer contracts from the cervix to the fundus.
- **Ovarian hyperstimulation syndrome:** This typically affects <5% of IVF cycles. <1% of IVF patients require hospitalization for severe OHSS.
- **Bleeding** or **infection** from egg retrieval occurs rarely.
- Elevated peak E_2 level (>3,450 pg/mL) on the day of hCG during IVF is associated with an increased risk of small for gestational age and preeclampsia (Imudia 2012; Nakashima 2013).
- Singleton babies born through IVF may have an increased risk for low birth weight and/or preterm delivery (Kalra 2011).

Cancer Risk to IVF Offspring

- There is a minimal increase risk from 1.4/1,000 to 2/1,000 cases; however, this is probably not attributable to ART but simply due to the women who undergo ART (Källén 2010).

Cancer Risk of Cancer in Women Undergoing Fertility Treatment

- Studies from the 1990s reported an increased risk of breast, endometrial and ovarian cancer with more recent studies refuting this. (Sergentanis 2013; Siristatidis 2013).
- By and large, infertility itself seems to be an important risk factor for ovarian cancer rather than infertility treatment increasing the risk.
- Retrospective cohort study in 87,403 Israeli women undergoing IVF found no significant increase in breast, endometrial or ovarian cancer in a ≤7 year time-span (Brinton 2013). Note: Borderline ovarian tumors were not included.
- Historical cohort study (with ~15 years of follow-up) in 19,146 women undergoing IVF compared to 6,006 subfertile women not treated with IVF (van Leeuwen 2011):

Possible Increased Risks of Ovarian Cancer with IVF

Excluding the 1st year of follow-up	HR, CI	Overall % increase
↑risk of ALL ovarian cancers	2.14 (1.07–4.25)	1.4% →3%
↑risk of borderline tumors	4.23 (1.25–14.33)	0.1% →0.4%

Note: Epithelial cancers account for 60% of all ovarian cancers of which the incidence of all ovarian cancers is 1.4% in a lifetime. Since borderline tumors account for 15% of the epithelial tumors this means epithelial cancers account for 0.84% of the 1.4% total and borderline would then be 0.13% risk in a woman's lifetime. (Adapted from van Leeuwen FE, Klip H, Mooij TM, et al. Risk of borderline and invasive ovarian tumours after ovarian stimulation for in vitro fertilization in a large Dutch cohort. *Hum Reprod.* Dec;26(12):3456-65, 2011).

Birth Defects

- Subfertile women should be aware that there is an increased risk of birth defects whether or not they undergo fertility treatment.

Risk of birth defects following IVF or IVF/ICSI (Davies 2012)

SINGLETON BIRTHS	AOR (CI)	# defects*	% defects*	Per 100
Spont and fertile	1.00	16,841/ 293,314	5.7%	6
Spont and infertility	**1.37** (1.02–1.83)	52/600	**8.7%**	**9**
IVF + ICSI	**1.28** (1.14–1.43)	361/4333	**8.3%**	**8**
IVF fresh ET	1.05 (0.82–1.35)	71/1005	7.1%	7
FET from IVF	1.08 (0.76–1.53)	34/479	7.1%	7
ICSI fresh ET	**1.73** (1.35–2.21)	76/713	**10.7%**	**11**
FET from ICSI	1.10 (0.65–1.85)	15/226	6.6%	7

*unadjusted
AOR, adjusted odds ratio
Source: Adapted from Davies MJ, Moore VM, Willson KJ, Van Essen P, Priest K, Scott H, Haan EA, Chan A. Reproductive technologies and the risk of birth defects. *N Engl J Med.* 10;366(19):1803-13, 2012.

Success Rates

- Success rates are IVF center–specific and depend on the patient's characteristics, quality of the ovarian stimulation, embryo culture system, and transfer technique. Center-specific pregnancy rates are published by the Centers for Disease Control and Prevention annually and can be found at http://www.cdc.gov/art/ARTReports.htm.
- High serum progesterone (>1.5 ng/mL or nmol/L) on the day of hCG is associated with a decreased pregnancy rate (31% vs. 19%) (Bosch 2010)
- Elevated progesterone (>2.25 ng/mL or 7.2 nmol/L) on day of trigger may be associated with lower fresh embryo transfer pregnancy rates but not when transferred later as a frozen embryo transfer (Xu 2012):

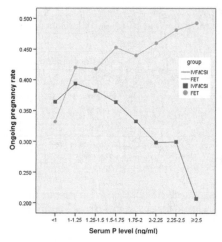

Source: Reproduced with permission from Xu B, Li Z, Zhang H, Jin L, Li Y, Ai J, Zhu G. Serum progesterone level effects on the outcome of in vitro fertilization in patients with different ovarian response: an analysis of more than 10,000 cycles. *Fertil Steril.* 97(6):1321-7, 2012.

- Cigarette smoking significantly lowers the live birth rate per cycle (OR 0.54, 95% CI 0.30–0.99), raises the odds of spontaneous miscarriage (OR 2.65, 95% CI 1.33–5.30) and raises the odds of an ectopic pregnancy (OR 15.69, 95% CI 2.87–85.76) (Waylen 2009)
- Pregnancy loss by age after documentation of fetal cardiac activity (in vitro fertilization, retrospective analysis).

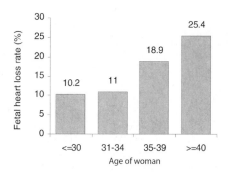

Source: Reproduced with permission from Spandorfer SD, Davis OK, Barmat LI, et al. Relationship between maternal age and aneuploidy in in vitro fertilization pregnancy loss. *Fertil Steril 81(5):1265, 2004.*

- Obesity
  - Cancellation rate based on BMI: (Dokras 2006)

BMI	% Cancellation
<25	11%
25-29.9	11%
30-39.9	8%
>40	25%*

*P<0.01 compared to <25 group (Source: Reproduced with permission from Dokras A, Baredziak L, Blaine J, Syrop C, et al. Obstetric outcomes after in vitro fertilization in obese and morbidly obese women. *Obstet Gynecol*. Jul;108(1):61–69, 2006.)

- Age-adjusted effect BMI on IVF live birth rate:
- Complementary and alternative medicine (CAM)

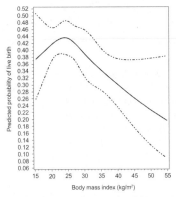

Predicted probability of live birth by body mass index. Cubic regression line of the predicted probability of live birth by body mass index, adjusted for age, among 1,721 women undergoing their first in vitro fertilization (IVF) cycle using fresh, autologous oocytes. Dashed lines represent 95% confidence intervals. (Source: Reproduced with permission from Shah DK, Missmer SA, Berry KF, et al. Effect of obesity on oocyte and embryo quality in women undergoing in vitro fertilization. *Obstet Gynecol*. Jul;118(1):63–70, 2011.)

  - Prospective observational cohort study (Boivin 2009):
    → Concurrent use of CAM during IVF was associated with a 30% lower pregnancy rate compared to non-CAM users
    → Could not ascertain which type of CAM was associated with this rate

- o RCT revealed no statistically significant difference if acupuncture were utilized compared with sham acupuncture (Moy 2011); further study is warranted (Meldrum 2013).
- Alcohol consumption (Rossi 2011)
  - o 16% lower live birth rate if a woman drank greater than 4 drinks/week compared with less than 4 drinks/week.
- Aspirin use (Groeneveld 2011; Siristaticlis 2012)

Impact of exercise on IVF

Exercise duration	Significant impact on IVF?
1-3 hours/week for 1-9 years	No effect
≥4 hours/week for 1-9 years	↓ OR 0.5 (95% CI, 0.3-0.9)
1-3 hours/week for 10-30 years	No effect
≥4 hours/week for 10-30 years	No effect

Source: Adapted from Morris SN, Missmer SA, Cramer DW et al. Effects of lifetime exercise on the outcome of in vitro fertilization. *Obstet Gynecol.* Oct;108(4):938–45, 2006.

- o Aspirin does not improve pregnancy rates after IVF although it may have beneficial effects in terms of preventing pre-eclampsia.
- Emotional stress coexisting with an IVF cycle did not compromise the success rate in a meta-analysis of prospective psychosocial studies (Boivin 2011).

Terminology

- **Pregnancy rate:** can have many definitions ranging from serum or urine positive for hCG to a live birth
- **Clinical pregnancy rate:** most common reported pregnancy rate from ART centers. This is the percentage of patients with at least one fetus in the uterine cavity with fetal cardiac activity at 7 weeks of pregnancy.
- **Live birth rate:** percentage of patients with a live birth from an ART cycle
- **Implantation rate:** This is the chance that each embryo transferred into the uterine cavity will result in a clinical pregnancy (intrauterine pregnancy with fetal cardiac activity at 7 weeks). Calculated by taking the number of clinical pregnancies divided by the number of embryos transferred.

LIVE BIRTHS PER TRANSFER FOR ASSISTED REPRODUCTIVE TECHNOLOGY CYCLES USING FRESH EMBRYOS FROM OWN EGGS, BY ASSISTED REPRODUCTIVE TECHNOLOGY PATIENT'S AGE, 2010

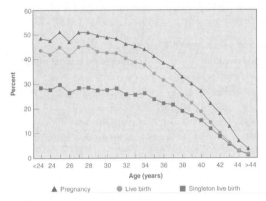

*For consistency, all percentages are based on cycles started.

Source: Reproduced from the Centers for Disease Control and Prevention (CDC). (http://www.cdc.gov/art/ARTReports.htm#5)

CUMULATIVE IVF LIVE-BRITH RATES STRATIFIED BY MATERNAL AGE

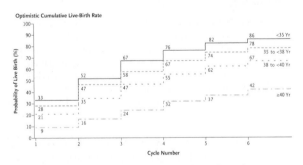

The plots illustrate the markedly reduced success rate of assisted reproductive technology in women aged >40 years. Increasing the number of intracytoplasmic sperm years but scarcely in older women. (Source: Reproduced with permission from Malizia BA, Hacker MR, Penzias AS. Cumulative live birth rates after in vitro fertilization. *N Engl J Med.* Jan 15;360(3):236–43, 2009.)

BLASTOCYST SCORING GRADE

- Any embryo with a grade of 3AA or better on day 5 should be considered suitable for a single embryo transfer.

Expansion Status	1 = Early blastocyst; blastocoel less than half the volume of the embryo, little or no expansion in overall size, zona pellucida (ZP) still thick
	2 = Blastocyst; blastocoel more than half the volume of the embryo, some expansion in overall size, ZP beginning to thin
	3 = Full blastocyst; blastcoel completely fills the embryo.
	4 = Expanded blastocyst: blastocoel volume now larger than that of the early embryo. ZP very thin
	5= Hatching blastocyst; trophectoderm has started to herniated through the ZP
	6 = Hatched blastocyst; the blastocyst has evacuated the ZP
ICM grading	A = ICM prominent, easily discernible and consisting of many cells, cells compacted and tightly adhered together
	B= Cells less compacted so larger in size, cells loosely adhered together, some individual cells may be visible
	C = Very few cells visible, either compacted or loose, may be difficult to completely distinguish from trophectoderm
	D = Cells of the ICM appear degenerate or necrotic
	E = No ICM cells discernible in any focal plane
Trophectoderm	a = Many small identical cells forming a continuous trophectoderm layer
	b = Fewer, larger cells, may not form a completely continuous layer
	c= Sparse cells, may be very large, very flat or appear degenerate

Source: Reproduced with permission from Cutting R, Morroll D, Roberts SA, et al. Elective single embryo transfer: guidelines for practice British Fertility Society and Association of Clinical Embryologists. *Hum Fertil (Camb).* Sep;11(3):131–46, 2008.

ALGORITHM OF EMBRYO MANAGEMENT

Patients are advised that embryo numbers and quality are assessed on Day 2

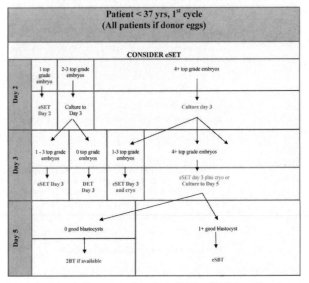

Source: Reproduced with permission from Cutting R, Morroll D, Roberts SA, et al. Elective single embryo transfer: guidelines for practice British Fertility Society and Association of Clinical Embryologists. *Hum Fertil (Camb)*. Sep;11(3):131–46, 2008.

23

Financially Efficient Fertility Care

BACKGROUND

- Without insurance coverage, financial obstacles pose a significant barrier to pursuit of fertility treatment.
- Costs for diagnostic testing and inefficient therapies can drain already limited resources.

FINANCIALLY EFFICIENT TESTING

- When patients can opt in/out of evaluation and treatment strategies, testing/therapy could be thought of in 3 levels: **mandatory, strongly recommended, and encouraged**
- Identify value in testing. Examples include:
  - Good Start Genetics provides patients with complete carrier screening services, including genetic counseling, for the most prevalent and severe diseases, as outlined by ACMG, ACOG and Jewish advocacy societies, such as cystic fibrosis and SMA. Using a single tube of blood, Good Start Genetics' next generation sequencing technology tests for 5–10 times more pathogenic mutations to provide higher detection rates and lower residual risks, minimizing the risk of missed carriers (http://www.goodstartgenetics.com).
  - The Counsyl test uses one tube of blood or saliva to detect over 100 recessive genetic diseases, including cystic fibrosis, spinal muscular atrophy, 18 Jewish genetic disorders, and Fragile X syndrome. The test is covered by insurance with minimal out-of-pocket costs. Complimentary genetic counseling is included for all tested patients. www.counsyl.com

FINANCIALLY EFFICIENT THERAPY

Optimizing Benefits

- A useful weblink on this topic is http://www.resolve.org/family-building-options/insurance_coverage/.
- Choose insurance plans or companies with unique plans that have fertility benefits
  - *Flexible health spending accounts* allow tax free dollars for fertility care.
  - The Federal Employee Retirement Income Security Act (ERISA) allows self-insured companies to opt out of state mandates, so even mandated states may have exceptions.
- If a patient does not have fertility benefits, it is still reasonable to submit claims relating to care that would be covered were she not desiring pregnancy (metabolic and other laboratory testing for PCOS evaluation, STI testing in the setting of concern over exposure, myomectomy for abnormal uterine bleeding, etc.)

Optimizing Therapy

- All other things being equal, increasing either follicle numbers or sperm improves pregnancy rates for a given cycle (Van Rumste 2008; Guzick 1999).
- Increased follicular recruitment improves pregnancy even with lower sperm counts except for when the inseminated motile count is <5 million (Guzick 1999; Khalil 2001; Van Voorhis 2001)
- These techniques in isolation have the greatest benefit when correcting an associated defect (ovulation induction for the anovulatory patient, inseminations for moderate male factor)
  - Oligoovulatory patients often have some degree of otherwise unexplained infertility and should be thought of as in a different category from truly anovulatory patients (Burgers 2010).
  - A patient who has not ovulated in 3 years has a different prognosis from a patient who has had an opportunity to conceive over the same timeframe with q45 day cycles and QOD coitus.
- In unexplained infertility, oral medications or insemination in isolation are unlikely to show dramatic benefit (Bhattacharya 2008) and one may need a clinical trial with over a thousand cycles to show a statistically significant improvement.

- However, combining **increased follicular recruitment with gonadotropins and insemination** does increase pregnancy rates meaningfully for unexplained infertility. Cycle fecundability increases 5 fold on average but at the risk of high order multiples.

Calculating Cost-Effective Therapy

- The following reflect some of the underlying assumptions for a cost-effectiveness fertility calculator; the factors are not exhaustive but provide a reasonable estimate of direct patient costs and value: www.umhc.com/fertility/costeffectivenesscalculator.
- 3 variables to consider: (1) what is the baseline pregnancy rate, (2) what is the relative increase with a particular therapy, and (3) what are the Costs of Treatment?
  - Age-based spontaneous monthly fecundity with 1 year of unexplained infertility (Gnoth 2003):
    → 18–25 yo = 4%
    → 26–30 yo = 3%
    → 31–35 yo = 2%
    → >35 yo = 1%
  - Fecundity associated with various negative conditions:
    → Stage I endometriosis (unstimulated cycles with therapeutic donor insemination): ~ ⅔ baseline live birth rate (LBR) of similarly aged women (Mattoras 2010)
    → Sonographically visible hydrosalpinx (ART cycles): ~½ baseline LBR of similarly aged women
    → Elevated BMI (ART cycles): 5% reduction for BMI 30–40, 15% reduction for BMI >40 (Luke 2011)
  - Relative increased fecundity with therapy
    → **Insemination:** ~1.5× if >100 million post-wash total sperm (multiple papers show benefit in the 1.2–1.8× range; however, the lower the baseline count, the greater the benefit, as in Guzick 1999, where the bottom two quartiles (0.4–126.9 million) for post-wash total sperm count saw benefit of 1.9-4.2× from IUI)

→ **Multifollicular recruitment with IUI:** ~60% beyond baseline for the second follicle recruited, and ~40% for each additional follicle—that is,

# Mature Follicles	~Pregnancy Rate	Improvement
1	8%	1x
2	13%	1.6x
3	16%	2x
4	19%	2.4x
5	22%	2.8x

This meta-analysis saw only an RR of 2 with four follicles, so data smoothing has been incorporated into the model. Note that accounting for follicular recruitment means that, with rare exception, FSH/IUI cycles are unlikely to be cost-effective relative to oral medications/IUI, as one typically increases costs 2–3x for a single extra follicle. (Source: Adapted from van Rumste MM, Custers IM, van der Veen F, et al. The influence of the number of follicles on pregnancy rates in intrauterine insemination with ovarian stimulation: a meta-analysis. *Hum Reprod Update.* Nov–Dec;14(6):563–70, 2008.)

Costs of Treatment

- Though inefficient, doing nothing is often the most "cost-effective," so the goal is balancing speed/benefit with cost.
  - Ultimately, therapy choices should be based on whether the increase in pregnancy rate exceeds the proportionate increase in cost, factoring in not just ultrasound, insemination, and medication costs, but time away from work, travel (gas) costs (as well as emotional costs), and so on.
- When does ART become more cost-effective?
  - Classically, many move on to IVF after 6 rounds of oral medication and insemination if <35 or 3 rounds if ≥35; however, with low ultrasound/insemination costs, it may be more cost effective to continue COS as opposed to IVF.
  - The FASTT study (Reindollar 2010) has shown that after three rounds of clomiphene/IUI, it is more cost-effective to progress directly to IVF than to attempt up to 3 cycles of gonadotropins/IUI before trying IVF.
  - The break-even point for this trial was $17,749 for IVF when CC is $500/cycle and FSH is $2,500/cycle; lower FSH costs (keeping IVF costs stable or higher) may favor FSH cycles.
    - → Common misinterpretations of this study include:
      - Applying it to clomiphene-resistant anovulation (the study looked primarily at **unexplained infertility**)

- Stating that one should never do more than 3 cycles of clomiphene and insemination (the study didn't compare 3 cycles with 6 cycles of oral medication)
- HYBRID cycles (letrozole + gonadotropins and IUI) were not studied

Maximizing Value in Services Provided

- Bundled services (a fixed fee for multiple IVF cycles and frozen embryo transfers with a 70–100% refund if not having a live birth) can simultaneously promote clinical success, profitability, and patient satisfaction.

APPENDIX A

ODDS OF PREGNANCY OVER MULTIPLE CYCLES

Baseline Chance of Pregnancy	Three Attempts
5%	14%
8%	22%
10%	27%
12%	32%
15%	39%
20%	49%
25%	58%
30%	66%
35%	73%
40%	78%
45%	83%
50%	88%

Equation: $1-(1-\%$ chance of conceiving)3, wherein $1-\%$ chance of conceiving is the probability of not getting pregnant in a month. One then calculates this probability of not getting pregnant the first month x the probability of not getting pregnant the following month, times the probability of not getting pregnant in the third month. This does not account for diminishing returns, which are increasingly important with improving effectiveness of therapy.

That is, if baseline chance of pregnancy is 15%, then: $(1 - 0.15)^3$
$= 0.85 \times 0.85. \times 0.85 = 0.61$
so,1 − 0.61= 39% chance of getting pregnant after 3 attempts

24

Ovarian Hyperstimulation Syndrome

INCIDENCE

- Iatrogenic complication of superovulation with gonadotropins (rarely clomiphene citrate) with a varied spectrum of clinical and laboratory manifestations
- Incidence in superovulation cycles:
  - Mild ovarian hyperstimulation syndrome (OHSS) → 33%
  - Moderate OHSS → 3–4%
  - Severe OHSS → 0.1–0.2%
- Risk factors:
  - <33 years old
  - Aggressive response to ovarian stimulation (≥18 follicles and/or E_2 ≥5000 ng/dL)
  - Anovulatory women with polycystic ovary syndrome (PCOS)
  - High antral follicle count
  - High basal anti-müllerian hormone (>3.36 ng/mL) (Lee 2008)
  - History of OHSS
  - hCG trigger

CLASSIFICATION

- Clinical, laboratory, and ultrasound findings:
- Symptoms typically start 3–4 days after hCG and peak 7 days after ovulation or follicle aspiration unless patient is pregnant, in which case symptoms persist/worsen.
- Pain is often the first presenting symptom.

	OHSS Stage		
Grade	*Mild*	*Moderate*	*Severe*
1	Abdominal distention/discomfort.		
2	Features of grade 1 + nausea and vomiting ± diarrhea. Ovaries enlarged to 5–12 cm.		
3		Features of mild OHSS + ultrasound evidence of ascites.	
4			Features of moderate OHSS + clinical evidence of ascites ± hydrothorax or shortness of breath.
5			All of the above + change in blood volume, ↑ blood viscosity due to hemoconcentration, coagulation abnormalities, and diminished renal perfusion and function.
6			All of the above plus respiratory distress, renal shutdown or venous thrombosis.

OHSS, ovarian hyperstimulation syndrome.
Source: Adapted from Golan A, Ron-El R, Herman A, et al. Ovarian hyperstimulation syndrome: an update review. *Obstet Gynecol Surv* 44:430, 1989.

PATHOPHYSIOLOGY

- Ovarian enlargement with multiple cysts
- Stromal edema
- ↑ Capillary permeability (marked arteriolar vasodilation) with acute fluid shift out of intravascular space
  - ○ ↑ Permeability secondary to a factor secreted by corpora lutea? *Factors:* Prostaglandins (PGs)? Endothelin-I? Vascular endothelial growth factor? Angiotensin-II?
- Shift of fluid from intravascular space into the abdominal cavity → massive 3rd spacing
- At time of oocyte retrieval, follicular aspirations of even smaller follicles offer partial protection against OHSS by removing granulosa cells.
- Early vs. late form (Papanikolaou 2004):
  - ○ **Early-onset OHSS** is related to exogenous hCG and is associated with a higher risk for preclinical miscarriage; presents 3–7 days after hCG administration.
  - ○ **Late-onset OHSS** is more likely associated with pregnancy and tends to be more severe with a relatively low risk for miscarriage; presents 12–17 days after hCG administration.

HYPERREACTIO LUTEINALIS

- Hyperreactio luteinalis (HL) can mimic OHSS (Foulk 1997) and may be viewed as entities in a continuum (Haimov-Kochman 2004).
- HL is the benign hyperplastic luteinization of ovarian theca-interna cells, leading to multicystic ovaries (bilateral though may occur unilaterally) and maternal virilization in 25% of women.
- Both may be managed conservatively.
- Comparison features of OHSS and HL:

Ovarian Hyperstimulation Syndrome	Hyperreactio Luteinalis
Superovulation therapy	Absence of ovulation induction
1st TM	Anytime during pregnancy (54%, 3rd TM; 16%, 1st TM)
Associated with polycystic ovary syndrome, hypothyroidism[a]	Associated with trophoblastic disease

TM, trimester.
[a]TM.

(Source: Nappi RG, Di Naro E, D'Aries AP, Nappi L. Natural pregnancy in hypothyroid woman complicated by spontaneous ovarian hyperstimulation syndrome. *Am J Obstet Gynecol.* Mar;178(3):610–611, 1998.)

MANAGEMENT

- Conservative management leading to spontaneous resolution with time:
  - 7 days in nonpregnant women
  - 10–20 days in pregnant women
- Have patient drink ≥1 L **fluid/day** (**Gatorade**).
- ↓ Physical activity
- Pelvic rest, in fact, bimanual examination may lead to ovarian rupture and hemorrhage
- Laboratory tests:
  - Electrolytes, creatinine (Cr)
  - Complete blood count (CBC) with platelets (PLTs)
  - Prothrombin time (PT)/partial thromboplastin time (PTT)
- Management scheme:

Classification	Clinical Characteristics/Biochemical Parameters	Management
A: Mild	Abdominal distention Inconvenience	Accept as inevitable
B: Moderate	**A** plus: Ascites on sonogram Variable ovarian enlargement	Instruct patient carefully Self-monitoring of body weight Bed rest Abundant fluid intake Frequent follow-up (outpatient basis)
C: Severe	**B** plus: Massive ascites Hypovolemia	Hospitalization Consider paracentesis IV fluids (crystalloids/ plasma expanders/ albumin) Monitoring fluid balance Low-dose heparin prophylaxis Diuretics only when hemodilution achieved Correction of electrolytes

(Continues on next page)

(Continued from previous page)

D: Critical	**C** plus: Hematocrit >55% Impaired renal perfusion Thromboembolism Impending multiorgan failure	**C** plus: Intensive care unit Continuous monitoring of hemodynamics Perform paracentesis/ transvaginal drainage IV heparin/SC heparin Consider termination of pregnancy

Source: Adapted from Beerendonk CC, van Dop PA, Braat DD, et al. Ovarian hyperstimulation syndrome: facts and fallacies. *Obstet Gynecol Surv* 53:439, 1998.

- Hospitalize **if:**
  - **Dehydration secondary to** intolerance of food/liquid and/ or persistant nausea/vomiting
  - severe abdominal pain
  - Physical **examination:**
    → Tachycardia
    → Hypotensive blood pressure (BP)
    → ↓ Breath sounds
    → Tense, distended abdomen
    → Peritoneal signs
  - **Blood tests:**
    → Hematocrit (Hct) >48% (more than 30% increment over baseline value)
    → Na^+ <135 mEq/L
    → K^+ >5.0 mEq/L
    → Cr >1.5mg/dL

TREATMENT

Oliguria Management

Urine output <600 mL/24 hours. See algorithm on following page.

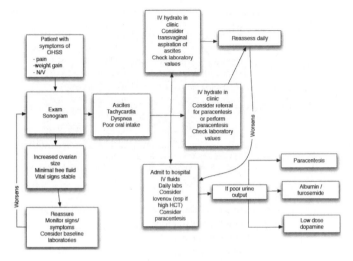

HCT, hematocrit; IV, intravenous; N/V, nausea and vomiting.

Hospital Management

Admission Orders for Severe Ovarian Hyperstimulation Syndrome

1. Daily weight
2. Strict intake and output (I&O)
3. CBC, PT/PTT, electrolytes, liver function tests (LFTs), and β-human chorionic gonadotropin (β–hCG) on admission and p.r.n.
4. Chest x-ray (CXR) and arterial blood gas (ABG) if short of breath
5. Bed rest with bathroom privileges
6. Enoxaparin* (Lovenox) if hemoconcentrated:
   ○ Prophylaxis: 40 mg SC once daily
   ○ Treatment: 1 mg/kg SC q12 hours
   * adjust dose if renal impairment: GFR < 30mL/min
7. Regular diet
8. Fluid replacement management (*remember* strict I&O)
   ○ Initial: 1 L of normal saline (NS) × 1 hr (Lactated Ringer solution [LR] not recommended, as patients with severe OHSS are hyponatremic)

- o Maintenance: D5NS at 125–150 mL/hr without added potassium (see below)
- o On diuresis: Restrict oral fluids to 1 L/day and stop IV fluid
9. Continue progesterone for luteal support.
10. Acetaminophen with narcotics as needed; avoid nonsteroidal anti-inflammatory drugs (NSAIDs).
11. Paracentesis/transvaginal aspiration for discomfort, shortness of breath (SOB), and/or persistent oliguria
12. If hypovolemic, oliguric (<30 cc/hr), see treatment algorithm on the previous page.
13. *Other management tips to consider:*
    - o No pelvic/abdominal examinations secondary to fragility of ovaries (can precipitate ovarian rupture and hemorrhage)
    - o CXR if SOB ensues
    - o White blood cell count (WBC) >22,000 is an ominous sign of imminent thromboembolism (Kodama 1995).
    - o K-exchange resins (i.e., Kayexalate) p.r.n.; no diuretics; electrocardiogram (ECG) p.r.n. for elevated K^+
    - o A falling Hct + diuresis is an *indication* of resolution, not hemorrhage.
    - o Patient may be given indomethacin, or perhaps captopril or antihistamines.
    - o Surgery if suspicion of intraperitoneal bleeding ($\downarrow$ Hct without diuresis) or torsion of ovarian cyst

Thrombosis Prevention in Patients with Severe Ovarian Hyperstimulation Syndrome

- 40 mg Lovenox SC once daily (treatment dosage → 1 mg/kg SC q 12 hr)
- Thigh-high venous support stockings

Ascites Management

- Indications for paracentesis:
  - o Severe discomfort/pain
  - o Pulmonary compromise
  - o Evidence of renal compromise unresponsive to fluid management
- Technique:
  1. Empty bladder and identify suprapubic target.
  2. Prep, drape, and inject local anesthetic.

3. Insert 18–20 gauge Angiocath with 1 ½-in. needle while aspirating until free flow is obtained, then advance catheter and withdraw needle. Ultrasound guidance may be helpful.
4. Connect Angiocath to evacuated IV bottle and tilt patient forward.

- Consider **indwelling "pig-tail"** catheter for extended drainage.

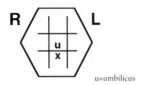

u=umbilicus

- Alternate management: early intervention with transvaginal aspiration of ascites

COMPLICATIONS

Tension Ascites

- Manifestation of capillary leakage
- Pleural effusions may be associated with tension ascites
- Treatment with paracentesis suggested by some

Thromboembolic Phenomena

- Coagulation abnormalities
- Hemoconcentration → arterial thromboemboli

Liver Dysfunction

- Hepatocellular and cholestatic changes

Renal Impairment

- Prerenal failure secondary to ↓ perfusion from hypovolemia
- Sign of recovery from OHSS = ↑ urine output
- Renal-dose dopamine after restoration of plasma volume

Acute Respiratory Distress Syndrome

- Due to ↑ capillary leakage
- Treat with positive end-expiratory pressure respiration

PREVENTION

- Choice of stimulation protocol may help avoid this situation.
- Dopamine agonist **cabergoline** can reduce the incidence of moderate OHSS (likely by ↓ VEGF-mediated vascular permeability) (Alvarez 2007; Youssef 2010).
  - Recommended protocol:
    - → Consider when E_2 >2,500 pg/mL, or >15 follicles >12 mm at the time of hCG, or >30 follicles >5 mm visualized at the time of hCG
    - → Start 0.5 mg cabergoline PO qhs the evening of hCG for a total of 8 days
- Cancel cycle, withhold hCG.
- Give hCG, aspirate, then cryopreserve all embryos (Imudia 2013; Maheshwari 2013).
  - Aspiration of follicles has a protective effect (decreasing volume of granulosa cells and subsequent vascular endothelial growth factor [VEGF] production for late-onset OHSS but not necessarily for early-onset OHSS)
- Induce ovulation/oocyte maturation with:
  - Minimal effective dose of hCG: 5,000 IU and avoid hCG in luteal phase
  - Gonadotropin-releasing hormone agonist (GnRH-a) (need to support the luteal phase with estradiol, 4 mg/day, and progesterone [micronized progesterone], 200 mg t.i.d.).
    - → Acceptable in cycles without GnRH agonist or in those using GnRH antagonist:
      - 4 mg SC leuprolide (= 80 units = 0.8 mL), some programs repeat dose in 12 hours; retrieval is done 36 hours later or
      - 3 puffs of nafarelin (Synarel GnRH agonist needs to be given > 12 hours after last antagonist) q8 hr, or
      - 50 μg intranasal buserelin
    - → Check serum LH and P_4 following day (should be LH ≥15 mIU/mL and P_4 ≥3 ng/mL to suggest an adequate response)
    - → Using GnRH agonist to trigger may be associated with lower pregnancy rates with fresh embryo

transfer but has a significantly lower rate of OHSS (Kolibianakis 2005; Melo 2009). So consider cryo-preservation of all embryos. Frozen embryo transfer may result in higher pregnancy rates (Roque 2013).
- Luteal phase support with progesterone rather than hCG
- Human albumin may prevent severe OHSS in high-risk women (meta-analysis odds ratio, **0.28; 95%** confidence interval [CI], 0.11–0.73); for every **18** women at risk of severe OHSS, albumin infusion **prevents one** more case (Aboulghar 2002).
  - 50 g IV albumin just before or immediately after oocyte retrieval

Obstetrical Outcome after OHSS during IVF (Case-Control Study) *(Courbiere 2011)*

	Control Group (n = 80)	**OHSS Group (n = 40)**
Miscarriages	16%	17.5%
Pregnancy-induced hypertension	9.2%	21.2%*
Preterm labor	10.7%	36%*
Premature delivery	18.5%	30.3%

*P<0.05 (Source: Adapted from Courbiere B, Oborski V, Braunstein D, Desparoir A, Noizet A, Gamerre M. Obstetric outcome of women with in vitro fertilization pregnancies hospitalized for ovarian hyperstimulation syndrome: a case-control study. *Fertil Steril.* Apr;95[5]:1629–632, 2011.)

25

Hyperemesis in Pregnancy

- Stimulus for nausea is produced by the placenta rather than the fetus
- Onset of nausea within 4 weeks of LMP with a peak at ~9 weeks of gestation
- 60% resolve by the end of the 1st trimester, 91% resolve by 20 weeks
- Nausea and vomiting are associated with a decreased risk of miscarriage (Weigel 1989)

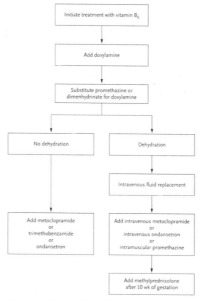

Pharmacologic Therapy for Nausea and Vomiting in Pregnancy. Ginger may be added to pharmacologic therapy at any time. At any step, enteral or parenteral nutrition may be considered if dehydration or persistent weight loss is noted; it should be limited to patients with persistent nausea and weight loss who do not tolerate enteral nutrition. (Source: Reproduced with permission from Niebyl JR. Clinical practice. Nausea and vomiting in pregnancy. *N Engl J Med.* Oct 14;363(16):1544–50, 2010.)

Pharmacologic Treatment of Nausea and Vomiting in Pregnancy*

Agent	Oral Dose	Side Effects	FDA Category[†]	Comments
Vitamin B$_6$ (pyridoxine)	10–25 mg every 8 hr		A	Vitamin B$_6$ or vitamin B$_6$–antihistamine combination recommended as first-line treatment
Vitamin B$_6$ (pyridoxine)–doxylamine combination (Diglegis)	2 tabs qhs; if symptoms persist after 2 days, increase to 1 tab PO qa.m. and 2 tabs qhs; may further increase to 1 tab qa.m., 1 tab every mid-afternoon and 2 tabs qhs; Max: 4 tabs/day; give on an empty stomach	Sedation	A	
Antihistamines		Sedation		
Doxylamine (Unisom SleepTabs)	12.5–25 mg every 8 hr		A	
Diphenhydramine (Benadryl)	25–50 mg every 8 hr		B	
Meclizine (Bonine)	25 mg every 6 hr		B	
Hydroxyzine (Atarax, Vistaril)	50 mg every 4–6 hr		C	
Dimenhydrinate (Dramamine)	50–100 mg every 4–6 hr		B	

(Continues on next page)

(Continued from previous page)

Pheno-thiazines		Extrapy-ramidal symptoms, sedation	
Promethazine (Phenergan)	25 mg every 4–6 hr	C	Severe tissue injuries with intravenous use (black-box warning); oral, rectal, or intramuscular administration preferred
Prochlorperazine (Compazine)	5–10 mg every 6 hr	C	Also available as buccal tablet
Dopamine antagonists		Sedation, anticholiner-gic effects	
Trimethobenza-mide (Tigan)	300 mg every 6–8 hr	C	
Metoclopramide (Reglan)	10 mg every 6 hr	B	Tardive dyskinesia (black-box warning) Treatment for more than 12 week increases risk of tardive dyskinesia
Droperidol (Inapsine)	1.25 mg to 2.5 mg intramuscu-larly or intrave-nously only	C	Black-box warn-ing regarding torsades de pointes
5-hydroxy-tryptamine3–receptor antagonist		Consti-pation, diarrhea, headache, fatigue	
Ondansetron (Zofran)	4–8 mg every 6 hr	B	Also avail-able as oral disintegrating tablet; more costly than oral ondansetron tablets

(Continues on next page)

(Continued from previous page)

Glucocorticoid

Methylprednisolone (Medrol)	16 mg every 8 hr for 3 days, then taper over 2 week	Small increased risk of cleft lip if used before 10 weeks of gestation	C	Avoid use before 10 weesk of gestation; maximum duration of therapy 6 weeks to limit serious maternal side effects
Ginger extract	125–250 mg every 6 hr	Reflux, heartburn	C	Available over the counter as food supplement

*This list of agents is not exhaustive. FDA denotes Food and Drug Administration.
†FDA categories are as follows: A, controlled studies show no risk; B, no evidence of risk in humans; C, risk cannot be ruled out; D, positive evidence of risk; and X, contraindicated in pregnancy.

26

Gamete Preservation

FEMALE GAMETE PRESERVATION

Medical indications
- Gonadotoxic therapies for cancer and other medical diseases
  - Radiotherapy
  - Autoimmune/collagen vascular disease
  - Oophorectomy for benign/malignant conditions (i.e., endometriosis, ovarian cancer)
- Genetic conditions
  - Women with BRCA mutations may undergo prophylactic oophorectomy
  - Mosaic Turner syndrome (efficacy of oocyte banking unknown)
  - Fragile X permutation (efficacy of oocyte banking unknown)
- Failure to obtain sperm for IVF on day of oocyte retrieval
- Those unable to cryopreserve embryos (moral or religious concerns)
- Elective cryopreservation to defer childbearing

Gonadotoxicity

- Chemotherapy damages the ovaries' steroid-producing cells (granulosa and theca cells) and oocytes → primary ovarian insufficiency (POI) → premature menopause → infertility
  - Chemotherapy drugs and their potential for gonadal damage: (alkylating agents have the highest risk)
    1. High potential: cyclophosphamide (RR between 4-9.3 (Sonmezer and Oktay 2004)), chlorambucil, melphalan, busulfan, nitrogen mustard and procarbazine
    2. Moderate potential: cisplatin and adriamycin

3. Mild or no potential: bleomycin, actinomycin D, vincristine, methotrexate and 5-fluorouracil
- Radiotherapy depletes the primordial follicle pool in a dose-dependent manner (Gosden 1997)
    → 6 Gy results in permanent ovarian failure (Howell and Shallet 1998)

OPTIONS FOR FEMALE GAMETE PRESERVATION

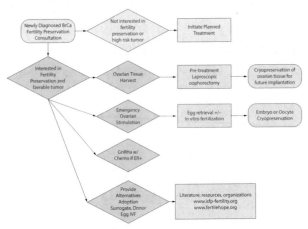

Source: Reproduced with permission from Kim SS, Klemp J, Fabian C. Breast cancer and fertility preservation. *Fertil Steril.* Apr;95(5):1535-43, 2011.

Embryo Cryopreservation

- Well-established technique
- Requires IVF protocol; therefore, controlled ovarian stimulation and egg retrieval may delay disease treatment
- Good option for women with a partner and time for an IVF cycle
- Not acceptable to single women who decline the use of donor sperm
- Not an option for pediatric/prepubertal females
- Ethical/legal concern: disposition of cryopreserved embryos in the case of the patient's death

Letrozole Protocol:

- For patients with estrogen-sensitive breast cancer, letrozole is a more desirable option (Kim 2011; Rodriguez-Wallberg 2010)
  - Letrozole 5 mg starting on cycle day 2 until day of trigger
  - FSH 150–300 IU/day starting on cycle day 4
  - 0.25 mg GnRH antagonist started when lead follicle reaches 14 mm or E_2 ≥250 pg/mL
  - 5,000-10,000 IU HCG or 250 µg recombinant HCG or 4 mg GnRH-agonist trigger
  - Restart letrozole on day of retrieval for 5 more days

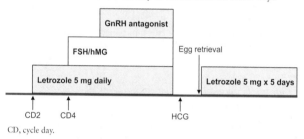

CD, cycle day.

Oocyte Cryopreservation

- This technique is no longer considered experimental (ASRM 2013).
- Requires IVF protocol; therefore, controlled ovarian stimulation and egg retrieval may delay disease treatment
- Does not require a male partner but not considered a routine procedure due to current pregnancy rates being significantly lower than those with embryo cryopreservation
- First report of successful pregnancy from thawed oocytes (Chen 1986) → more than 900 babies born to date
- Freezing techniques utilize theoretically eliminating ice crystal formation and growth
- Post-thaw survival rates in vitrified oocytes have improved and fertilization rates are similar to those of fresh oocytes (Cobo 2010; Rienzi 2010).
- Online age-specific individualized oocyte freezing live birth success rates: http://www.i-fertility.net/probability-calc

Ovarian Tissue Cryopreservation & Transplantation

- Experimental, under auspices of IRB; an area of extensive research with great potential (Donnez 2013)
- Future applications include patients with cancer and those who decline donor oocytes.
- Tissue ischemia and risk for reintroduction of cancerous cells are two crucial issues (Kim 2006; Dolmans 2013).

Oophoropexy (Ovarian Transposition)

- Technique involves dividing the utero-ovarian ligament and laterally transposing the ovary (Tulandi 1998).
- Pelvic irradiation at doses > 300 cGy can result in loss of ovarian function.
- Total lymph node irradiation in patients with Hodgkin's lymphoma exposes the ovaries to 2,000–4,000 cGy, invariably causing POF (Williams 1999).

Gonadotropin-Releasing Hormone (GnRH) Agonists/Antagonists

- Administered to downregulate hypothalamic-pituitary-ovarian (HPO) axis to decrease susceptibility to gonadotoxicity although no GnRH receptor has been identified as yet on human primordial follicles or oocytes
- Efficacy is controversial.
- Possible mechanism(s) include mediation of antiproliferative effects by GnRH receptors on ovarian cells (Volker 2002), a decrease in gonadotropin concentrations, decreased ovarian perfusion due to hypoestrogenic milieu, antiapoptotic effect mediated by sphingosine-1-phosphate, and germline stem cell preservation
- Blumenfeld et al.'s (Blumenfeld 1996) study of young women with lymphoma who received chemotherapy: in GnRH-agonist-treated group, 94% had spontaneous menses within 3–8 months of completing chemotherapy treatment; in the control group, 61% had POI.
- Randomized trial of 281 patients with breast cancer who received chemotherapy (anthracycline, cyclophosphamide, methotrexate, fluorouracil) (Del Mastro 2011)
  - 3.75 mg GnRH-agonist administered at least 1 week before the start of chemotherapy and then every 4 weeks for the duration of chemotherapy

- 8.9% premature menopause in GnRH-agonist treated group compared with 25.9% in the control group (P<0.01) with NNT=6.
- One protocol adapted from ClinicalTrials.gov #NCT01257802:
  - 3.75 mg GnRH-agonist monthly throughout course of chemotherapy with transdermal E_2 add-back (0.05-1 mg) beginning 1 month into the Lupron.

Fertility Preservation Options

	Timeframe for Referral/Initiation	Potential for Success
Male Patients		
Sperm cryopreservation[1]	Anytime before cancer treatment	Established
Testicular tissues/ spermatogonial cryopreservation[16]	Anytime before cancer treatment	No clinical experience
Hormonal therapy	Anytime before cancer treatment	Unsuccessful
Female Patients		
Embryo cryopreservation	Before chemotherapy begins	Established
Surgical transposition[8]	Before pelvic radiation begins if no chemotherapy administered	Established
Oocyte cryopreservation[19]	Needs minimum of 2 weeks for stimulation	Over 200 live births; success rates lower than with fresh oocytes
Transplantation of cryopreserved ovarian tissue[21,22]	Can be performed at any time before, and sometimes after, chemotherapy	Successful return of ovarian function and fertility shown in case studies
Ovarian stimulation with aromatase inhibitors[18]	Requires minimum of 2 weeks	Controlled studies show equal success rates to standard IVF; no increase in recurrence in short-term follow-up
GnRH agonist administration[23,24]	During chemotherapy treatment	Mixed results; no benefit in women undergoing high-dose chemotherapy with HSCT

GnRH, gonadotropin-releasing hormone; HSCT, hematopoietic stem cell transplant; IVF, in vitro fertilization.

Source: Modified from Oktay K, Meirow D. Planning for fertility preservation before cancer treatment. *Sexuality, Reproduction and Menopause*, 5(1):17–22, 2007.

MALE GAMETE PRESERVATION

Indications

- Chemotherapy - affects germinal epithelium
- Radiotherapy - affects germinal epithelium, Leydig cell function and sperm DNA integrity
- Retroperitoneal surgery
- Postmortem

Options

Sperm Cryopreservation

- Most reliable option for adolescent and adult males
- If time before treatment allows, 3 samples are produced at least 48 hours apart (Holoch 2011).
- For azoospermic men, testicular extraction of sperm for future IVF/ICSI.

Embryo Cryopreservation

- Viable option for reproductive-aged male and partner
- Requires IVF

27
Luteal Phase Deficiency

DEFINITION

- Historical definition: >2-day lag in endometrial histologic development (Noyes criteria [Noyes 1950]; updated by Murray 2004)
  - However, it is no longer recommended to obtain endometrial biopsies, because histologic endometrial dating is neither accurate nor precise (Murray 2004; Coutifaris 2004).

DIAGNOSIS

- Controversial, ambiguous diagnosis without a definitive diagnostic criteria.
- Consider search for luteal phase deficiency (LPD) if:
  - Normal cycles and unexplained infertility
  - >35 years old
  - Short luteal phases (<13 days from positive LH peak to menses)
  - History of recurrent losses (28% associated with LPD) (Vanrell and Balasch 1986).

INCIDENCE

- Perhaps 30% of isolated cycles in fertile women; 30–40% of infertile women

ETIOLOGY

- Plausible etiologies:
  - ↓ Hormone production by corpus luteum
  - ↓ Follicle-stimulating hormone (FSH) in follicular phase (FSH stimulates granulosa cell proliferation and luteinizing hormone [LH] receptors on granulosa cells)

- o Abnormal patterns of LH secretion
- o ↓ Levels of LH and FSH at the time of ovulatory surge
- o ↓ Response of the endometrium to pregnancy
- o Hyperprolactinemia leading to abnormal gonadotropin-releasing hormone (GnRH) pulsatility

DIAGNOSTIC CRITERIA

Luteal Phase Duration

- Short luteal phase duration (<13 days) as defined by the interval from midcycle LH surge to the onset of menses may define LPD.

Mid–Luteal Phase Progesterone Level

- Insufficient evidence because serum P_4 is subject to variation associated with pulsatile LH secretion and poor correlation with histologic stage of endometrium (i.e., endometrial inadequacy can be found in the presence of normal progesterone [P_4] levels)
  - o Pulsatile, mid-luteal P_4 is higher in the a.m. (Syrop and Hammond 1987).
  - o Historically, a P_4 level <10 ng/mL (32 nmol/L) or the sum of three serum P_4 levels that is <30 ng/mL (Jordan 1994) 7 days before menses → LPD.
  - o Argument for measuring P_4 8 days after a positive LH-kit change: Mid–luteal phase P_4 <9.4 ng/mL is associated with a lower pregnancy rate (Hull 1982).
  - o Argument for mid-luteal P_4 supplementation: LPD successfully treated if P_4 <6.6 ng/mL (receiver operator curve) (Daya 1988)

Does serum progesterone predict luteal phase dysfunction?

LH, luteinizing hormone. Source: Reproduced with permission from Wuttke W. Regulation of steroid production and its function within the corpus luteum. *Steroids*, 63:299–305, 1998.

Endometrial Biopsy

- Historically performed 5–7 days before menses, with dating reference being the **subsequent** menses.
- Timed endometrial biopsy with histologic dating provides no clinically useful information as a subfertility screening test:
  - Out-of-phase biopsy results poorly discriminated between women from fertile and subfertile couples (in either mid-luteal or late luteal phase) (Coutifaris 2004).
  - Out-of-phase biopsy found in approximately 20–30% of normal cycles
  - Randomized, observational study concluded that there is poor accuracy and reproducibility in histologic endometrial dating (Murray 2004).

TREATMENT

- Treat hyperprolactinemia and hypothyroidism (see Chapters 28 and 29)
- Aromatase inhibitor: letrozole 5 mg days 3–7 (or 20 mg single dose on day 3 [Mitwally and Casper 2005]), ultrasound day 12, human chorionic gonadotropin (hCG) booster and intrauterine insemination.
- Clomiphene citrate (CC):
  - 50 mg q.d. × 5 days beginning on cycle day 3, 4, or 5

- o Drawbacks:
  - → 10% chance of multiple gestation
  - → Occasional hot flashes
  - → Occasional severe mood changes
  - → Rare visual changes (*palinopsia* = prolonged afterimages or shimmering of the peripheral field) that may be irreversible (Purvin 1995)
  - → Potential for inducing LPD (Manners 1990), although this may just reflect underlying anovulation (Hecht 1990)
- Gonadotropin superovulation:
  - o risk of OHSS
  - o risk of multiples
  - o increased cost
- Progesterone:
  - o 25–100 mg P_4 suppositories b.i.d., Crinone 8% every evening, or Prometrium, 200 mg b.i.d. per vagina starting 3 days after ovulation (i.e., after 3 days of temperature rise >97.8°F); treatment is maintained until menses, or if pregnant, continue until 11th week, although literature support is weak for use past 9 weeks (Csapo and Pulkkinen 1978).
  - o Drawback: can prolong the luteal phase and thus delay menses (causes patient frustration!)
  - o No difference in outcome between CC vs. P_4 treatment of LPD (Huang 1986; Murray 1989)

LUTEAL PHASE SUPPORT IN CONTROLLED OVARIAN STIMULATION CYCLES FOR WOMEN WITH UNEXPLAINED INFERTILITY:

- Clomiphene citrate 50 mg with IUI:
  - o RCT with vaginal micronized progesterone (Prometrium 200 mg 3× daily) beginning 1 day after insemination (196 women) vs. control group without luteal phase support (204 women): 8.7 vs. 9.3% ongoing pregnancy rate respectively, P = 0.82 (Kyrou 2010)
- FSH with IUI:
  - o RCT with vaginal progestin gel (Crinone 8%) daily beginning 2 days after insemination (109 women) vs. control group without luteal phase support (105 women): 17.5% vs. 9.3% live birth rate per cycle respectively, P=0.16 (Erdem 2009)

LUTEAL PHASE SUPPORT IN IN VITRO FERTILIZATION CYCLES

- Clearly necessary
- Need may reflect:
  - GnRH agonist down-regulation
  - Removal of granulosa cells with oocyte retrieval/poor corpus luteum function

Regimens

- **hCG:** 2,500 IU IM 4 days after embryo transfer, then every 4 days
- **P_4:** (treat through luteal-placental shift)
  - **Oral:** micronized 300–800 mg/day
  - **Vaginal:** micronized P_4, 200 mg b.i.d.—t.i.d.; compounded suppositories, 200–600 mg/day; Crinone, 90 mg q.d.-bid; Endometrin, 100 mg bid-t.i.d.
  - **IM:** P_4 in oil, 50–100 mg/day; 17α–hydroxyprogesterone caproate, 341 mg q3d
- Meta-analysis: IM hCG and IM P_4 better than no treatment; IM P_4 better than oral and vaginal P_4 (Pritts 2002); others report vaginal supplementation as effective as IM (Yanushpolsky 2010)
- The addition of oral **estrogen** (estradiol, 2–6 mg PO/day) to luteal support regimens may improve the implantation rate, but it has not been shown to improve the clinical pregnancy rate (Pritts 2002)
- hCG booster is associated with ↑ incidence of ovarian hyperstimulation syndrome.

28

Hyperprolactinemia and Galactorrhea

DEFINITION

- Consistently elevated fasting serum prolactin in the absence of pregnancy or postpartum lactation; nonpuerperal lactation

PROLACTIN

- Little PRL = polypeptide hormone of 198 amino acids, but there are several different circulating forms:
- Circulating big PRL can be converted to little PRL by disulfide bond reduction
- In the vast majority of cases, big-big PRL (bbPRL) consists of a complex of PRL and an anti-PRL IgG autoantibody and is referred to as macroprolactin. Less commonly, big-big PRL is composed of either covalent or noncovalent polymers of monomeric PRL. This may account for 10% of hyperprolactinemia but this is not symptomatic (Gibney 2005).
- Macroprolactin (or bbPRL) should be suspected when the clinical history or MRI findings are inconsistent with the elevated PRL (D'Ercole 2010).

Name	Molecular Weight	Biologically Active	Immunologically Active
Little PRL	22 kd	Yes	Yes
Glycosylated little PRL	25 kd	Yes, but decreased	No
Big PRL	50 kd	No	Yes
Big-big PRL	>100 kd	No	Yes

PRL, prolactin.

- Synthesized and stored in the pituitary gland in lactotrophs (also synthesized in decidua and endometrium, although not under dopaminergic control)
- Mean levels of 8 ng/dL in adult women; $t_{1/2}$ = 20 minutes
- Cleared by the liver and kidney (hence ↑ PRL with renal failure)
- Functions:
  - Mammogenic → stimulates growth of the mammary tissue
  - Lactogenic → stimulates mammary tissue to produce and secrete milk

PHYSIOLOGY

- Synthesis and release controlled by central nervous system (CNS) neurotransmitters (usually inhibitory)
- Dopamine (DA; PRL-inhibiting factor) and cannabinoids inhibit secretion through D2 DA receptors (DA-Rs) on lactotrophs (Pagotto 2001).
- PRL-releasing peptide (PrRP), thyrotropin-releasing factor, and estrogen stimulate release (Rubinek 2001).
- FSH may be suppressed by ↑ PRL through GnRH suppression; in addition to a direct action on GnRH neurons, PRL may modify these neurons through afferent pathways via GABAergic and kisspeptin neurons in the arcuate nucleus (Anderson Endo 2008; Kokay 2011))
- Episodic secretion varying throughout the day and cycle (↑ PRL at time of luteinizing hormone [LH] surge) (Djahan-bakhch 1984)
- No clinically relevant changes over the menstrual cycle, although there is a significant albeit subtle midcycle peak in PRL (Fujimoto 1990).
- Hypertrophy and hyperplasia of lactotrophs in pregnancy in response to ↑ estrogen
- PRL:
  - Steadily ↑ during pregnancy, reaching 200 ng/mL in the 3rd trimester (TM)
  - Return to normal in nonlactating women 2–3 weeks postpartum
  - Return to normal in lactating women 6 months postpartum ↑ With breast stimulation, exercise, sleep, stress

PREVALENCE OF INCREASED PROLACTIN WITH THE FOLLOWING SIGNS AND SYMPTOMS

Sign/Symptom	Chance of ↑ Prolactin (%)
Anovulation	15
Amenorrhea	15
Galactorrhea	30
Amenorrhea + galactorrhea	75
Infertility	34

Source: Adapted from Molitch ME, Reichlin S. Hyperprolactinemic disorders. *Dis Mon* 28(9):1, 1982.

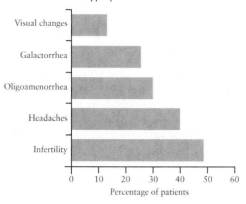

Most Commonly Reported Symptoms in Patients with Hyperprolactinemia

Source: Adapted from Bayrak A, Saadat P, Mor E et al. Pituitary imaging is indicated for the evaluation of hyperprolactinemia. *Fertil Steril.* 2005;84(1):181–185.

- ↑ PRL induces a dose-dependent ↑ DA secretion, which in turn inhibits GnRH pulsatile release through the D_1 receptor on GnRH neurons and by the activation of the β-endorphin neuronal system that further inhibits GnRH release (Seki 1986).
- Autopsy: pituitary adenomas in 27% of women (Burrow 1981) (**PRL-secreting** incidence in autopsies: 11%)

Potential Causes of Hyperprolactinemia

Cause	Example	Mechanism
Physiological	Pregnancy	Increasing estrogen levels
	Breast stimulation	Inhibition of dopamine via the autonomic nervous system
	Breastfeeding	
	Stress	Reduced dopamine stimulation
	Exercise	
	Sleep	
Pituitary disorders	Pituitary tumors: micro- or macroprolactinoma, adenoma, hypothalamic stalk interruption, hypophysitis (inflammation)	Disruption of dopamine delivery from the hypothalamus and/or secretion of growth hormone and prolactin
	Acromegaly	Prolactin secretion from a growth hormone adenoma
	Cushing syndrome	Prolactin secretion from a corticotroph adenoma
	Empty sella syndrome	Damage to/regression of the pituitary
	Rathke cysts	Compressed pituitary
	Infiltrative diseases (tuberculosis, sarcoidosis)	Infiltration of pituitary
Hypothalamic disorders	Primary hypothyroidism	Increased hypothalamic thyrotrophin-releasing hormone and decreased metabolism
	Adrenal insufficiency	
Medications	Anti-psychotics (phenothiazines, haloperidol, butyrophenones, risperidone, monoamine oxidase inhibitors, fluoxetine, sulpiride)	Inhibition of dopamine release
	Anti-emetics (metoclopramide, domperidone)	
	Antihypertensives (methyldopa, calcium channel blockers, reserpine)	
	Tricyclic antidepressants	
	Opiates	Stimulation of hypothalamic opioid receptors
	Estrogens	Positive action on lactotrophs
	Verapamil	Unknown
	Protease inhibitors	

(Continues on next page)

(Continued from previous page)

Neurogenic	Chest wall injury Spinal cord lesions	Peripheral triggers of autonomic control that interrupt central neurogenic pathways that attenuate dopamine release into the hypophyseal portal circulation; may act via the same nerves affected by nipple stimulation
Increased prolactin production	Polycystic ovary syndrome	Usually transient
Reduced prolactin elimination	Renal failure Hepatic insufficiency	Less rapid clearance of prolactin from the systemic circulation plus central stimulation of prolactin
Abnormal molecules	Macroprolactinemia	Polymeric form of prolactin formed following binding of prolactin to immunoglobulin G antibodies that cannot bind to the prolactin receptor
Idiopathic	Unknown	Unknown

Source: Adapted with permission from Crosignani PG. Current treatment issues in female hyperprolactinemia. *Eur J Obstet, Gynecol and Reprod Biol.*;125:152–164, 2006.

Prolactinoma (Most Common)

- Even with normal values or only mildly elevated PRL, patient may have a large tumor (Bayrak 2005)
- Arise most commonly from the lateral wings of the anterior pituitary where the lactotrophs predominate.
- Islands of pituitary lactotrophs may be released from the normal tonic inhibitory effect of DA through spontaneous or estradiol (E_2)-dependent generation of arteriolar shunts (Elias and Weiner 1984).
- Found in 10% of general population (most asymptomatic)
- Found in 50% of women with hyperprolactinemia
- Incidence increases with (a) increasing PRL levels and (b) severity of symptoms.
- Microadenoma <1 cm
  - Prevalence of up to 27% in autopsy series (Burrow 1981)

- ○ Enlargement uncommon (≤5%) (Schlechte 1989)
- ○ Most regress spontaneously.
- Macroadenoma >1 cm and usually PRL >200 ng/mL

*Correlation between the Pituitary Size
and Serum PRL Level (ng/mL)*

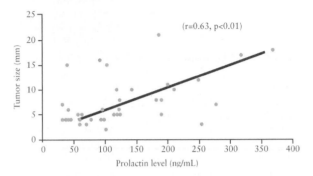

Source: Reproduced with permission from Bayrak A, Saadat P, Mor E et al.
Pituitary imaging is indicated for the evaluation of hyperprolactinemia. *Fertil Steril.*
2005;84(1):181–185.

- The risk of diminished secretion of other pituitary hormones due to the presence of a prolactinoma is based on their proximity to the prolactinoma mass and their overall cell number: mnemonic for the adenohypophyseal hormones with the greatest to least propensity to be affected → **GnTAG** (% relates to the number of cells):
  - ○ Gonadotropins (Gns) (5%, close to lactotrophs), thyroid-stimulating hormone (TSH) (5%), adrenocorticotropic hormone (ACTH) (20%), growth hormone (GH) (50%), antidiuretic hormone (ADH) (rare, posterior pituitary)

Acromegaly

- GH-secreting pituitary adenoma
- Associated symptoms: acral changes, macrognathia (enlarged jaw), macroglossia, spread teeth, sweaty palms, carpal tunnel syndrome
- Affected patients experience symptoms of the disease ~7 years before diagnosis.
- GH can bind to PRL receptors (but PRL does not bind to GH receptors).

- ~20% of GH-secreting pituitary adenomas secrete PRL (Vance 2004).
- Check serum insulin-like growth factor-I (IGF-I) (need age-adjusted and sex-adjusted IGF-I levels) as GH-secreting pituitary adenomas may not be visible on magnetic resonance imaging (MRI); IGF-I is produced primarily by the liver in response to GH. GH levels may appear normal since this hormone is released in pulses.
- Diagnosis: Elevated basal fasting GH and IGF-I; 1-hr glucose (75 mg) challenge reveals GH concentration >1 ng/mL in patients with acromegaly.
- Currently, surgery is the 1st choice for acromegaly; if the adenoma is not fully resectable then utilize a long-acting somatostatin analog (i.e., octreotide).

Cushing's Disease

- Diagnosis: elevated 24-hr urinary free cortisol excretion and failure of cortisol to suppress with dexamethasone suppression tests:
  - **Low-dose dexamethasone suppression test**: differentiates patients with Cushing's syndrome of any cause from patients without Cushing's syndrome:
    - → Overnight 1 mg test —1 mg dexamethasone at 11 p.m. to 12 a.m., measurement of serum cortisol at 8 a.m. the next day. Cushing's syndrome if > 1.8 μg/dL (50 nmol/L)
    - → At least one other test should be performed to confirm the diagnosis
  - **High-dose dexamethasone suppression test**: differentiates patients with Cushing's disease (pituitary hypersecretion of ACTH) from those with ectopic ACTH syndrome:
    - → Two-day 2 mg test—0.5 mg dexamethasone every 6 hours × 8 doses, measurement of serum cortisol either 2 or 6 hours after the last dose. Cushing's disease if > 1.8 μg/dL (50 nmol/L)
- Adenoma secretes ACTH.
- Patients present with hypertension, hirsutism, weakness and proximal muscle wasting, coarse facial features, arthritis, and ↑supraclavicular/posterior dorsal fat
- 10% secrete PRL.

Other Pituitary Tumors

- Clinically nonfunctioning microadenoma (~80% are gonadotroph adenomas), lymphocytic hypophysitis, craniopharyngioma, Rathke's cleft cyst, TSH-pituitary adenoma (rarest)

- Growth of nonfunctioning pituitary adenomas: ~13% of microadenomas and ~50% of macroadenomas over 5 years (for review please see Dekkers 2008)

Lactotroph Hyperplasia

- 8% of pituitary glands at autopsy
- Can only be distinguished from microadenoma by surgery
- Follistatin is a specific marker.

Empty Sella Syndrome

- Congenital or acquired defect in the sella diaphragm
- Intrasellar extension of the subarachnoid space results in compression of the pituitary gland and an enlarged sella turcica.
- 5–10% have hyperprolactinemia (usually <100 ng/mL).
- Diagnose with MRI.
- Benign course, although headaches (mostly localized anteriorly) are a frequent symptom (Catarci 1994).

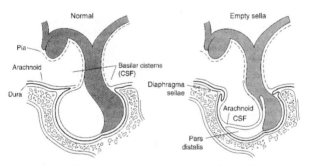

CSF, cerebrospinal fluid. (Source: Reproduced with permission from Jordan RM, Kendall JW, Kerber CW. The primary empty sella syndrome: analysis of the clinical characteristics, radiographic features, pituitary function and cerebrospinal fluid adenohypophysial hormone concentrations. *Am J Med* 62[4]:569, 1977.)

Hypothalamic Disease

- Alters normal portal circulation of DA
- Craniopharyngioma (most common)
- Infiltration of hypothalamus by sarcoidosis, histiocytosis, leukemia, carcinoma

Pharmacologic Agents

- Interfere with DA production, action, uptake, or receptor binding
- PRL levels range from 25–100 ng/mL.

- Return to normal level within days after the cessation of the offending drug (Rivera 1976)
- Examples:
  - Neuroleptics (phenothiazines, haloperidol)
  - Antidepressants (selective serotonin reuptake inhibitors, not tricyclics)
  - Opiates
  - Antihypertensives (α-methyldopa, reserpine, verapamil)
  - Metoclopramide (a DA-R blocker)
  - H-2 blockers (intravenous cimetidine)

Hypothyroidism

- Found in 3–5% of patients with hyperprolactinemia; 20–30% of patients with primary hypothyroidism have ↑PRL.
- Galactorrhea secondary to ↑ thyroid-releasing hormone (TRH) → ↑ PRL
- Primary hypothyroidism: ↓ thyroxine (T_4) → ↑ TRH → pituitary → ↑ TSH and ↑ PRL
- Secondary hypothyroidism (from a pituitary tumor): given circadian rhythm of TSH and variable set-points. TSH can be in the low to normal range: therefore, need to check T_4.

Chronic Renal Disease

- ↓ PRL clearance and ↑ production rate

Chronic Breast Nerve Stimulation

- Status post-thoracic surgery, herpes zoster, chest trauma

Stress Idiopathic Hyperprolactinemia

- PRL levels later return to normal in ⅓.
- Unchanged PRL levels in nearly ½
- 10% will develop radiographic evidence of a pituitary tumor during a 6-year follow-up (Sluijmer and Lappohn 1992).

EVALUATION OF ELEVATED PROLACTIN

Magnetic Resonance Imaging with Gadolinium Enhancement

- Preferred technique with resolution down to 1 mm
- Accurate soft-tissue imagery without radiation exposure

LABORATORY STUDIES

Fasting a.m. laboratory tests: PRL, IGF-I, T_4, TSH

IGF-I obtained because 25% of acromegalics secrete ↑ PRL.

T_4 obtained to rule out *other* pituitary tumor leading to low-normal TSH and low T_4.

Cortisol, LH, FSH, α-subunit, if hyperprolactinemia and no response to medication, especially in cases with hypertension

Routine breast examination does not acutely alter serum PRL levels in normal women (Hammond et al. 1996).

If PRL values are <200 ng/mL, and a macroadenoma (>1 cm) is seen on MRI, it is most likely not a prolactinoma (probably gonadotroph tumor or nonsecretory).

Three Caveats on the PRL Assay

1. The upper limit of PRL detection is usually between 180 and 200 ng/mL, so if the sample is not diluted, the value may be misleadingly reported as "200 ng/mL" when, in reality, with adequate dilution, the actual value is 2,000 ng/mL or higher.
2. When present in very high concentrations, prolactin saturates both the capture and signal antibodies, blocks formation of the capture antibody-prolactin-signal antibody "sandwich," and results in falsely decreased prolactin results (referred to as the high-dose hook effect). Dilution of the sample eliminates the analytic artifact in these cases.
3. Macroprolactin due to immunoglobulins can be screened for with polyethylene glycol serum precipitation.

Management

- Microadenoma or functional hyperprolactinemia: risk of progression for PRL secreting tumors to macroadenomas is <7% (Gillam 2005).
  - Most patients with microadenomas verified by MRI may be monitored by serial PRL as it is very rare for a prolactinoma to grow significantly without an increase in PRL (Hofle 1998).
- Macroadenomas should be treated no matter the severity of symptoms.
- Without treatment of microadenomas, there is a 24% chance of PRL normalization within 5 years, and 95% do not grow (Schlechte 1989).
- Microadenoma follow-up: measure PRL yearly and do not repeat an MRI unless there is a marked rise in PRL or there are clinical signs of tumor expansion.

- Macroademona follow-up: repeat MRI 2-3 years after PRL normalized to confirm tumor suppression (Schlechte 2007)

GOALS OF TREATMENT

IF Low E$_2$ (<40 pg/mL)

Estrogen treatment or oral contraceptives (OCs) (no ↑ size of microadenoma or ↑ [serum PRL])

Yearly PRL levels

IF Normal E$_2$

Normal cycles

Yearly PRL levels

IF Oligomenorrhea or amenorrhea and E$_2$ >40 pg/mL

Progestin withdrawal or OCs

Yearly PRL levels

TREATMENT ENDPOINTS (EFFECTS OF MEDICAL THERAPY)

- Bromocriptine (Parlodel) or cabergoline is used to achieve desired fertility (80% restored), relieve intolerable galactorrhea (60% eradicated), and reduce mass effect (reduced tumor size in 80–90%).
- Cardiac valvular regurgitation seen with very high doses of cabergoline (3 mg, ~10–20× higher than the maximal dose used for prolactinomas); not reported for bromocriptine

Dopamine Agonists Commonly Used in the Treatment of Hyperprolactinemia

	Bromocriptine	**Cabergoline (Dostinex)**	**Quinagolide (Norprolac)[a]**
Dopamine receptor target sites	D$_1$ and D$_2$	D$_1$ (low affinity) and D2 (high affinity)	D$_2$
Duration of action	8–12 hours	7–14 days	24 hours
Half-life (hours)	3.3	65	22
Available doses	1.0 and 2.5 mg scored tablets; 5 and 10 mg capsules	0.5 mg scored tablets	25, 50, 75, and 150 µg tablets

(Continues on next page)

((Continued from previous page))

	Bromocriptine	**Cabergoline (Dostinex)**	**Quinagolide (Norprolac)**[a]
Typical dose	2.5 mg/day in divided doses	0.5 mg/week or 0.25 mg twice weekly	75 μg/day
Dosing regimens, starter packs, dosage	Start at 1.25–2.5 mg/day at bedtime. Gradually increase to a median of 5.0–7.5 mg/day and a maximum of 15–20mg/day	Start at 0.25–0.5 mg twice weekly. Adjust by 0.25 mg twice weekly up to 1 mg twice weekly every 2–4 months according to serum prolactin levels	Start at 25 μg/day. Increase over 1 week up to 75 μg/day. Starter pack (3× 25 μg tablets + 3× 50 μg tablets) allows quick and convenient titration
Advantages	Long history of use; does not appear to be teratogenic; inexpensive	Good efficacy; low frequency of adverse events; may be useful in bromocriptineresistant patients; weekly or twice-weekly dose	Good efficacy and tolerability; once-daily dosing; simple titration; pituitary selective; use to the time of confirmed pregnancy
Disadvantages	Tolerance; recurrence; resistance; multiple daily dosing	Not yet indicated for use during pregnancy	Not currently available in the United States or Japan
Common side effects	Nausea, headache, dizziness, abdominal pain, syncope, orthostatic hypotension, fatigue	Milder and less frequent compared with bromocriptine	Milder and less frequent compared with bromocriptine

[a]Quinagolide is not approved for treatment of hyperprolactinemia in the United States or Japan. (Source: Adapted with permission from Crosignani PG. Current treatment issues in female hyperprolactinemia. *Eur J Obstet, Gynecol and Reprod Biol.*;125:152–164, 2006.)

NOTES ON MEDICAL THERAPY

- Bromocriptine
  - DA agonists do not restore bone mass to a clinically meaningful degree (Colao 2000).
  - Discontinue after 2 years in patients treated for galactorrhea to assess for remission (11% after 1 year, 22% after 2 years) (Ciccarelli and Camanni 1996).
  - Measure PRL 4–6 weeks after initiating treatment.
  - No risk for pituitary insufficiency (including diabetes insipidus [DI]) as opposed to surgical or radiation treatment
  - Response occurs in 6 weeks in ⅔ and can take up to 6 months in ⅓.
  - No need to repeat MRI if microadenoma and ↓ PRL; if macroadenoma, if ↑ PRL, repeat MRI after 3 months of treatment, if PRL normalized then repeat MRI in 2–3 years.
  - Follow PRL every 6–12 months once stabilized—no need to repeat MRI scans; visual field testing is more sensitive than MRI for detecting tumor shrinkage.
  - Advise patients to take medicine in the middle of a bulk meal.
  - Alternate route: 2.5 mg **per vagina** q.d. (fewer side effects) (Jasonni 1991)
  - Depot form (q month injection) not yet available
- Cabergoline is a more specific D_2 agonist; approximately ½ of those who do not respond to bromocriptine respond to cabergoline (Verhelst 1999).
  - Follow-up after cabergoline withdrawal (Colao 2003):
    - → 2–5 years after normalization of hyperprolactinemia:
      - ↑ PRL in 24% of nontumoral hyperprolactinemia
      - ↑ PRL in 31% with microadenomas
      - ↑ PRL in 36% with macroadenomas
      - 22% showed gonadal dysfunction.
      - 0% renewed tumor growth
      - Rate for recurrence of hyperprolactinemia was 19% for each mm increment in the maximal tumor diameter.
      - Before discontinuation of cabergoline, decrease by 0.25 mg of the weekly dose in 3-month intervals, check PRL after each dose reduction and obtain an MRI 6 months after initiation of tapering (Schlechte 2007).

Pregnancy and Prolactinomas

- 70% increase in pituitary size during normal pregnancy due to lactotroph hypertrophy.

Microadenoma: 1.6%
Macroadenoma: 15.5%; check visual-field testing, a.m. cortisol, and TSH every trimester.

- Complete remission of hyperprolactinemia occurs in 17-37% of women after pregnancy
- Risk of symptomatic tumor enlargement during pregnancy (Molitch 1985):

Operative Approach

Transsphenoidal Microsurgical Resection

- Mortality: <0.5%
- Pituitary insufficiency rate of 19%
- Temporary DI, 10–40%; permanent DI, <2%
- 3.9% require glucocorticoid replacement therapy (Feigenbaum 1996)
- 3% chronic sinusitis; 2% septal defect (i.e., epistaxis) (Feigenbaum 1996)
- Initial cure rate (Amar 2002):
  - Microadenoma: 65–91%
  - Macroadenoma: 20–40%
- Effect on reproductive function (those actively attempting postoperatively):
  - 6 months: 82% pregnancy rate
  - 12 months: 88% pregnancy rate
- Better prognosis: PRL <100 ng/mL
- Poor prognosis: PRL >200 ng/mL, >26 years old, amenorrhea >6 months
- Cure rates based on pre- and postoperative PRL levels (Feigenbaum 1996):
  - Preoperative levels <100 ng/mL: 69% cure rate
  - Preoperative levels <200 ng/mL: 60% cure rate
  - Immediate postoperative levels <5 ng/mL: 84% cure rate
  - Immediate postoperative levels <20 ng/mL: 74% cure rate
- Recommended after failure of medical treatment (i.e., cabergoline) or if patient is intolerant of side effects
- Transsphenoidal approach provides a decompression of the bony confines of the sella turcica, so that recurrence of the

tumor tends to follow the path of least resistance into the sphenoid sinus rather than the intracranial compartment.

Radiation Therapy

- Cobalt, proton beam, heavy particle therapy, or brachytherapy
- Inconsistent results; takes years to ↓ tumor growth
- Delay in symptom resolution
- Only used in adjunctive management with surgery for large tumors

Other Possible Therapies

- Gamma knife: inconclusive data but may be preferred over conventional radiation treatment for patients not responding to DA with residual tumor after surgery

NOTES

- Oral contraceptives are safe in women with hyperprolactinemia, but they do not normalize bone density (they can prevent progressive bone loss) (Corenblum and Donovan 1993).
- Prospective data suggest that higher PRL levels are associated with an ↑ risk of breast cancer in postmenopausal women (Hankinson 1999).
- Osteoporosis: ↓ bone mineral density in women with hyperprolactinemia; although bone density may ↑ when prolactin levels are normalized, it typically remains subnormal, continuing the risk of vertebral and hip fractures.
- Hirsutism: PRL receptors have been found on the human adrenal gland, thereby influencing the secretion of androgens (Glasow 1996).

APPENDIX A

Clinically Nonfunctional Pituitary Mass

- Hormonal assessment to rule out:
  - Pituitary hormone excess from clinically silent adenoma
  - Pituitary hormone deficiency attributable to a pituitary tumor/infiltrative disease with mass effects

Axis	Hypersecretion Assessment	Reserve Assessment
Somatotropic	100 mg oral glucose suppression test	GH level does not decrease to <2 ng/mL if there is a GH-producing adenoma.
PRL	a.m. PRL (normal range, 1.4–24.2 ng/mL)	TRH stimulation test → PRL should ↑ 2× 15–30 minutes after TRH.
Gonadotropic	LH, FSH, E$_2$, free α-subunit	E$_2$ should be >30 pg/mL; TRH stimulation test with 500 µg TRH → abnormal result if there is more than a 2-fold increase in free alpha-subunit at 30 to 60 minutes
Corticotropic	Low-dose dexamethasone test (normal if cortisol <1.8 µg/dL)	Metyrapone test (normal if 11-deoxycortisol >10 µg/L).
Thyrotropic	Free T$_4$, free T$_3$, TSH	Free T$_4$, free T$_3$, TSH; TRH stimulation test.

E$_2$, estradiol; FSH, follicle-stimulating hormone; GH, growth hormone; LH, luteinizing hormone; PRL, prolactin; T$_3$, triiodothyronine; T$_4$, thyroxine; TRH, thyroid-releasing hormone; TSH, thyroid-stimulating hormone.

29
Hypothyroidism

PREVALENCE

- ↑ Thyroid-stimulating hormone (TSH) is found in 4–10% of all adult women (Hollowell 2002).

THYROID FUNCTION

- Most of the released hormone is thyroxine (T_4), which is then peripherally converted to triiodothyronine (T_3).
- T_3 is more biologically active than T_4.

SIGNS AND SYMPTOMS

- Fatigue
- Dry or rough skin
- Irritability
- Weakness
- Hair loss
- Myalgia
- Memory loss
- Weight gain
- Cold intolerance
- Constipation
- Abnormal menses
- Coarse or dry hair
- Depression
- ↓ Libido
- Primary thyroid failure → abnormal uterine bleeding
- Hyperthyroidism → oligomenorrhea

DEFINITIONS

- Subclinical hypothyroidism: asymptomatic; normal T_4, T_3 but ↑ TSH ± thyroid antibodies (Abs); incidence, 4–10% of the general population
- Progression to overt hypothyroidism is dependent on the magnitude of TSH elevation.
- **Antithyroperoxidase Abs** (APA) = antimicrosomal Abs (AMA)
- Antithyroglobulin Abs (<1:1,600 titer → no progression seen) (Vanderpump 1995)

FERTILITY AND PREGNANCY *(Lincoln 1999)*

- Screening for hypothyroidism useful in women with ovulatory dysfunction
- Prepubertal hypothyroidism → short stature, delay in sexual maturity
- Infertility from anovulation and abnormal uterine bleeding from estradiol (E_2)-withdrawal bleed
- Increased pregnancy loss rate (6.1 vs. 3.6%, P = 0.006) if TSH is between 2.5–5 mIU/L (n = 4123) (Negro 2010)
- During pregnancy, T_4 requirements increase approximately 45% (secondary to [a] ↑ thyroxine-binding globulin and [b] ↓ free thyroid hormone concentrations as pregnancy progresses)

As soon as pregnancy is confirmed (Toft 2004):

↑ Levothyroxine (LT4) 25–50 µg daily

Recheck TSH in 4 weeks

SCREENING

- Non-fertility patient: TSH >5 mIU/L, start LT4
- Check TSH at age 35 years and then every 5 years; yearly for fertility patients.

- Fertility patient: TSH >2.5 mIU/L ⟶ start LT4

- Subclinical hypothyroidism has been associated with adverse maternal and fetal outcomes, so universal treatment of all patients with TSH >2.5 mIU/L, regardless of TPOAb status, seems reasonable and may reduce pregnancy loss (see page 333).

- The American Thyroid Association recommends LT4 treatment for all patients with TSH >2.5 mIU/L who are TPOAb positive but has no recommendation regarding those who are TPOAb negative (Stagnaro-Green 2011).
- Reassessment of TSH in pregnant patients with prior TSH >2.5 mIU/L who are not treated is reasonable.

Table Probability of a Miscarriage Based on TSH Level

TSH mIU/L	SAB
<2.5 (n = 3481)	3.6%*
2.5-5 (n = 642)	6.1%

*P<0.01; NNT = 40
Source: Adapted from Negro R, Schwartz A, Gismondi R, Tinelli A, Mangieri T, Stagnaro-Green A. Increased pregnancy loss rate in thyroid antibody negative women with TSH levels between 2.5 and 5.0 in the first trimester of pregnancy. *J Clin Endocrinol Metab.* Sep;95(9):E44–48, 2010.

TREATMENT GOALS *(Cooper 2001)*

- Fertility Patient: 50–75 µg/day initially; recheck in 4 weeks, ↑ by 25 µg p.r.n.
- Goal of treatment based on trimester-specific pregnancy reference range (Stagnaro-Green 2011):

Trimester	Serum TSH goal (mIU/L)
1	0.1–2.5
2	0.2–3.0
3	0.3–3.0

- Nonfertility patient: 1.6 mg/kg/day starting dose, once stable (TSH 0.45–4.5 mIU/L), the TSH can be monitored annually.

30

Recurrent Pregnancy Loss

FAST FACTS

- Fetal viability is only achieved in 30% of all human conceptions, 50% of which are lost before the first missed menses (Edmonds 1982).
- 15–20% of clinically diagnosed pregnancies are lost in the 1st or early 2nd trimester (TM) (Warburton and Fraser 1964; Alberman 1988).
- Risk of loss:
  - 12% after one successful pregnancy
  - 24% after two consecutive losses
  - 30% after three consecutive losses
  - 40% after four consecutive losses
- Risk of a 4th loss after three prior losses depends on past reproductive history:
  - If no prior live birth → 40–45%
  - If ≥1 prior live birth → 30%
- ↑ Rate of pregnancy loss with advanced maternal age (most common cause is isolated nondisjunction)

Incidence of SM or RM Occurring by Chance and of RM in Total, in Women of Different Age Groups

Age Groups (years)	Sporadic Mis-carriage (%)[a]	Rm Occurring by Chance[b], % (CI)	RM Occurring in Total (%)
20–24	11	0.13 (0.13–.013)	-
25–29	12	0.17 (0.17–0.17)	~0.4
30–34	15	0.34 (0.34–0.34)	~1
35–39	25	1.56 (1.56–1.56)	~3
40–44	51	13.3 (13.29–13.31)	-

CI, confidence intervals for binomial proportions.
[a]Data from Nybo Anderson et al. (2000).
[b]Calculated based on the assumption that if sporadic miscarriage rate = μ, recurrent miscarriage rate occurring by chance = μ^3

- 80% of spontaneous abortions (SABs) occur within first 12 weeks of pregnancy, and 60–75% of these are due to chromosome abnormalities.
- Recurrent pregnancy loss (RPL) is a risk factor for ectopic pregnancy (2.5%), complete molar gestation (5 in 2,500), and neural tube defects (Adam 1995).

Prognostic Value of Transvaginal Ultrasound Observation of Embryonic Heart Activity

Maternal Age (Years)	Risk of Loss (%)
≤35	<5
36–39	10
≥40	29
History of recurrent pregnancy loss	15–25

Source: Adapted from Van Leeuwen I, Branch DW, et al. First-trimester ultrasonography findings in women with a history of recurrent pregnancy loss. *Am J Obstet Gynecol* 168(1 Pt 1):111, 1993; Laufer MR, Ecker JL, et al. Pregnancy outcome following ultrasound-detected fetal cardiac activity in women with a history of multiple spontaneous abortions. *J Soc Gynecol Investig* 1(2):138, 1994; and Deaton JL, Honore GM, et al. Early transvaginal ultrasound following an accurately dated pregnancy: the importance of finding a yolk sac or fetal heart motion. *Hum Reprod* 12(12):2820, 1997.

- Advanced paternal age may be associated with spontaneous abortion: For fathers age 40 years or older there is a ~3-fold increase in SAB compared with women conceiving with men <25 years old (Kleinhaus 2006).

INCIDENCE

- RPL (≥2 spontaneous losses ≤20 weeks) occurs in **approximately 1–4%** (Salat-Baroux 1988). Chemical pregnancies and ectopic pregnancies are not considered part of RPL.
  - The risk of RPL in sisters of patients with RPL is ~11% (Christiansen 1990)
  - **Abortion:** pregnancy loss before 20 weeks gestation or a fetal weight of <500 g
  - **Primary RPL:** refers to a woman who has never carried a pregnancy to viability
  - **Secondary RPL:** refers to a history of ≥1 viable term pregnancy before a series of losses
  - **Early pregnancy loss:** refers to a loss <12 weeks estimated gestational age (EGA)
  - **Late pregnancy loss:** refers to a loss between 12 and 20 weeks EGA

- ~ 5% of women attempting to conceive experience 2 consecutive losses
- ~ 1% of women attempting to conceive experience ≥3

ETIOLOGY

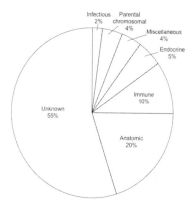

Etiologies of recurrent pregnancy loss.

Genetic Factors

Parental Chromosome Abnormality

- Approximately 4% in couples with RPL (vs. 0.2% in normal population)
- The maternal to paternal ratio is 3 to 1.
- One aneuploid SAB ↑ the risk of a subsequent loss to aneuploidy (Golbus 1981).
- 4% probability that either parent is a carrier of a balanced translocation if there are ≥2 SABs or one SAB + a malformed fetus.
- Majority of abnormalities are balanced translocations (no DNA is lost and phenotype of the parent is normal), resulting in an unbalanced translocation in the fetus. However, with no intervention there is still a 70% chance of a live birth.
- Breakdown of prevalence of balanced translocations found in RPL couples:
  o 40% Robertsonian (any)
  o 60% Reciprocal (any)

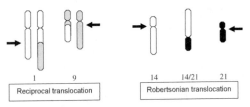

Source: Reproduced with permission from PROLOG. *Reproductive Endocrinology and Infertility.* 4th ed. Washington, DC: American College of Obstetricians and Gynecologists, 2000.

- o **Reciprocal translocation:** even exchange of chromatin between two nonhomologous
- o **Robertsonian translocation:** involves group D (13–15) and G (21 and 22) chromosomes (i.e., 14/21 translocation = long arms join up, but some short-arm material may be lost; breakage occurs close to the centromere; there are 45 chromosomes present (one normal 14 and 21, along with the balanced 14/21)
- o Gamete permutations for parent with reciprocal or Robertsonian balanced translocation:
  - → Reciprocal translocation: ½ of gametes are normal (including balanced). (bal, balanced; nl, normal)

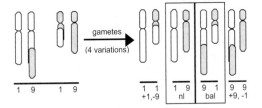

  - → Robertsonian translocation: ⅓ of gametes are normal (including balanced). (bal, balanced; nl, normal)

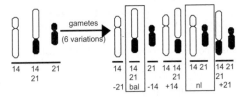

Risk of an Abnormal Live Birth

	Risk for Live Birth Trisomy
Reciprocal translocations	**0–30%**, varies depending on chromosomes involved, break-points and amount of material translocated
Robertsonian translocations as a group	**<1%**
t(13,14) = 75% of all Robertsonian translocations	**<0.4%**
t(14;21) = 10% of all Robertsonian translocations	**10%** (21') if mother is carrier **1%** (21') if father is carrier

21', trisomy 21

- → Robertsonian translocation of homologous chromosomes (incidence of 1 in 2,500 with RPL) necessitates donor gametes for the affected partner.
  - o *De novo* translocations (Warburton 1991):
    - → Reciprocal translocation: 1 in 2,000
    - → Robertsonian translocation: 1 in 9000
- Turner mosaics are more susceptible to spontaneous miscarriages (Tarani et al. 1998):
  - o Out of 160 pregnancies:
    - → 29%: spontaneous loss
    - → 20%: malformed babies (Turner syndrome [TS], trisomy 21, and so forth)
    - → 7%: perinatal death

Fetal Chromosomal Abnormality

- Approximately 60–75% of SABs (Fritz 2001)
- Karyotyping of the conceptus may reveal need for parental karyotype testing.
  - o The survival rate of 45,X embryos is ~1 in 300
  - o Chromosomally normal embryos tend to abort later in gestation (~12–13 weeks) than aneuploid embryos
- It is generally held that fetal chromosomal abnormalities play a prominent role in affecting single pregnancy losses but not recurrent losses; in fact, as the number of losses increases, the chance of a fetal chromosomal aberration decreases (Ogasawara 2000; Christiansen 2002).

- The greater the number of previous miscarriages, the greater the chance the embryo had a normal karyotype (Ogasawara 2000).

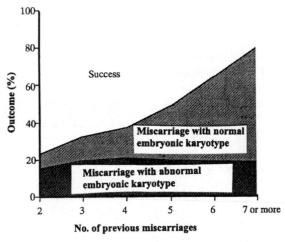

No. of previous miscarriages

Source: Reproduced with permission from Ogasawara M, Aoki K, et al. Embryonic karyotype of abortuses in relation to the number of previous miscarriages. *Fertil Steril* 73(2):300, 2000.

Algorithm for Estimating the Probability of a Miscarried Embryo/Fetus with Normal Karyotype According to the Number of Previous Miscarriages (11) and Maternal Age (8)

Miscarriages, n	Maternal age, %			
	18–29	30–35	36–39	>40
≥7	**79**	**77**	**57**	**50**
6	**73**	**71**	**51**	44
5	**63**	**61**	41	34
4	47	45	25	18
3	43	41	21	14

Bold figures: high risk of miscarriage of a karyotypically normal embryo.
Source: Reproduced with permission from Christiansen OB, Steffensen R, Nielsen HS, et al. Multifactorial etiology of recurrent miscarriage and its scientific and clinical implications. *Gynecol Obstet Invest.* 66(4):257–67, 2008.

- As a group, the trisomies are the most common anomaly, and of these, trisomy 16 is the *most common trisomy* found in abortuses, although the *single most common aneuploidy* for 1st TM losses is 45,XO.

Anatomic Factors

Congenital Uterine Anomalies

Prevalence (%) of Uterine Anomalies

	Fertile	Subfertile	RPL (≥3 losses)
Didelphys	0.03	0.2	0.1
Unicornuate	0.03	0.4	0.4
Bicornuate	0.3	0.8	1
Septate	2	3.5	5
Arcuate	**6.7**	**7.3**	**16.1**

Source: Adapted from Saravelos SH, Cocksedge KA, Li TC. Prevalence and diagnosis of congenital uterine anomalies in women with reproductive failure: a critical appraisal. *Hum Reprod Update.* Sep–Oct;14(5):415–29, 2008.

Reproductive Performance of Different Uterine Malformations

	Spontaneous Abortion (%)	Preterm Delivery (%)	Live Birth (%)
Didelphys	32.2	28.3	55.9
Unicornuate	36.5	16.2	54.2
Bicornuate	36.0	23.0	55.2
Septate	**44.3**	22.4	50.1
Arcuate	25.7	7.5	66.0

Source: Adapted from Grimbizis GF, Camus M, Tarlatzis BC, et al. Clinical implications of uterine malformations and hysteroscopic treatment results. *Hum Reprod Update.* Mar–Apr;7(2):161–74, 2001.

- A bicornuate uterus may not be associated with RPL (Proctor and Haney 2003).
- Incomplete caudal to cephalad septum reabsorption, type V (**septate**) anomaly, is associated with a 60% rate of RPL (Buttram 1983).
- The vascular density in uterine septa removed at the time of metroplasty is similar to that of the normal uterine wall (Dabirashrafi 1995).
- Pregnancy loss is more common among women with diethylstilbestrol (DES) exposure (Kaufman 2000).
- Benefit of metroplasty on pregnancy outcome is currently being assessed by an RCT study in the Netherlands.
- Repair of a uterine septum for a nulligravid women is not recommended (Branch 2010).

Acquired Uterine Anomalies

- Intrauterine synechiae (also known as *Asherman syndrome*) from vigorous uterine curettage have been found to occur in 5% of women with RPL.

- Submucosal leiomyomas may cause an unfavorable implantation site by interfering with vascularization or by reducing the intrauterine cavity size; likewise, subserosal and intramural fibroids may cause reproduction failure if they distort the uterine cavity.
- Pregnancy losses are reduced after removal of large intramural fibroids (>5 cm) (Bajekal 2000).
- Uterine polyps may induce an inflammatory milieu that may be unfavorable for implantation.

Diagnosis

- Hysterosalpingogram/hysteroscopy/hysterosonography/laparoscopy/magnetic resonance imaging (MRI); 3D transvaginal sonography
- Imaging for septate uterus (Pellerito 1992):
  - *Transvaginal sonography (TVS)* has a sensitivity of 100% and specificity of 80%; addition of 3D transvaginal scanning may increase accuracy.
  - *MRI* has a sensitivity and specificity of 100%.

Treatment

- **Primary method of treatment in all cases is corrective surgery.** In the case of congenital anomalies, unification procedures such as the Strassman procedure are rarely undertaken. Septum resection may be warranted. In the case of Asherman syndrome, hysteroscopy to lyse adhesions is advisable. Hysteroscopic myomectomy, when feasible, is recommended for submucosal fibroids.
- IVF with gestational carrier should be considered as effective treatment

Endocrinologic Factors

Luteal Phase Deficiency

- A large multicenter study is underway to assess the benefit of progesterone supplementation for unexplained RPL (PROMISE, http://www.medscinet.net/promise).
- The insufficient level of progesterone, presumably from a deficient corpus luteum in the 2nd half of the menstrual cycle, is hypothesized to prevent implantation of conceptus or impair maintenance of pregnancy; luteal phase deficiency (LPD) is more clearly associated with RPL than subfertility; histologic differences between fertile and infertile women are not significant (Coutifaris 2004); consider LPD if duration of

luteal phase is <13 days (from positive luteinizing hormone [LH] kit to start of menses).

- o Normal women have endometrial histology suggestive of LPD in up to 50% of single menstrual cycles and 25% of sequential cycles (Davis 1989).
- o If progesterone deficiency is the cause of a miscarriage, the pregnancy is usually lost before the sixth week of gestation.
- o Suggested treatment options include aromatase inhibitor, clomiphene citrate, recombinant human follicle-stimulating hormone (rhFSH), human chorionic gonadotropin (hCG), and progesterone supplementation (beginning 3 days after positive ovulation prediction kit [OPK] until 10 weeks EGA).
- o **Hyperprolactinemia** has been shown to induce luteal phase insufficiency (possibly by ↓ progesterone from luteal cells).

Polycystic Ovary Syndrome

- Sonographic evidence of polycystic-appearing ovaries (PCAOs) in women with RPL does not predict worse pregnancy outcome than in women with RPL without PCOS (Rai 2000).

Insulin

- ↑ Prevalence of **insulin resistance** in women with RPL (Craig 2002):
  - o 27.0% vs. 9.5%; odds ratio (OR), 3.55; 95% confidence interval (CI), 1.40–9.01
- Insulin resistance confers >8-fold risk of miscarriage during IVF than those without insulin resistance (Tian 2007); intervention with appropriate **insulin sensitizing therapy** has been suggested to reduce miscarriage risk among women with PCOS (Glueck 2002). A free androgen index (FAI) <5 was associated with a significantly higher miscarriage rate and women with PCOS are more prone to have elevated FAI (Cocksedge 2008).

Thyroid

- **Hyper-** and **hypothyroidism** have been associated with ↑ pregnancy loss; no direct causal relationship specifically known toward RPL.
- Euthyroid women with TSH > 2.5 mIU/L have increased pregnancy loss rates when compared to those with TSH < 2.5 mIU/L (see the following table):

Table Probability of a Miscarriage Based on TSH Level

TSH mIU/L	SAB
<2.5 (n = 3,481)	3.6*
2.5–5 (n = 642)	6.1

*P<0.01; NNT=40
Source: Adapted from Negro R, Schwartz A, Gismondi R, et al. Increased pregnancy loss rate in thyroid antibody negative women with TSH levels between 2.5 and 5.0 in the first trimester of pregnancy. *J Clin Endocrinol Metab.* Sep;95(9):E44–48, 2010.

Probability of a Miscarriage and Live Birth After IVF with or without Levothyroxine: Prospective Randomized Trial of Women Referred for Mild Thyroid Failure

Age (years)	SAB	LBR
Synthroid (n = 35; mean TSH = 1.1)	9[a]	26[b]
Placebo (n = 35; mean TSH = 4.9)	13[a]	3[b]

[a]P = 0.44
[b]P = 0.0001
NNT for LB = 2
Source: Adapted from Abdel Rahman AH, Aly Abbassy H, Abbassy AA. Improved in vitro fertilization outcomes after treatment of subclinical hypothyroidism in infertile women. Endocr Pract. Sep–Oct;16(5):792–97, 2010.

Obesity

- Obesity (body mass index >30 kg/m^2) is associated with ↑ risk of 1st TM and recurrent miscarriage (Lashen 2004).
  - Early miscarriage OR 1.2; 95% CI, 1.01–1.46
  - RPL OR 3.5; 95% CI, 1.03–12.01

Microbiologic Factors

- Several infectious agents have been implicated as etiologic factors in sporadic pregnancy loss, but no infectious agent has been clearly proven to cause RPL.
- Studies of women with RPL show an increased colonization with *Ureaplasma urealyticumas* well as evidence of chronic endometritis (9.3% incidence for RPL) in the endometrium (Kundsin 1981; Kitaya 2011).
- Other commonly linked infections include *Toxoplasma gondii*, rubella, herpes simplex virus (HSV), measles, cytomegalovirus (CMV), coxsackie virus, *Listeria monocytogenes*,

and *Mycoplasma hominis*, although none has been convincingly associated with RPL.

- Bottom line: more cost effective and time efficient to empirically treat each partner with azithromycin (1 g × 1 dose) or doxycycline (100 mg b.i.d. × 10 days) than to pursue multiple and repeated cultures.
- Reasonable to omit infectious testing or treatment

Inherited Thrombophilia

- Who should be tested? (Lockwood 2011)
  - Screening is appropriate for non-RPL indications that would lead to altered management decisions (see below). There is insufficient evidence of a causal relationship between inherited thrombophilia and RPL. Also, there is insufficient evidence of anticoagulant therapy efficacy.
    → Personal history of venous thromboembolism (VTE) associated with a nonrecurrent risk factor
    → 1st degree relative having a VTE before age 50
    → 1st degree relative with a history of a high risk thrombophilia (AT deficiency; double heterozygous for prothrombin G20210A mutation and factor V Leiden; factor V Leiden homozyous or prothrombin G20210A mutation)
- Factor V Leiden (FVL) and prothrombin G20210A (ProG) mutation, found in approximately 9% (1% of these are homozygous for the FVL mutation) and 3%, respectively, of white women in the United States; these mutations are associated with ~25% of isolated thrombotic events and ~50% of familial thrombosis.
- Although all who carry the FVL mutation show phenotypic resistance to activated protein C (PC), approximately 15% of all cases of activated PC resistance are not related to FVL mutation.
- The majority of large prospective studies have not found an association between fetal loss and inherited thrombophilia (Lockwood 2011).
- Bottom line: there is no evidence-based benefit of universal hereditary thrombophilia screening for early RPL.
- Other less common thrombophilias include autosomal-dominant deficiencies of the anticoagulants PC, protein S (PS; bad if <60%, then test antigenic levels of PS), and antithrombin deficiency.
- It is believed that women with inherited thrombophilia may be susceptible to local microthrombosis affecting syncytiotrophoblast invasion of maternal vessels at the site

of implantation; however, since maternal blood does not perfuse the intervillous space until later in the 1st trimester, implantation failure cannot be explained solely on a thrombophilia disorder. (Stern 2006)

VTE Risk in Pregnancy with Various Thrombophilias

	% Prevalence	% VTE Risk/Pregnancy (no history of VTE)	% VTE Risk/Pregnancy (previous history of VTE)	Percentage of all VTE in Pregnancy
No Thrombophilia	0.0	0.25	0.1	
Factor V Leiden heterozygote	1–15	<0.3	10	40
Factor V Leiden homozygote	<1	1.5	17	2
Prothrombin G20210A heterozygote	2–5	<0.5	>10	17
Prothrombin G20210A homozygote	<1	2.8	>17	0.5
Factor V Leiden/ prothrombin G20210A double heterozygote	0.01	4.7	>20	1–3
Antithrombin deficiency	0.02	3-7	40	1
↓Protein C activity	0.2–0.4	0.1–0.8	4–17	14
↓Protein S free antigen	0.03–0.13	0.1	0–22	3

Source: Reproduced with permission from ACOG Practice Bulletin no. 124. Inherited thrombophilias in pregnancy. *Obstet Gynecol.* 118:730, 2011.

TREATMENT

- Hereditary thrombophilia and thrombophilia:

Clinical Scenario	Antepartum Management
Low-risk thrombophilia[a] without previous VTE	Surveillance without anticoagulation therapy or prophylactic LMWH or UFH
Low-risk thrombophilia[a] with a single previous episode of VTE — not receiving long-term anticoagulation therapy	Prophylactic or intermediate-dose LMWH/UFH or surveillance without anticoagulation therapy
High-risk thrombophilia[b] without previous VTE	Prophylactic LMWH or UFH
High-risk thrombophilia[b] with a single previous episode of VTE — not receiving long-term anticoagulation therapy	Prophylactic, intermediate-dose or adjusted-dose LMWH/UFH regimen

LMWH, low molecular weight heparin, UFH, unfractionated heparin, VTE, venous thromboembolism.
[a] Low-risk thrombophilia: factor V Leiden heterozygous; prothrombin *G20210A* heterozygous; protein C or protein S deficiency.
[b] High-risk thrombophilia: antithrombin deficiency; double heterozygous for prothrombin *G20210A* mutation and factor V Leiden; factor V Leiden homozygous or prothrombin *G20210A* mutation homozygous.
Source: Adapted from ACOG Practice Bulletin #123. Thromboembolism in pregnancy. Obstet Gynecol 118:718, 2011.

Immunologic Factors

Endometriosis

- Although few clinical data support a direct association of endometriosis with RPL (Vercammen and D'Hooghe 2000; Balasch 1988), several underlying pathophysiological features are common to the two conditions (Somigliana 1999).

Autoimmunity (Self-Antigens) or Acquired Thrombophilia

- **Antiphospholipid-Ab syndrome** (APS or Hughes syndrome) is present in approximately 5% of women with RPL; fetal loss more commonly occurs >10 weeks of gestation (Simpson 1998). It is characterized by
  - ↑Antiphospholipid antibodies (Abs) (anticardiolipin- or anti-β2 glycoprotein-immunoglobulins (IgG or IgM)

[Katsuragawa 1997]) or **lupus anticoagulant** with one or more clinical features:

→ RPL, thrombosis, autoimmune thrombocytopenia

o APS is actually composed of two syndromes:

→ Not associated with another illness (*primary APS*)

→ Additional burden of systemic lupus erythematosus or other rheumatic disease (*secondary APS*)

o ⅓ of patients with lupus have antiphospholipid Abs.

o Possible mechanism: uteroplacental thrombosis and vasoconstriction secondary to immunoglobulin binding to platelets and vascular endothelial membrane phospholipids

→ Note: True blood flow through placental vasculature does not occur until 9 to 10 weeks' EGA (Jaffe 1997).

REVISED CLASSIFICATION CRITERIA FOR THE ANTIPHOSPHOLIPID SYNDROME

- Diagnosis:
  o APS if **one** from A and **one** from B:

A: Clinical criteria

1. ≥1 Clinical episode of arterial, venous, or small-vessel **thrombosis**

2. **Pregnancy morbidity:**
   (a) ≥1 SAB morphologically normal fetus ≥10 weeks' EGA, or
   (b) ≥1 Premature birth morphologically normal neonate <34 weeks because of severe preeclampsia or severe placental insufficiency, **or**
   (c) ≥3 SABs <10 weeks' EGA (without maternal anatomic or hormonal abnormalities; no maternal/paternal chromosomal causes)

B: Laboratory criteria (on ≥2 occasions 12 weeks apart)

1. **Lupus anticoagulant**
   (a) Dilute RVVT (Russell's viper venom time) ≥1.2 = prolonged phospholipid-dependent coagulation

2. **Anticardiolipin antibody** >40 GPL or MPL or >99th percentile

3. **Anti-β2 glycoprotein-I antibody** (IgG or IgM) >99th percentile

TREATMENT OF APS

- **Low-molecular-weight heparin (LMWH) may be an effective alternative to unfractionated heparin** (Rai et al. 1997; Greer 2002); initiate along with low dose asprin (81 mg/day)at positive pregnancy test, should stop at 36 weeks and potentially convert to unfractionated heparin to reduce risk of epidural hematoma.
  - Efficacy: Low dose asprin (81 mg/day) and unfractionated heparin (with a positive BhCG) compared to asprin alone led to decreased pregnancy loss by 54% (RR 0.46, 0.29–0.71) (Empson 2002)
- Some experts (Branch 2011) believe that unfractionated heparin therapy is superior to LMWH: head to head comparisons are recommended.

Unfractionated heparin, 5,000 U SC every 12 hours

Enoxaparin (Lovenox), 1 mg/kg/day SC every 12 hours

Dalteparin (Fragmin), 100 IU/kg SC every 12 hours

- Monitoring
  - Consider anti-factor Xa levels: goal = 0.6–1 U/mL 4 hours after injection (LMWH only)
  - Check PLTs monthly
- **Risk of thrombosis presumably highest first 6 weeks postpartum.** Continue anticoagulation through 6–12 weeks postpartum; some recommend long-term anticoagulation.
  - Initiating heparin before conception is potentially dangerous because of the risk of hemorrhage at the time of ovulation.
  - Need close maternal and fetal surveillance secondary to high risk for complications (i.e., preeclampsia, fetal distress, intrauterine growth restriction [IUGR], preterm labor [PTL], and so forth)
  - If surgery planned while on LMWH, stop 18–24 hours before procedure and restart 12 hours postprocedure. If emergent, may try to reverse with **protamine sulfate** (1 mg/100 anti-Xa units of LMWH; though not as effective as with UFH); **slow infusion, no need to reverse if >18 hours from last dose.** For enoxaparin, use *mg/mg*, for dalteparin, *50 mg/5,000 IU.*
- If surgery planned while on UFH, stop 12 hours preprocedure, restart 8–12 hours after the procedure. UFH can be rapidly reversed with protamine sulfate (1 mg protamine sulfate/100 units heparin; not greater than 20 mg/minute and no more than 50 mg over any 10 minute period).

Alloimmunity

- A controversial entity with uncertain diagnosis or history.
- Refers to all causes of recurrent abortion related to an abnormal maternal immune response to antigens on placental or fetal tissues (i.e., T-helper [Th] 1 immunity)
- Progesterone-induced Th1 immunodystrophism: a dichotomous **Th1** (↑) and **Th2** (↓) cytokine profile directed toward trophoblasts (Hill 1995); although an aberrant cytokine profile by peripheral blood mononuclear cells was not seen in RPL patients in a more recent report (Bates 2002).
- Aberrant cytokine profile not detected in peripheral serum
- Treatment: immunosuppressive doses of progesterone vaginal suppositories (200 mg b.i.d., beginning 3 days after ovulation)
- It has been proposed that maternal production of blocking factors may prevent maternal rejection of fetus, and RPL mothers do not make this blocking factor (Sargent 1988):
  - Immunotherapy to stimulate maternal immune tolerance of fetal material is **not effective** (Stephenson 2010).
  - Proposed treatments: IVIg, paternal lymphocyte isoimmunization, glucocorticoid therapy, anticoagulation, humira, intralipid.
  - No datum to demonstrate that any clinical intervention increases implantation rate or reduces the risk of pregnancy loss.
  - Furthermore, agammaglobulinemic women are not at ↑ risk for fetal loss.

Ovarian Reserve Factors

- Prevalence of elevated FSH in women with RPL is the same as for an infertility population (Hofmann 2000).
- Women with **unexplained** RPL have a greater incidence of ↑ day 3 serum FSH than women with a known cause of RPL (Trout 2000).

	Day 3 Follicle-Stimulating Hormone ≥10 mIU/mL (%)
57 Women with ≥3 spontaneous abortions	
36 Unexplained RPL	31
21 Explained RPL	5

RPL, recurrent pregnancy loss.
Source: Adapted from Trout SW, Seifer DB. Do women with unexplained recurrent pregnancy loss have higher day 3 serum FSH and estradiol values? *Fertil Steril.* Aug;74(2):335-7, 2000.

Environmental Factors

- Exposure to nonsteroidal anti-inflammatory drugs and risk of miscarriage (note: small numbers):

Use of NSAIDs	Hazard Ratio (95% confidence interval)
Nonsteroidal anti-inflammatory drug use	**1.8** (1.0–3.2)
First used at time of conception	**5.6** (2.3–13.7)
Duration of use >1 week	**8.1** (2.8–23.4)

Source: Adapted from Li DK, Liu L, Odouli R. Exposure to non-steroidal anti-inflammatory drugs during pregnancy and risk of miscarriage: population based cohort study. *BMJ.* Aug 16;327(7411):368, 2003.

- Folate ≤2.2 ng/mL (≤4.9 nmol/L) associated with ↑ SAB; OR. 1.47; CI, 1.01–2.14 (George 2002)
- Smoking, alcohol (>2 oz/week), and heavy coffee (caffeine) consumption are associated with a slight, but statistically significant, ↑ in absolute risk of recurrent abortion.
  - The ingestion of caffeine may ↑ risk of an SAB among nonsmoking women carrying fetuses with normal karyotypes (Weng 2008, Cnattingius 2000).
  - The half-life of caffeine is halved in smokers and doubled in women taking OCs.

Caffeine/Day (mg)	Spontaneous Abortion Adjusted Hazard Ratio (confidence interval)
<200	1.42 (0.93–2.15)
≥200	2.23 (1.34–3.69)

Quantity	Caffeine (mg)
150 mL coffee	If brewed, 115
	If boiled, 90
	If instant, 60
150 mL tea	If tea bag, 39
	If herbal tea, 0
150 mL soft drink	15
(soda can = 355 mL)	(~36)
1 g chocolate bar	0.3

Note: 150 mL = 5.2 oz.

- Exposure to anesthetic gases, tetrachloroethylene (used in dry cleaning), lead, and mercury is linked to abortion.
- Isotretinoin (Accutane) definitely associated with ↑ incidence of SAB.

HLA Antigens

- Reproductive failure may result from aberrant expression of HLA antigens during any stage of pregnancy (Choudhury 2001).

Sperm DNA Damage

- Increased sperm DNA fragmentation may lead to an increased risk for spontaneous pregnancy loss; options for management include sperm washing and/or testicular sperm extraction (TESE) as the DNA fragmentation is thought to be a post-testicular phenomenon (Zini 2008).

Uteroplacental Microthromboses

- RPL (2 losses) is associated with homozygous polymorphisms in the angiotensin I-converting enzyme (ACE) and plasminogen activator inhibitor-1 (PAI-1) genes although no evidence for efficacy of LMWH as therapy (Buchholz 2003).

DIAGNOSIS

- Possible karyotype of conceptus to help decide if parental karyotyping is worthwhile
- Evaluation begun after 2nd consecutive loss, because (a) the risk of RPL after two successive abortions (30%) is similar to the risk of recurrence among women with ≥3 consecutive abortions (33%) and (b) the prevalence of abnormal results does not differ with 2 or more losses (Jaslow 2010).

History

- Maternal age
- Paternal age >40 has a 1.6 (CI 1.3–2) risk of abortion compared to men aged 25–29.
- Current medical illnesses and medications
- Pattern, timing, and characteristics of prior pregnancy losses
- Exposure to environmental toxins, occupation, recent travel
- Gynecologic and/or obstetric infections
- Previous diagnostic tests
- Family history
  - Cycle regularity
  - Spontaneous pregnancy losses
  - Maternal use of DES
  - Genetic syndromes
  - Thrombotic complications

Physical Examination

- General physical and gynecologic examination

DIAGNOSTIC TESTS

Nocturnal gonadotropin-releasing hormone (GnRH) pulses begin 4 weeks postpartum. Therefore, wait at least 1 month after pregnancy loss before obtaining hormonal serum tests (Liu 1983).

Genetic

- Parental Karyotyping
  - selective karyotyping may be reasonable when an unbalanced abnormality is seen in a conceptus
  - expensive and not always covered by insurance.
- Conceptus Karyotyping
  - aneuploid conceptus indicates a more favorable outcome for subsequent pregnancy.

Anatomic

- **Sonohysterogram, hysterosalpingogram, hysteroscopy, or 3D transvaginal sonography**
  - Intrauterine cavity assessment
  - MRI p.r.n.

Endocrine

- **Luteal phase duration** (positive kit until 1st day of menses):
  - <13 days → LPD
- **Anti-müllerian hormone or day 3 FSH** ovarian reserve testing
- **Thyroid-stimulating hormone (TSH)**
- **PRL**
- Hemoglobin A1c (if suspect insulin resistance or diabetes)

Thrombophilia

Not recommended due to lack of evidence of a causal relationship and lack of evidence of treatment efficacy; see page 345 for exceptions

Immunologic

(Note: Low or unsustained, moderately positive values are clinically meaningless.)

- Russell's viper venom time (RVVT) (**lupus anticoagulant**)
- aCL (**anticardiolipin antibodies, immunoglobulin [Ig] G or IgM**)
- **anti-β-2 glycoprotein-I antibodies, IgG or IgM**

TREATMENT

- Antiphospholipid antibody syndrome and history of RPL: ASA + LMWH or UFH
- Patients with RPL are anxious and desperate to have a "take-home baby." Support and counseling are important.
- Remember, 60–70% of women with unexplained RPL have a successful subsequent pregnancy (Jeng 1995).
- Oocyte donation has been efficacious in treating RPL (Remohi 1996).
- In vitro fertilization (IVF) with preimplantation genetic screening (PGS) may eventually prove to benefit RPL patients although studies to date do not indicate that PGS improves the live birth rate (Fanssen 2011).
  - If, however, the goal is to minimize recurrence of a loss then PGS may be an option while pointing out that the LBR is not necessarily improved.
  - There may be single gene defects present that are not detected by karyotyping; consider offering IVF/ICSI and preimplantation genetic diagnosis; the parents should be referred to genetic counseling/prenatal diagnosis.

RPL (number of prior losses)	Loss Rate with Subsequent Pregnancy				
	20 yo	25 yo	30 yo	35yo	40 yo
2	8%	11%	16%	23%	31%
3	10%	14%	20%	27%	36%
4	12%	18%	24%	32%	42%
5	15%	21%	29%	29%	48%

RPL, recurrent pregnancy loss; yo, years old.
Source: Adapted from Brigham SA, Conlon C, Farquharson RG. A longitudinal study of pregnancy outcome following idiopathic recurrent miscarriage. *Hum Reprod.* Nov;14(11):2868–71, 1999.

- Prognosis for viable birth (derived from >1,000 cases at Brigham and Women's Hospital):

Status	Intervention	Viable Births (%)
Genetic factors	Timed intercourse and supportive care	20–90
Anatomic factors	Surgery and supportive care	60–90
Endocrine factors		
Luteal phase deficiency	Progesterone ± ovulation induction and supportive care	80–90
Hypothyroidism	Thyroid replacement and supportive care	80–90
Hyperprolactinemia	Dopamine agonist	80–90
Infections	Antibiotics and supportive care	70–90
Antiphospholipid syndrome	Aspirin, heparin, and supportive care	70–90
Unknown factors	Timed intercourse and supportive care	60–90

Source: Adapted from Hill JA. *Recurrent Pregnancy Loss: Male and Female Factor, Etiology and Treatment.* Frontiers in Reproductive Endocrinology. Washington, DC: Serono Symposia USA, Inc., 2001.

31

Management of Early Pregnancy Failure

- **Early pregnancy failure (EPF):** broader term describing 1st trimester pregnancy failures; preferred term by many
- Incidence of pregnancy loss:
  - 15–20% of all clinically diagnosed pregnancies
  - Mortality for spontaneous abortions: approximately 0.4 in 100,000 (Creinin 2001)
  - If bleeding occurs before 6 weeks of gestation, there is no increase in adverse pregnancy outcomes; bleeding >7 weeks, even with cardiac activity, indicates a risk for pregnancy loss ~10% as opposed to 5% if there is no bleeding (Jauniaux 2005; Juliano 2008).

DEFINITIONS

Anembryonic pregnancy: Double decidual sign sac without an embryo

Blighted ovum: literally "bad egg"; often used to mean *anembryonic pregnancy* but not currently the preferred terminology

Embryonic demise: demise of an embryo between 4 and 15 mm in length; lack of cardiac activity documented by ultrasound

Fetal demise: demise of a fetus >15 mm in crown-rump length; lack of cardiac activity documented by ultrasound

Incomplete abortion: passage of some but not all fetal or placental tissue <20 weeks gestation

Inevitable abortion: uterine bleeding at gestational age <20 weeks, with cervical dilation but without passage of any fetal or placental tissue

Threatened abortion: uterine bleeding at <20 weeks gestation, without cervical dilation or effacement

> **Missed abortion:** historic terminology describing a nonviable pregnancy (<20 weeks gestation) that has been retained in the uterus without spontaneous passage for at least 8 weeks (terminology evolved before availability of ultrasound; **based on size less than expected by date and no fetal heart tones** via fetoscope)

TREATMENT OPTIONS

Surgical Options

- Historically, surgical intervention was standard management and is the most frequently used.
  - **Sharp curettage:** Higher complication rate with sharp curettage as compared to suction curettage; should be avoided (Foma and Gulmezoglu 2003)
  - **Electric suction curettage**
  - **Manual vacuum aspiration** (see page 361): Handheld suction device that generates suction pressure equivalent to electric suction devices until the syringe is almost full
- **Anesthesia options:** general, regional, or local (paracervical block)
- **Surgical setting:** Operating room or office
- **Complications (1st trimester evacuations):** 0–10% postprocedural infection; 2–3% incomplete evacuation; up to 15% intrauterine adhesions (many are mild adhesions); <1% hemorrhage, uterine perforation, or cervical laceration (Creinin 2001; Friedler 1993)

Expectant Management

- Two studies have suggested that surgical intervention may result in fewer complications (bleeding, infection, etc.) with gestational sac >10 mm (Hurd 1997), but these studies were small and not randomized (Jurkovic 1998).
- Complete expulsion of 1st trimester losses occurs in 25–80% and may be related to the amount of tissue (Nielsen and Hahlin 1995; Chipchase and James 1997).
- Complications: 1–3% infection, 3% hemorrhage
- A decline of ≥ 12% in 2 days is adequate to defer immediate intervention (Chung 2006)

Medical Management *(Note: The following applies to nonviable pregnancies only.)*

- 800 μg vaginal misoprostol for early pregnancy failure has an approximately 84% success rate (Zhang 2005)
- **Vaginal misoprostol** appears to have higher efficacy than oral administration.

Failure to achieve abortion at 24 hours

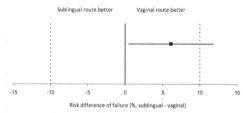

Source: Reproduced with permission from von Hertzen H, Piaggio G, Wojdyla D, et al. Comparison of vaginal and sublingual misoprostol for second trimester abortion: randomized controlled equivalence trial. *Hum Reprod.* Jan;24(1):106-12, 2009.

- Use of misoprostol is an off-label indication.
- Probably faster than expectant management but not as fast as surgical intervention
- No clear consensus on best regimen: misoprostol alone vs. mifepristone and misoprostol
  - Multiple trials using different regimens are published based on completion at 14–21 days.
  - Definition of success differed in many studies (from absence of gestational sac to retained products).
  - Efficacy differs by dose and route of administration (see table below).

Regimen	Success (%)	Comments
Misoprostol, 400–600 μg PO	42–95	Side effects include nausea, vomiting, and diarrhea.
Misoprostol, 400–800 μg per vagina	75–85	**Vaginal administration has fewer side effects and, in randomized trials, had greater efficacy than oral routes.**
Mifepristone 400 mg PO + misoprostol 400–600 μg PO 48 hours later	52–95	Mifepristone has not been consistently shown to increase efficacy.

Source: Adapted from Creinin MD, Schwartz JL, et al. Early pregnancy failure—current management concepts. *Obstet Gynecol Surv* 56(2):105, 2001.

- Reasonable regimen (Bagratee 2004):
  - Document intrauterine pregnancy (IUP)
  - Exclusion criteria:
    → Prostaglandin allergy
    → Cardiac, respiratory, hepatic, renal, or adrenal disease
    → Hypertension (HTN), coagulopathy, deep venous thrombosis (DVT), diabetes

Day 0

Misoprostol, 4 × 200 µg per vagina in recumbent position, then wait 15 minutes.
Doxycycline, 100 mg PO b.i.d. × 5 days (meta-analysis of randomized controlled trials of periabortal antibiotics →↓ 42% risk of infection [Sawaya 1996]).

Day 1

Repeat misoprostol (800 µg) if there is no bleeding.
If it's complete, return in 14 days for hCG.

Day 2

If there is still no bleeding, discuss evacuation of retained products.

Days 3-7

Repeat Ultrasound

hCG, human chorionic gonadotropin.

- Pain medications such as Tylenol No. 3 and nonsteroidal anti-inflammatory drugs (NSAIDs).
- <42 days (6 weeks EGA) from last menstrual period (LMP) → 96% effective; 42–56 days (6–8 weeks EGA) → 86%

Outcome Measures	Misoprostol	Placebo
Overall success	88.5%	44.2%[a]
For early pregnancy failure	86.7%	28.9%[a]
For incomplete miscarriage	100.0%	85.7%
Cumulative success rate over time:		
Day 1	32.7%	5.8%[a]
Day 2	73.1%	13.5%[a]
Day 7	88.5%	44.2%[a]

[a]Statistically significant.
Source: Adapted from Bagratee JS, Khullar V, et al. A randomized controlled trial comparing medical and expectant management of first trimester miscarriage. *Hum Reprod* 19(2):266, 2004.

Office Manual Vacuum Aspiration

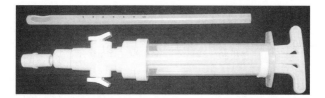

- Conduct a medical history, physical examination, and any indicated laboratory tests.
- 400 μg misoprostol by mouth × 1 the evening before the procedure.
- Oral pain medications, such as 800 mg of ibuprofen
- Bimanual examination to determine the size and position of the uterus
- Place the speculum and cleanse the cervix with an antiseptic.
- If dilatation is needed, administer a paracervical block and apply a tenaculum.
- Dilate the cervix as needed and then gently insert the cannula.
    - Cannula size = gestational age
    - Size of Pratt dilator needed = 3 × cannula size + 1
- Place the cannula through the cervix to just past the internal os, then attach the prepared aspirator to the cannula.
- Release the pinch valve to transfer the vacuum pressure into the uterus.
- Evacuate the uterine contents by rotating and moving the cannula gently back and forth within the uterine cavity.
- Check for signs of completion, including
    - Red or pink foam passing through the cannula
    - Gritty sensation
    - Contraction of the uterus
    - Products of conception are visible
    - Increased cramping
- If patient is Rh negative, administer Rh immune globulin.
- Menses usually returns ~6 weeks after evacuation of spontaneous loss.

How to Administer a Paracervical Block (Modification of Glick Technique)

Use 10–20 CC of Lidocaine or Bupivicaine

Agent	Concen-tration*	Onset (min)	Dura-tion (hr)	Max Dose	Max Dose in 60-kg Adult
Lidocaine	1%	1	0.5–1	4.5mg.kg or 0.45 mL/kg	270 mg or **27 mL**
Lidocaine + Epinephrine	1%	1	2–6	7 mg/kg or 0.7 mL/kg	420 mg or **42 mL**
Bupivicaine	0.25%	5	2–4	2 mg/kg or 0.8 mL/kg	120 mg or **48 mL**
Bupivicaine + Epinephrine	0.25%	5	3–7	3 mg/kg or1.2 mL/kg	180 mg or **72 mL**

*percent (%) = grams/100 mL; % solution x 10 = mg/mL.

- 23-Gauge 1.5-in. needle or a spinal needle facilitates placement.
- Inject 1–2 cc at tenaculum site (usually at 12 or 6 o'clock).
- Place tenaculum.
- Inject lidocaine at junction between the vaginal wall and cervix (5 o'clock on one side and 7 o'clock on the other)

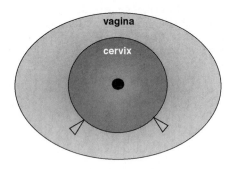

- Always aspirate to avoid intravascular injection (do not inject if blood in aspirate).
- Lack of resistance means that you are not in the uterus, but excessive resistance means that you are too close to the internal os.
- Inject to a depth of 1.0–1.5 in.

Rh Immune Globulin (Jabara 2003)

- Fetal RBCs can express Rh(D) antigen as early as 52 days from the LMP.
- 0.25 mL of fetal blood is needed to cause isoimmunization.
- Standard of care is to give at least **50 µg of Rh immune globulin** IM to all unsensitized women with an early-trimester loss (or ectopic pregnancy).
- There is weak evidence to support this but there is little risk involved.

32

Primary Ovarian Insufficiency/Primary Ovarian Failure

DEFINITION *(Rebar and Connolly 1990)*

- <40 years old
- Follicle stimulating hormone (FSH) > 30 mIU/mL × 2 at least 1 month apart
  - E_2 < 50 pg/mL signifies nonfunctioning follicles
- Amenorrhea ≥4 months*
  *more likely there is > 4 months of disordered menses (amenorrhea, oligomenorrhea, polymenorrhea, metrorrhagia) (Nelson 2009)

- Primary ovarian insufficiency (POI) = hypergonadotropic amenorrhea
- Oocyte physiology: The acme in number of oocytes is reached by 20 weeks of gestation when the number reaches 6 million. By birth, this number is down to 2 million, and approximately 400,000 follicles are present at the onset of puberty. Through the process of apoptosis, no responsive oocytes are found by the time of menopause. The timing of ovarian failure is determined by both the original oocyte quantity and the rate of apoptosis.
- The above dogma has recently been challenged by data indicating the presence of **germ stem cells** in ovaries (White 2012).

INCIDENCE *(Coulam 1986; Luborsky 2003)*

- **1.1%**
  - 0.1% by age 30 years
  - 1.1% by age 40 years
  - 10–28% of those with primary amenorrhea

- o 4–18% of those with secondary amenorrhea
- o 10-15% have an affected first-degree relative.
- FMR1 premutation (Fragile X syndrome)
  - o 2% incidence with isolated spontaneous POI
  - o 14% incidence with familial spontaneous POI
- Autoimmunepolyglandular syndrome comorbidity:
  - o 15% rate of POI with type I (hyperparathyroidism, chronic mucocutaneous candidiasis, Addison disease)
  - o 5% rate of POI with type II (Addison disease, autoimmune thyroid disease, diabetes)

	Primary Amenorrhea*	Secondary Amenorrhea
Karyotypic abnormalities	56%	13%
Y-chromosome present	**10%**	**None**
Symptoms of estradiol deficiency	22%	85%
Progesterone withdrawal bleed	22%	51%
Ovulation after diagnosis	None	24%
Pregnancy after diagnosis	**None**	8%

*Primary amenorrhea may be the presenting feature in ~10% of cases.
Source: Adapted from Rebar RW, Connolly HV. Clinical features of young women with hypergonadotropic amenorrhea. *Fertil Steril* 53(5):804, 1990.

CHARACTERISTICS

- Both groups show diminished bone densities, although ⅔ of women with karyotypically normal POI have a bone mineral density (BMD) one standard deviation below the mean of similar aged women despite having taken standard hormone replacement therapy (Anasti 1998).
- Progesterone withdrawal bleed is a poor screening test unless patient fails to withdraw after initial response.
- Increased incidence of dry eyes (Smith 2004)

ETIOLOGY

Ovarian Follicle Depletion

- Deficient initial follicle number
  - o Pure gonadal dysgenesis
  - o Thymic aplasia/hypoplasia
  - o Idiopathic

- Accelerated follicle atresia
    - X-chromosome related
        - → X mosaics, for example, most common anomaly (45,XO/46,XX; 46,XX/47,XXX)
        - → Turner syndrome
        - → X deletions
    - Galactosemia
    - Iatrogenic (chemotherapy, e.g., cyclophosphamide; radiation treatments ≥600 cGy)
    - Viral agents
    - Autoimmunity
    - Oocyte-specific cell-cycle regulation defect
    - Surgical extirpation (need 40% of one ovary to maintain normal ovulatory function)
    - Idiopathic
    - Fragile X

Ovarian Follicle Dysfunction

- Enzyme deficiencies
    - 17α-Hydroxylase
    - 17–20 Desmolase
    - Cholesterol desmolase
    - Galactose-1-phosphate uridyltransferase

- Autoimmunity
- Lymphocytic oophoritis
    - Gonadotropin receptor–blocking immunoglobulin (Ig) G antibodies
    - Antibodies to gonadotropins
- Signal defects
    - Abnormal gonadotropin
    - Abnormal gonadotropin receptor
    - Abnormal G protein
- Gene mutations: specific inhibin alpha subunit promoter haplotypes may predispose to POI (Harris 2005)
- Iatrogenic
    - previous ovarian surgery
- Idiopathic (resistant ovary syndrome)

DIAGNOSTIC TESTS *(Lieman and Santoro 1997)*

- In 90% of POI the cause remains a mystery
- History and physical
- Karyotype

- o **Y chromosome necessitates** gonadectomy to prevent gonadoblastoma; 50% of **gonadoblastomas** give rise to dysgerminomas.
- o X-chromosome mosaicism accounts for 11% of POI and these women may have cardiac defects similar to XO (Gunther 2004)
- ~14% of women with familial POI will have a premutation in the **fragile X mental retardation 1** (FMR1) gene compared with 2% of women with isolated POI (Wiltenberger 2007). Note: "premutation" signifies 61–200 triplet repeats of cytosine-guanine-guanine and means that the person is usually phenotypically normal. Possible associations include:
  - o Premutation may expand during meiosis and be transmitted in the oocytes; the potential risk for having a child with Fragile X syndrome could be as high as 40%
  - o Increased risk of a late-onset neurodegenerative disorder characterized by tremor and ataxia.
  - o Increased frequency of autism in children with a premutation.
- Progression of deficits (in general): TPA = *t*hyroid, *p*ancreas, *a*drenal

ALL PATIENTS

Karyotype (may identify Turner mosaic that can influence counseling)

FMR1 genetic testing

Thyroid-stimulating hormone (TSH)

Dual-energy x-ray absorptiometry (DXA) scan for bone densitometry

Adrenal antibody test (titer <1:10 is normal)
- If positive adrenocorticotropic hormone (ACTH) stimulation test to confirm diagnosis (**Addison disease**; signs and symptoms: hyperpigmentation of gums and hand skinfolds, loss of pubic/axillary hair): 1 µg cosyntropin IM (cortisol should be >18 µg/dL at 30 or 60 minutes) (Bakalov 2002)

Based on Symptomatology
- **Hemoglobin A1c**
- **Complete blood cell count (CBC)** (pernicious anemia)
- **Ca^{2+}, PO_4** (hypoparathyroidism)

If Signs and Symptoms Warrant

- Total serum protein; albumin/globulin ratio (**IgA deficiency**, if frequent respiratory tract infections)

- Magnetic resonance imaging (MRI) of sella turcica if signs and symptoms of central nervous system (CNS) mass lesion (rule out **pituitary tumor**)
  - 20% of POI associated with hypothyroidism
  - 2.5% associated with diabetes;
  - 4% associated with adrenal cortex autoantibodies* (Bakalov 2005). (If adrenal antibodies is positive, evaluate annually with corticotropin stimulation test.)

TREATMENT

Prepubertal patient: *(ACOG 2011; see page 53 for an alternate regimen)*

- Daily estrogen until break through bleeding occurs (but no longer than 2 years)
  - 25 μg estradiol-17β-transdermal patch
  - 0.3 mg conjugated etrogen orally
  - 0.2–0.5 mg micronized estradiol orally; then add progestin
- Daily progestin:
  - 100 mg/day oral micronized progesterone for 12–14 days every 30–60 days
    Note: Combined hormonal contraception should not be used until puberty has been completed in order to ensure normal breast development.

Postpubertal Patient

- Combined oral contraception if patient has reached Tanner stage 5 breast development
- Estrogen treatment: begin with 0.3 mg Premarin for 1 year or once patient has bleeding, then add progestin; may become pregnant, therefore offer 20 μg ethinyl estradiol oral contraceptive (OC) (Mircette, Alesse) (Taylor 1996).
- Pregnancy may occur in 5-10% of patients with POF (secondary amenorrhea), as there is episodic ovarian function in approximately 50% (as judged by elevated estradiol levels) and approximately 20% of these women will ovulate (as noted by serum progesterone >5 ng/mL).
- Resumption of ovarian function:
  - ~25% of POI patients recovered ovarian function or conceived within 2 years (Bidet 2011)
- Fertility counseling:
  - Adoption
  - Donor egg IVF

- o FSH rebound (Tartagni 2007) using ethinyl-estradiol 0.05 mg 3-times-a-day for 2 weeks to get FSH ≤15 mIU/mL; if FSH <15 ok to undergo controlled ovarian stimulation with Menopur 225 IU daily; continue ethinyl-estradiol administration until day of hCG trigger; need to add luteal phase support:
  - → Follicle development was obtained only in women with a serum FSH ≤15 mIU/mL.
  - → Ovulation rate 32% vs. 0 for control group.
  - → Pregnancy rate 16% vs. 0 for control group.

33

Genetic Testing

There are many genetic screening tests that may be appropriate for couples considering pregnancy. These include: carrier screening, diagnostic testing for male factor (Y chromosome microdeletion) and female factor infertility (Turner syndrome, fragile X syndrome), and testing during pregnancy for high-risk aneuploidies.

CARRIER SCREENING

- Testing to identify individuals/couples at risk to have a child with a genetic disorder.
- Typically ordered based on ethnic background, prior affected child and/or family history.
- Based on results of genetic testing, patients should be offered genetic counseling to discuss their reproductive risks and options.

Autosomal Recessive Inheritance

- Most disorders screened are autosomal recessive. Two carriers of the same disorder have a 25% risk with each pregnancy to have an affected child.

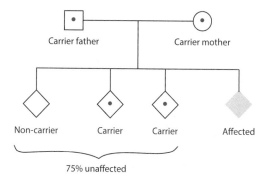

Possible Results of Carrier Screening

- Positive: The individual tested is a carrier.
  - Next step: Test the reproductive partner.
  - Exception: Fragile X syndrome, if a woman is a carrier, her pregnancies are at risk, no need to test her reproductive partner unless clinically indicated.
- Negative: The individual is at reduced risk to be a carrier.
  - There is a small residual risk to be a carrier even after a negative test.
  - No additional testing is recommended.
- Indeterminate/inconclusive
  - Test results may be indeterminate (e.g., Tay-Sachs enzyme).
  - May be due to specimen quality or quantity or failure of test due to other reasons; sample rerun may clarify

Benefits and Limitations of Carrier Screening

- Benefits
  - Identify at-risk couples.
  - Provide reassurance of reduced risk to have an affected child.
- Limitations
  - No test detects 100% of mutations; there is always a residual risk.

Guidelines/Recommendations

The American Congress of Obstetricians and Gynecologists (ACOG), American College of Medical Genetics and Genomics (ACMG), and several national advocacy organizations publish guidelines for carrier screening. Additional testing may be appropriate based on the patient's family history.

Pan Ethnic Carrier Screening

- Involves screening for a panel of common mutations in many disorders, regardless of ethnicity.

- Especially useful for individuals with mixed ethnicity or those unaware of their ethnicity

Disorder (Gene)	Ethnicity	Carrier frequency	Recommendation
Cystic fibrosis (CFTR)	African American	1 in 61	ACOG & ACMG: recommended for **all women of reproductive age**, regardless of ethnic background
	Ashkenazi Jewish	1 in 23	
	Asian	1 in 94	
	Caucasian	1 in 25	
	Hispanic	1 in 58	
Fragile X syndrome (FMR1)	All ethnicities	1 in 178 women	Recommended based on medical and/or family history
Spinal muscular atrophy (SMN1)	African American	1 in 72	ACMG: recommended for **all women of reproductive age**, regardless of ethnic background
	Ashkenazi Jewish	1 in 67	
	Asian	1 in 59	
	Caucasian	1 in 47	
	Hispanic	1 in 68	

- **Cystic fibrosis (CF)**: an **autosomal recessive**, chronic disorder affecting epithelia of the respiratory, gastrointestinal, genitourinary, and hepatobiliary systems. Symptoms include but are not limited to: obstructive lung disease, recurrent lung infection, meconium ileus, pancreatic insufficiency, recurrent pancreatitis, malnutrition, and male infertility. In severe cases, lung transplant may be necessary; pulmonary disease is the major cause of mortality. Average lifespan is into the late 30's.
  - Cystic Fibrosis Transmembrane Conductance Regulator (CFTR) on chromosome 7 encodes a chloride channel in the epithelia.
    - → >1900 known variants reported in CFTR (Cystic Fibrosis Mutation Database http://www.genet.sickkids.on.ca). Not all are pathogenic.
  - Incidence in the United States: ~1/3,700, regardless of gender; varies by ethnic background (see carrier frequencies above) (CDC and Prevention 2004)
  - Genitourinary symptom include male infertility, specifically congenital bilateral absence of the vas deferens (CBAVD), presenting as **obstructive azoospermia** (see Male Subfertility, p. 240).

○ Odds of *CFTR* mutations in a man with CBAVD

% of Men with CBAVD	*CFTR* Mutations on Both Alleles
46%	2
28%	1
26%	0

Source: Adapted from Yu J, Chen Z, Ni Y, Li Z. CFTR mutations in men with congenital bilateral absence of the vas deferens (CBAVD): a systemic review and meta-analysis. *Hum Reprod.* Jan;27(1):25–35, 2012.

- **Carrier screening for CF:** molecular testing. ACOG recommends screening for at least 23 of the most common disease-causing mutations. **Detection of more mutations will increase the detection rates.**
  - **Genotyping-based tests** detect the most common mutations via SNP-based testing; limited to only pre-defined set of known, common mutations.
  - **Sequencing-based tests** detect a greater number of disease-causing mutations, including novel, pathogenic mutations, increasing sensitivity (detection rate). Depending on the application of the technology, it may identify variants of unknown significance.
- Genotype-phenotype correlation
  - Nomenclature:
    → ΔF508: denotes a deletion ("delta") of phenylalanine ("F") at amino acid position 508.
    → c.1521_1523delCTT: denotes a deletion ("del") of nucleotides "CTT" at positions 1521 through 1523 in the cDNA sequence.
    → R117H: denotes an amino acid change from arginine ("R") to histidine ("H") at amino acid position 117.
  - Mutation information
    → Some provide reliable genotype-phenotype correlations for pancreatic function; however, the severity of pulmonary disease is more difficult to predict.
    → Inheritance of any two disease-causing mutations, one from each reproductive partner, can result in cystic fibrosis. It is <u>not</u> necessary to inherit two copies of the same mutation in order to have the disease.

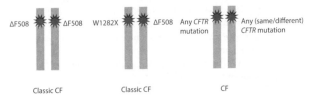

ΔF508 ⚡ ΔF508   W1282X ⚡ ΔF508   Any *CFTR* ⚡ Any (same/different)
                                    mutation   *CFTR* mutation

Classic CF   Classic CF   CF

- ΔF508 is the most common mutation in northern Europeans (75% of all CF mutations); known to cause severe/classic CF
- W1282X accounts for 46% of all CF mutations in Ashkenazi Jews
- If positive for R117H **reflex** tests performed on the same proband looking for poly T tract (5T/7T/9T)
    → R117H is considered a classic disease-causing mutation <u>only</u> when in cis (same chromosome) with the 5T variant AND if there is a CF mutation on the other chromosome.
    → While 5T is known to be associated with CBAVD, other genetic modifiers (e.g., the TG tract in CFTR), make it difficult to predict the exact phenotype.

R117H + 5T in *cis* (same chromosome) **AND** ΔF508 in *trans* (on opposite chromosome)	Classic CF
Other permutations in a MALE fetus:	CBAVD only
R117H + ΔF508 on opposite chromosomes	
R117H + 5T on opposite chromosomes	
R117H + 7T on opposite chromosomes	
5T/5T homozygosity (5T on each chromosome)	

Source: Adapted with permission from: Wenstrom KD, Cystic fibrosis: Prenatal genetic screening. In: UpToDate, Basow DS (Ed), UpToDate, Waltham, MA, 2013. Copyright © 2013 UpToDate, Inc. For more information visit www.uptodate.com.

- **Fragile X syndrome:** most common cause of inherited intellectual disability.
    - Fragile X Mental Retardation 1 (*FMR1*) encodes a protein (FMRP) that is found in many tissues throughout development and abundantly in neurons.
        → Large **expansions of CGG repeats** cause methylation and reduced/no expression of FMRP.
    - X-linked inheritance: Fragile X syndrome is inherited from the mother. CGG repeats may expand when passed through the maternal line (maternal anticipation).

# CGG Repeats	Type of Allele	Presentation in Proband	Risk of Expansion in Next Generation	
< 45	Normal	n/a	n/a	
45–54	Intermediate	n/a	16% to expand to intermediate/premutation	
55–200	Premutation	FXPOI & FXTAS	Increases with premutation size[a]	
			55–59	very low*
			60–69	2%
			70–79	32%
			80–89	74%
			90–99	94%
			100–200	98%
>200	**Full Mutation**	**Fragile X syndrome**	**~100%**	

[a]Nolin et al., 2011.
*There have been occasional reports of expansion from 56 and 59 repeats to full mutations in one generation (Fernandez-Carvajal 2009).

- → AGG interruptions
  - In 45–69 length CGG repeats, the presence of AGG interruptions may decrease the risk of expansion in offspring (Nolin 2013).
- o Full mutations (>200 CGG repeats) cause fragile X syndrome. Symptoms include but not limited to:
  - → Developmental: delayed motor/verbal milestones, intellectual disability.
  - → Behavioral: autistic-like behaviors, hyperactivity, anxiety, and autism.
  - → Physical: long face, prominent forehead and jaw, large ears, macroorchidism, joint hyperextensibility, mitral valve prolapse, and smooth skin.
  - → Incidence
    - ■ Males: 1 in 4,000 to 6,250 (de Vries 1997)
    - ■ Women with a full mutation can be asymptomatic, mildly affected, or have fragile X syndrome. The prevalence of females with fragile X syndrome is presumed to be approximately one half the male prevalence.

- Premutation (55–200 CGG repeats) carriers:
  → Fragile X-associated Premature Ovarian Insufficiency (FXPOI).
    - 21% of premutation carriers develop POI (Sherman 2005).
  → Fragile X-associated Tremor Ataxia Syndrome (FXTAS).
    - Late-onset, progressive ataxia and intention tremor; includes memory loss, muscle weakness, and autonomic dysfunction
    - 8–16% risk in females (Saul 2012).
    - Up to 45% risk in males (Saul 2012).
- Intermediate (45–54 CGG repeats) carriers:
  → Clinically asymptomatic; not at risk for FXPOI or FXTAS.
  → 16% risk for expansion to intermediate/premutation, depending on repeat size.
    - Unlikely to expand to a full mutation in one generation (Saul 2012)
- **Carrier screening for fragile X:** triplet repeat analysis with Southern blot for confirmation.
  → Recommended for individuals with a personal or family history of premature ovarian insufficiency (POI), diminished ovarian reserve, unexplained intellectual disability, unexplained autism, or fragile X syndrome.

- **Spinal muscular atrophy (SMA):** autosomal recessive neuromuscular disorder characterized by degeneration of anterior horn cells (lower motor neurons), resulting in progressive muscle weakness; the bulbospinal variety of SMA is a triplet repeat (CAG) expansion disorder of the androgen receptor gene on the X chromosome.
  - Survival Motor Neuron 1 (*SMN1*) encodes a protein involved in small nuclear ribonuclear protein (snRNP) biogenesis and function.
    → *SMN2*, directly adjacent to *SMN1*, differs by eight nucleotides. Also encodes SMN protein, at reduced levels compared to *SMN1*. *SMN1* is the disease-causing gene. Increased copy number of *SMN2* can decrease severity of SMA.
  - Incidence 1/10,000, regardless of gender. Varies by ethnic background, see carrier frequencies above.
  - Symptoms and severity vary by age of onset, however intellect and appearance are not affected.

Types of SMA

Classification	% of Cases	Onset	Clinical Presentation
SMA type 1 Werdnig-Hoffman	60%[a]	< 6 months	Symmetric hypotonia; lack of motor development; unable to sit unsupported; difficulty sucking, swallowing, and breathing; death by age 2
SMA type 2 Dubowitz disease	27%[a]	6–12 months	Slow attainment of motor milestones, can sit unsupported, loss of skills with time, majority live into 20s
SMA type 3 Kugelberg-Welander	rare	>12 months	Independent walking, frequent falls, lose walking in teens or 30s, poor weight gain, sleep problems, scoliosis, normal life expectancy
SMA type 4	rare	Adult onset	Muscle weakness develops in teens or 20s, poor weight gain, sleep problems, scoliosis, normal life expectancy

[a]Ogino 2004

- o 95–98% of disease is caused by a deletion in *SMN1*.
  - → 2–5% of affected individuals are compound heterozygotes.
  - → Carrier screening looks at exon 7 of *SMN1* to determine gene copy number.
- o Limitations of carrier screening specific to SMA:
  - → ~6% of parents of an affected child will have a negative carrier screen.
    - *De novo* mutations: Approximately 2% of affected individuals are born to a non-carrier parent. *De novo* mutations are typically paternal in origin (Wirth 1997; Smith 2007).
    - While most individuals have one copy of *SMN1* on each chromosome, about 4% of people have two copies of *SMN1* on one chromosome (Ogino 2004)
      - ❖ "2+0" silent carrier: normal carrier screening results because the carrier screen identifies 2 copies of the *SMN1* gene. However, this person is at risk for passing on the chromosome with no copies of the *SMN1* gene and is therefore at risk for having an affected child.

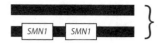

Two Copies of *SMN1*
Normal carrier screening result
• increased risk to have an affected child

❖ 3 copies: reduced residual risk

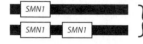

Three Copies of *SMN1*
Normal carrier screening result
• very reduced risk to have an affected child

- o **Routine carrier screening for SMA:** copy number analysis of *SMN1*.
  - → Copy number of *SMN1* (determined by the copy number of exon 7) is done by a PCR-based assay, such as multiplex ligation-dependent probe amplification (MLPA).

Ethnic-Specific Carrier Screening

Disorders typically recommended based on a patient's ethnic background. Disorders may occur outside of high-risk ethnicities.

Ethnic Background	Disorder	Carrier Frequency
African American	Alpha thalassemia	1 in 30
	Beta thalassemia	1 in 75
	Sickle cell disease	1 in 10
Ashkenazi Jewish	Ashkenazi Jewish panel*	1 in 5
Asian	Alpha thalassemia	1 in 20
	Beta thalassemia	1 in 50
Cajun	Tay-Sachs disease	Increased
French Canadian	Tay-Sachs disease	1 in 251
Irish	Tay-Sachs disease	1 in 522, 3
Hispanic	Alpha thalassemia	Variable
	Beta thalassemia	1 in 32–75
	Sickle cell	1 in 30–200
Mediterranean	Alpha thalassemia	1 in 30–50
	Beta thalassemia	1 in 20–30
	Sickle cell disease	1 in 30–50
Middle Eastern	Alpha thalassemia	Variable
	Beta thalassemia	1 in 50
	Sickle cell disease	1 in 50–100
Sephardic Jewish	Alpha thalassemia	1 in 4–100
	Beta thalassemia	1 in 5–7
	Sephardic Jewish panel**	Increased

[1]Andermann 1977. [2]Van Bael 1996 [3]Branda 2004

- **Ashkenazi Jewish disorders:** recommended for Jewish individuals from Eastern Europe. Disorders range in severity and symptoms; however, all can have a serious impact on quality of life and life expectancy. May occur outside the Ashkenazi Jewish population at a reduced frequency. The 1-in-5-carrier frequency is based on the full extended screening panel.
- **Sephardic Jewish disorders:** recommended for Jewish individuals from Spain, Portugal, the Middle East, or North Africa. Disorders range in severity and symptoms; however, all can have a serious impact on quality of life and life expectancy. May occur outside the Sephardic Jewish population at a reduced frequency.
  - Disorders at increased frequency (not all appropriate for routine carrier screening) include: alpha-thalassemia, ataxia telangiectasia, beta-thalassemia, corticosterone methyloxidase type II deficiency, Costeff optical atrophy, cystic fibrosis, hereditary inclusion body myopathy, familial Mediterranean fever, glucose-6-phosphate-dehydrogenase (G6PD) deficiency, limb girdle muscular dystrophy, metachromatic leukodystrophy, polyglandular syndrome, pseudocholinesterase deficiency, spinal muscular atrophy, Wolman syndrome.

Ashkenazi Jewish Disorders

Disorder	Gene	Ashkenazi Jewish Carrier Frequency
Bloom's syndrome[2, 3]	BLM	1 in 134
Canavan disease[1, 2, 3]	ASPA	1 in 55
Cystic fibrosis[1, 2, 3]	CFTR	1 in 23
Dihydrolipoamide Dehydrogenase Deficiency[3]	DLD	1 in 107
Familial dysautonomia[1, 2, 3]	IKBKAP	1 in 31
Familial hyperinsulinism[3]	ABCC8	1 in 68
Fanconi anemia C[2, 3]	FANCC	1 in 100
Gaucher disease[2, 3]	GBA	1 in 15
Glycogen storage disease type 1a[3]	G6PC	1 in 64
Joubert syndrome type 2[3]	TMEM216	1 in 92
Maple syrup urine disease A/B[3]	BCKDHB/A	1 in 97
Mucolipidosis type IV[2, 3]	MCOLN1	1 in 89

(Continues on next page)

(Continued from previous page)

Disorder	Gene	Ashkenazi Jewish Carrier Frequency
Nemaline myopathy[c]	NEB	1 in 168
Niemann-Pick disease type A/B[b, c]	SMPD1	1 in 115
Spinal muscular atrophy[b, c]	SMN1	1 in 67
Tay-Sachs disease[a, b, c]	HEXA	1 in 27
Usher syndrome type 1F[c]	PCDH15	1 in 147
Usher syndrome type III[c]	CLRN1	1 in 120
Walker-Warburg syndrome[c]	FKTN	1 in 150

[a]ACOG recommended disorder.
[b]ACMG recommended disorder.
[c]Jewish advocacy organization recommended disorder.

- **Hemoglobinopathies:** inherited disorders that affect the quantity or quality of hemoglobin. Severe disease may result in transfusion dependency. **Carrier screening for hemoglobinopathies can be done with a complete blood count (CBC) with ferritin and a hemoglobin electrophoresis with quantitative A2.**

Alpha-Thalassemia

- Caused by mutations in the alpha-globin genes (*HBA1* & *HBA2*).
- **Molecular testing, typically deletion/duplication analysis of *HBA1* and *HBA2*, may be appropriate for the partner of an alpha-thalassemia trait carrier.**
- Severity depends on number of working alpha-globin genes.
  - Silent carrier (–α/αα) one mutation; asymptomatic. Normal MCV/MCH. Only detected by molecular analysis.
  - Alpha-trait (–α/–α) or (––/αα) two mutations; mild anemia. Low MCV/MCH.
  - Carriers of mutations in *trans* (–α/–α) are more common in African American and Mediterranean populations. They are not at risk for having a child with Hb Barts hydrops fetalis.
  - Carriers of mutations in *cis* (––/αα) are more common in Southeast Asian populations and are at risk for Hb Barts hydrops fetalis.

- Hemoglobin H disease (- -/-α) three mutations: moderate anemia. Symptoms include splenomegaly, increased risk of infection, pregnancy complications. Low MCV/MCH.
- Hb Barts Fetalis (- -/- -) four mutations: not compatible with life. Maternal complications with an affected pregnancy.

Beta-Thalassemia

- Caused by mutations in the beta-globin gene (*HBB*).
- **Carriers typically have a low mean corpuscular volume (MCV) on CBC and elevated hemoglobin A2 on electrophoresis.**
  - Partners of beta-thalassemia carriers should be screened for beta-thalassemia and sickle cell disease; heterozygous beta-thalassemia and sickle cell mutations cause sickle-beta-thalassemia, which could be clinically severe.
- Severity ranges from mild to severe, depending on residual beta-globin production.
  - Symptoms may include: poor growth, skeletal abnormalities, risk for infection, and shortened lifespan.

Sickle Cell Disease

- Caused by mutations in the beta-globin gene (*HBB*).
- **Carriers have an abnormal (HbS) peak on hemoglobin electrophoresis. Molecular testing can identify the causative mutation, a point mutation changing the sixth amino acid, glutamic acid, to valine (Glu6Val).**
  - Partners of sickle cell carriers should be screened for beta-thalassemia and sickle cell disease; heterozygous beta-thalassemia and sickle cell mutations cause sickle-beta-thalassemia, which could be clinically severe.
- Sickle-shaped red blood cells clog arteries causing vaso-occlusive events, which can result in pain, stroke, cardiomyopathy, bone and joint complications, etc.
- Symptoms may be exacerbated by dehydration, alcohol consumption, high altitudes, extreme temperatures, and stress.
  - Sickle cell disease carriers may become symptomatic under these conditions.

GENETIC CAUSES OF INFERTILITY

There are many causes of infertility including genetic, environmental, a combination of both, and idiopathic. The genetic risks differ based on male or female factor, and the physiological cause of infertility (CBAVD, POI, etc).

<u>Male factor:</u> 19–24% of men with azoospermia or severe oligo-zoospermia ($<5 \times 106/mL$) have some genetic abnormality (Dohle 2002; Ghorbel 2012).

- *CFTR* / Congenital Bilateral Absence of the Vas Deferns (CBAVD).
    - 10–15% of men with obstructive azoospermia have *CFTR* mutations.
- Y chromosome microdeletion (YCMd).
    - Most common genetic cause of male infertility due to spermatogenic failure. Important to delineate before testicular sperm aspiration (TESA) or intracytoplasmic sperm injection (ICSI) (Foresta 2001; McElreavey 2000; Stahl 2012).
    - YCMd are too small to be detected on a karyotype but can be identified with molecular techniques (i.e., azo-ospermic factor c (AZFc) deletion).

YCMd Incidence Based on Subgroup (*Ghorbel 2012*)

Type of Infertility	YCMd Incidence	AZFc Deletion
Severe oligospermia	7–10%	6%
Non-obstructive azoospermia	10–15%	13%

- Most deletions occur on the long arm of the Y chromo-some (Yq11) in the azoospermic factor (*AZF*) region.
    - → Nonoverlapping segments in *AZF* region: *AZFa*, *AZFb*, and *AZFc*; these contain multiple genes important for spermatogenesis;
    - → **DAZ** (deleted in azoospermia) is in *AZFc*.
    - → Distribution of frequencies for *AZF* deletions:
- Phenotype defined on the basis of semen analysis and testis histology:

Type of AZF Microdeletion for Men with YCMd

	YCMd Incidence
AZFa	5%
AZFb	10–16%
AZFc	60%
2–3 deletions	14%
Not involving a, b, or c	5%

→ *AZFa–c* deletions →**absent spermatozoa**
→ *AZFa* deletions: poor prognosis for sperm retrieval
→ *AZFb* deletions: poor prognosis for sperm retrieval
→ *AZFc* deletions: may have sperm in ejaculate with severe oligozoospermia; others may be azoospermic but produce sufficient numbers to allow sperm recovery from testicular biopsy.

o Y microdeletions currently not associated with other health problems, although limited information is available regarding phenotypes of sons of affected males.

→ Males with Y microdeletion may be at higher risk for 45,X/46,XY offspring due to instability of the deleted Y chromosome (see page 387) (Siffroi 2000).

- Chromosome abnormalities
  o 7% of infertile males have a karyotypic abnormality (McLachlan 2010).
  o Klinefelter's Syndrome
    → 47,XXY or 46,XY/47,XXY (mosaic) accounts for 2/3 of chromosome abnormalities in infertile males.
    → Reduced testicular size, need for testosterone supplementation, risk of infertility and gynecomastia.
    → Excess of 24XX/24XY sperm; if sperm are aspirated for IVF, increased risk for chromosome abnormalities in offspring. PGS may reduce this risk.
  o Other chromosomal abnormalities
    → ~4% of couples with recurrent pregnancy loss (RPL) have a chromosome abnormality, most commonly a translocation.
      ■ Can be Robertsonian or reciprocal; both increase risk for chromosome abnormalities in the fetus.
    → Other chromosome problems (e.g., inversions) can lead to infertility / RPL
  o Karyotyping is appropriate for:
    → A couple after two miscarriages.
    → Males with severe oligozoospermia.
- Other genetic and non-genetic factors may contribute to male infertility. Consider testing based on physiological cause of infertility and/or additional findings.

Female Factor

- Fragile X Syndrome
  o Testing is appropriate for a woman with low AMH or high FSH, especially if she has a family history of early menopause, fragile X syndrome or unexplained mental retardation in the family.

- ○ Fragile X associated Premature Ovarian Insufficiency (FXPOI)
  - → Premutation carriers at 21% risk of FXPOI
  - → ~4–6% of idiopathic POI may be due to fragile X syndrome premutations. (Sullivan 2011)
- Chromosomal abnormalities

CGG Repeats	Odds Ratio for POI
59–79	6.9
80–99	25.1
>100	16.4

Source: Adapted from Sherman S, Pletcher BA, Driscoll DA. Fragile X syndrome: Diagnostic and carrier testing. *Genet Med.* 7(8): 584–587, 2005.

- ○ Turner syndrome (45,XO) or mosaic Turner syndrome (46,XX/45,XO)
  - → Women with Turner syndrome (45,XO) have ovarian dysgenesis that rarely produce eggs. They can carry a pregnancy so egg or embryo donation is an option. Thorough prenatal screening is obligatory (i.e., pre-conceptional cardiac evaluation).
  - → Mosaic Turner syndrome may or may not cause fertility issues, however there may be an increased risk for chromosome abnormalities.
    - Risk depends on degree of mosaicism, specifically in gonads. Has been reported up to 15.9% risk for chromosome abnormalities (Sybert 2002).
- ○ Other chromosomal abnormalities
  - → ~4% of couples with recurrent pregnancy loss (RPL) have a chromosome abnormality, most commonly a translocation.
    - Can be Robertsonian or reciprocal; both increase risk for chromosome abnormalities in the fetus.
  - → Other chromosome problems (e.g., inversions) can lead to infertility / RPL.
- ○ Karyotyping is appropriate for:
  - → A couple after two miscarriages.
  - → A woman with infertility and short stature.
- Other genetic and non-genetic factors may contribute to female infertility. Consider testing based on physiological cause of infertility and/or additional findings.

CHROMOSOME ABNORMALITIES IN THE FETUS

The vast majority of aneuploidies are due to errors in chromosome segregation at the first meiotic division in the oocyte (thus, they are maternal in origin).

- Incidence of chromosome abnormalities
  - Miscarriages / SAB
    → 60–70% of all 1st trimester spontaneous abortions.
    → 6–11% of all stillbirths.
  - During pregnancy

Incidence of Chromosome Abnormalities, by Maternal Age

Maternal Age at Delivery	Risk of Trisomy 21		Risk of Any Chromosome Abnormality	
	2nd Trimester	At Birth	2nd Trimester	At Birth
25	1 in 906	1 in 1250	-	1 in 476
30	1 in 610	1 in 840	-	1 in 385
35	1 in 256	1 in 356	1 in 141	1 in 179
40	1 in 75	1 in 94	1 in 44	1 in 63
45	1 in 22	1 in 24	1 in 14	1 in 19

Note: Does not include mosaicism, translocations, or marker chromosomes.
Source: Greenwood Genetics Center Counseling Aid.

→ The recurrence risk of a chromosomal trisomy in a subsequent pregnancy is increased (de Souza 2009)

Previous Trisomy (T)	Risk of Same Trisomy	Risk of Other Viable Trisomy
T13	0.5%	0.8%
T18	0.3%	0.7%
T21 (<30 years)	0.7%	0.3%
T21 (30–34 years)	0.5%	0.8%
T21 (35–39 years)	1.8%	0.8%
T21 (40+ years)	4.2%	0.8%

- Sex chromosome abnormalities
  - Incidence: 1 in 400 (Nielson 1990).
    → 2.5% recurrence risk after previous sex chromosome aneuploidy (Warburton 2005).
    → No increased recurrence risk after 47,XYY or 45,XO.

Features of Common Chromosome Abnormalities

Trisomy 21 Down syndrome	Incidence: 1/650 to 1,000 live births (exact risk depends on maternal age; see table above)
	Clinical presentation: Short, broad hands with single palmar crease, decreased muscle tone, mental retardation, broad head with characteristic features, open mouth with large tongue, up-slanting eyes.
Trisomy 13	Incidence: 1/10,000
	Clinical presentation: Multiple congenital malformations of many organs, low-set malformed ears, receding mandible, small eyes, mouth and nose with general elfin appearance, severe mental deficiency, congenital heart defects, horseshoe or double kidney, short sternum, posterior heel prominence. Typically results in fetal loss or early neonatal death.
Trisomy 18	Incidence: 1/3,000 to 8,000
	Clinical presentation: Severe mental deficiency, failure to thrive, cardiac anomalies, hypertonia, clenched fists, "rocker-bottom feet" with prominent heel bone, prominent occiput, micrognathia, low-set malformed ears, short palpebral fissures. Typically results in fetal loss or early neonatal death.
47,XXY Klinefelter syndrome	Incidence: 1/500 to 1,000 newborn males
	Clinical presentation: normal pregnancy, birth, childhood. Reduced testicular size, need for testosterone supplementation beginning in adolescence and through adulthood. Risk of infertility and gynecomastia. Risk of learning disabilities (reading), expressive language deficits, 50% have dyslexia
47,XXX Trisomy X	Incidence: 1/1,000 newborn females
	Clinical presentation: increased risk for early menopause and poor ovarian function. Risk of learning disability, hyperactivity, depression, and variable menses.

(Continues on next page)

(Continued from previous page)

45,XO Turner syndrome	Incidence: 1/1,500 to 2,500 newborn females
	Clinical presentation: Pre/neonatal: lymphedema, risk for cardiac malformations, webbed neck, kidney malformations. Short stature, ovarian dysgenesis, hormone supplementation needed in adolescence. Additional risks include: otitis media, hypertension, diabetes, thyroid disease, learning disabilities, depression. Risk of pregnancy: increased maternal cardiovascular mortality in women with XO. If there is a documented cardiac abnormality, pregnancy is an **absolute contraindication**; if no documented cardiac abnormality, pregnancy is a **relative contraindication**.
47,XYY	Incidence: 1/10,00 newborn males
	Clinical presentation: appearance typically unaffected; most males have normal sexual development and are able to father children. Increased risk of learning disability, speech delay, hyperactivity.
Triploidy 69, XXY/69, XYY /69,XXX	Incidence: 1–3% of recognized conceptions; 1/10,000 livebirths
	Clinical presentation: Typically results in early fetal loss; clinical presentation depends on diandric or digynic origin. If liveborn, high risk of ambiguous genitalia, rapid demise and neonatal death.
Translocations: Exchange of segments of DNA between two chromosomes.	Reciprocal translocations: 1/600 newborns.
	Non-homologous chromosomes exchange material and the total chromosome number remains the same. If balanced, can be phenotypically normal; however, increased risk of infertility, RPL, and chromosome abnormalities in the fetus.
	Robertsonian translocations
	Two acrocentric chromosomes fuse, resulting in loss of the short arms. Results in balanced karyotype with 45 chromosomes. Most common is 13q14q, with frequency of 1/1,300 people. Increased risk of infertility, RPL, and chromosome abnormalities in the fetus.

TESTING

- Chromosome aberrations (e.g., aneuploidy, translocations, large deletions/duplications)
  - Detected by karyotype and/or chromosome microarray analysis.
- Microdeletions (e.g., Y chromosome microdeletions)
  - Detected by PCR and/or microarray analysis.
- Small mutations (i.e., single gene disorders such as cystic fibrosis)
  - Detected by DNA analysis methods such as genotyping and sequencing.
    - → Genotyping can cost-effectively detect the most common disease-causing mutations in a gene.
    - → Sequencing provides increased detection rates by detecting any disease-causing mutation within a gene (with the exception of large deletions/duplications), however traditional applications of sequencing also detect variants of unknown significance (VUS).

REPRODUCTIVE OPTIONS

Preconception

- Preimplantation Genetic Diagnosis (PGD)
  - Allows for genetic testing to be performed on a cell or cells from a developing embryo created through IVF.
  - Biopsy/testing can take place at various stages of development: polar bodies, blastomeres and blastocysts can be biopsied and analyzed; current trends appear to favor trophectoderm biopsy of 5–10 cells per embryo (Forman 2013)
  - Healthy embryos, free of the tested disorder are selectively transferred.
  - **Can be performed for all single gene disorders as long as the DNA mutations are known.** Can also test embryos for HLA matching, chromosome rearrangements, aneuploidy screening. Testing for multiple indications is often possible.
  - Limitations
    - → Not 100% accurate and prenatal testing is still recommended.
    - → Biopsy is an invasive procedure that can damage embryos.
- Gamete / embryo donation
  - Using gametes from a donor reduces the risk of passing on a genetic disorder. This is an option for dominant, X-linked and recessive genetic disorders.

- For recessive disorders, the donor would need to undergo screening for the disorders prior to undergoing treatment.
- Egg donation can decrease the likelihood of aneuploidy due to age-related risks.
- Limitations
  - → Donation reduces the risk but does not guarantee an embryo/pregnancy free of genetic disorders or birth defects.

During Pregnancy

- **Non-Invasive Prenatal Testing** (NIPT)
  - Detects common aneuploidies (i.e., trisomies 13, 18, 21) by sequence analysis of cell-free fetal DNA in maternal serum.
  - Performed as early as **10 weeks gestation**.
  - Limitations: positive screens currently require follow-up with diagnostic test (CVS or amniocentesis); cannot detect open neural tube defects (e.g., spina bifida)
- **Maternal serum screening** (MSS)
  - Screens for common aneuploidies by analysis of pregnancy analytes in maternal serum. May include fetal features observed on ultrasound (nuchal translucency, nasal bone).
  - Performed from **10 to 18 weeks of pregnancy**.
  - 85–96% detection rates, for combined first/second trimester assessments (ACOG 2007).
  - Limitations: high false-positive rate; positive screens require follow-up with diagnostic test (CVS or amniocentesis).
- **Chorionic Villus Sampling** (CVS)
  - Detects chromosome abnormalities or single gene disorders by analysis of fetal cells from placental tissue.
  - Performed between **10–12 weeks of gestational age**.
  - Risk of complication, including pregnancy loss: 1/1,000 (Caughey 2006).
  - Risk of placental mosaicism: 1/100 (1%).
- **Amniocentesis**
  - Detects chromosome abnormalities or single gene disorders by analysis of fetal cells from amniotic fluid.
  - Performed between **15–20 weeks of gestation**; may be done later with increased risk of preterm labor.
  - Risk of complication, including pregnancy loss: < 1/1,000 (<0.1%) (Eddleman 2006).

Other Options

- Testing after birth
  - Newborn screening can detect children with cystic fibrosis and numerous other genetic disorders. Screening panels vary by state.
    (see http://www.cdc.gov/newbornscreening/)
  - Symptomatic testing, once a child has symptoms of a disorder.
- Adoption
  - Can reduce the risk of having a child with a genetic disorder when reproductive partners are known carriers.

34

Androgen Replacement Therapy

ANDROGENS

- The majority of androgens are synthesized by the adrenal glands and ovaries:
  - Pro-hormones: A, androstenedione; DHEA, dehydroepiandrosterone; DHEA-S, dehydroepiandrosterone sulfate
  - Potent androgens: T, testosterone and the non-aromatizable dihydrotestosterone (DHT)

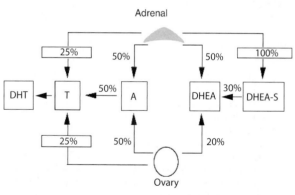

Adrenal

Ovary

Source: Adapted from Fritz MA, Speroff L. Normal and Abnormal Growth and Pubertal Development. In: *Clinical Gynecologic Endocrinology and Infertility*. 8th ed. Philadelphia: Lippincott Williams & Wilkins, 2011.

- Relative binding affinity of hormones to sex hormone–binding globulin (SHBG): DHT > testosterone (T) > androstenedione (A) > estradiol (E$_2$) > estrone (E$_1$) (Dunn 1981). Only free (i.e., unbound to SHBG) hormones are biologically active. Insulin and androgens decrease SHBG production, whereas estrogens, thyroxine, and growth hormone increase SHBG production. Conditions with low SHBG include polycystic ovary syndrome, diabetes, and hypothyroidism. Conditions with high SHBG include pregnancy and hyperthyroidism.

	Relative Potency
Dihydrotestosterone	300
Testosterone	100
Androstenedione	10
Dehydroepiandrosterone sulfate	5

- Controversies: Does androgen-supplementation improve libido or sexual function and, if so, in which women (i.e., premenopausal, postmenopausal, status post bilateral oophorectomy)? Effects of androgens on energy level, muscle mass and strength, and bone mineral density (BMD)/ fracture risks are also being studied.
- Androgen levels decline by 50% from ages 18 to 54, and decline more slowly throughout later life (↓ production from both the ovaries and adrenal glands). This progressive decline in androgen production occurs independent of the menopausal transition but appears to be exacerbated by oophorectomy in pre- and postmenopausal women, suggesting that the postmenopausal ovary could produce androgens even decades beyond menopause (this is controversial, see the following) (Davison 2005).

- Alterations in testosterone levels from premenopausal to postmenopausal (natural/surgical):

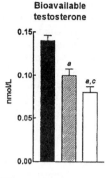

Bioavailable testosterone

■ Intact
▨ Hysterectomy with ovarian conservation
□ Hysterectomy with bilateral oophorectomy

Source: Adapted from Laughlin GA, Barrett- Connor E, et al. Hysterectomy, oophorectomy, and endogenous sex hormone levels in older women: the Rancho Bernardo Study. *J Clin Endocrinol Metab* 85[2]:645, 2000.)

	↓ **Testosterone (%)**	**Testosterone (µg/day)**
Pre-MP	—	250
Natural MP	28	180
Surgical MP	50	125

MP, menopausal.
Source: Adapted from Snyder PJ. The role of androgens in women. *J Clin Endocrinol Metab* 86(3):1006, 2001.

	Testosterone (µg/ day) % ↓	**Androstenedione % ↓**
Pre-MP ovariectomy	50	50
Natural MP	28	50
Post-MP ovariectomy	50	50

MP, menopausal.
Source: Adapted from Snyder PJ. The role of androgens in women. *J Clin Endocrinol Metab* 86(3):1006, 2001.

- In premenopausal women, oophorectomy results in equal decline in T and A (50%), suggesting that these two androgens come equally from the ovaries and adrenal glands in premenopausal women.
- In postmenopausal women, the T concentration drops more after oophorectomy (50%) compared with natural menopause with ovaries intact. Therefore, the secretion

of T may be maintained in the menopausal ovary of some women.

- In two studies examining the relation of remote hysterectomy ± oophorectomy to endogenous sex hormone levels in older women, bilateral salpingo-oophorectomy had no effect on circulating estradiol (E_2) levels but was associated with a substantial and sustained reduction in bioavailable T levels (as was hysterectomy alone!). Although T levels were low around the time of menopause, an apparent slight ↑ in ovarian T production and a return to perimenopausal levels occurred in women with intact ovaries in their seventh and eighth decades of life (Laughlin 2000; Davison 2005). These data argue for some measure of ovarian androgen production from the postmenopausal ovary.

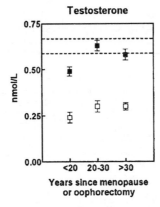

Testosterone

Body mass index–adjusted mean (± standard error) testosterone levels in 438 intact women (closed squares) and 123 bilateral salpingooophorectomy women (open squares) stratified by years since menopause for intact women and years since surgery. Dotted lines indicate the mean (± standard error) testosterone level for premenopausal women. (Source: Reproduced from Laughlin GA, Barrett-Connor E, et al. Hysterectomy, oophorectomy, and endogenous sex hormone levels in older women: the Rancho Bernardo Study. *J Clin Endocrinol Metab* 85[2]:645, 2000.)

- Controversy: does the postmenopausal ovary generate clinically meaningful concentrations of androgens?
  - Evidence in favor of postmenopausal androgen production from the ovary:
    → Oophorectomy reduces androgen levels in postmenopausal women (Laughlin 2000; Davison 2005).
  - Evidence against postmenopausal androgen production from the ovary:
    → Free androgen levels remain at the limit of detection in postmenopausal women, regardless of whether they retain or lack ovaries. The significance of

statistically significant changes in what amounts to exceedingly low free androgen levels before and after oophorectomy remains to be established in post-menopausal women.

→ In the absence of adrenal function, postmenopausal women have no circulating androgens. Homogenized postmenopausal ovaries lack T, androstenedione (A), detectable levels of most steroidogenic enzymes, follicle-stimulating hormone (FSH) receptors, and luteinizing hormone (LH) receptors (Couzinet 2001; Jabara 2003).

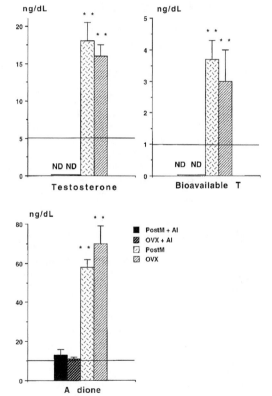

A dione, androstenedione; AI, adrenal insufficiency; PostM, postmenopausal; ND, no difference; OVX, ovariectomized women; T, testosterone. (Source: Reproduced with permission from Couzinet B, Meduri G, Lecce MG, et al. The postmenopausal ovary is not a major androgen-producing gland. *J Clin Endocrinol Metab* 86[10]:5060, 2001.)

- Oophorectomy may reduce adrenal androgen production via uncertain mechanisms, arguing for a principally adrenal source of androgens in postmenopausal women (Davison 2005).

FOR DECREASED LIBIDO: TREAT WITH ESTRADIOL FIRST

- Offer E_2 first: 90% reported a return of desire after 3–6 month of E_2 treatment. Clitoral sensitivity returned, and there was return of orgasmic capacity (Sarrel 1999). Adding androgens did not differ from E_2 alone.

INDICATIONS FOR ANDROGEN THERAPY

- Indications for androgen supplementation in estrogen replete women remain controversial. Problems include ill-defined clinical syndromes (i.e., hypoactive sexual desire disorder/female androgen deficiency) for which androgen might be indicated, concerns regarding androgen assay specificity, sensitivity, reproducibility, and normative values in women, and concerns regarding long-term safety (notably with respect to effects of testosterone on breast and other cancers, cardiovascular disease, and stroke) (Wierman 2006).
- Liquid chromatography/mass spectrometry assays will be the future standard for measuring T and E_2 at the low ranges (i.e., menopause and pediatric populations).
- No androgen therapies are FDA approved for the treatment of female androgen deficiency or menopausal symptoms.
- No relationship between a specific (or low) free T level and diminished sexual function has ever been established (Dennerstein 2002; Santoro 2005; Davis 2005). In perimenopausal patients undergoing hysterectomy, the retention or removal of ovaries had no measurable effect on female sexual function when estrogen therapy was appropriately provided (Aziz 2005; Farquhar 2006).
- Androgen therapy will not address established correlates of woman's sexual satisfaction which include her mental health status, positive feelings for her partner, history of past abuse, and her partner's sexual function (Lutfey 2009).
- The considerable evidence in support of androgen therapy is for premenopausal women after oophorectomy, and after failing estrogen therapy (for references see Somboonporn 2005).
  - Consider treatment in premenopausal patients with recognized androgen deficiency such as women with premature ovarian failure, hypopituitarism, adrenal

insufficiency, bilateral oophorectomy, and receiving glucocorticoid therapy.

- In postmenopausal women not receiving estrogen therapy, treatment with a patch delivering 300 µg of testosterone per day resulted in a modest but meaningful improvement in sexual function (Davis 2008). T therapy decreased HDL levels while increasing acne and unwanted hair.
- There is emerging evidence that adding testosterone to menopausal hormone therapy (HT) has a beneficial effect on sexual function in postmenopausal women (Shifren 2006, and Panay 2010).
- Clinical profile of E_2-replete women most likely to respond to androgen therapy:
  ○ Persistent inexplicable fatigue
  ○ Blunted motivation
  ○ ↓ Libido
  ○ ↓ Well-being
  ○ ↓ Free T (in the lower ⅓ range)

CONTRAINDICATIONS

- Moderate to severe acne
- Liver disease
- Cardiovascular disease
- Clinical hirsutism
- Androgenic alopecia
- Known or suspected androgen-dependent neoplasia

POTENTIAL SIDE EFFECTS

- Virilization/hirsutism
- Hoarseness
- Alopecia
- Fluid retention
- Acne
- Unknown if there is a relationship between androgen treatment and breast/uterine cancers
- Adverse lipoprotein/lipid effects
- Clitoromegaly

ANDROGEN THERAPY

- Oral form: methyltestosterone (MT) (0.625 mg E_2 + 1.25 mg MT or 1.25 mg E_2 + 2.5 mg MT)
  ○ MT is at least as potent as T.

- Alternative formulations: no topical testosterone creams/gels or transdermal patches are FDA-approved for use in women, although compounding pharmacies will produce testosterone creams of uncertain purity, dosage, and safety in women. Theoretical but unproven advantages reside with parenteral androgen delivery via avoidance of first pass metabolism of oral preparations.
  - Oral androgen therapy decreases high-density lipoprotein (HDL), increases triglycerides and may increase low-density lipoprotein (LDL) levels (Wang 2011)
  - Further studies are needed to assess the overall cardiovascular (CV) effects of androgen therapies.
  - If treating to improve sexual function, the goal is to restore T levels to at least the upper end of the normal physiologic range for premenopausal women (notably, MT levels cannot be measured and MT is not metabolized to T).
  - Studies have demonstrated that androgen therapy increases the bioavailability of androgens and estrogens by decreasing SHBG.

Pros and Cons for Androgen Therapy

- Possible advantages of androgen therapy: ↑ libido ↑ sexual function ↑ well-being ↑ bone density and ↓ breast tenderness
- Disadvantages of androgen therapy: Masculinizing effects (hirsutism, acne, alopecia, deepening of voice, clitoromegaly), possible hepatic, cancer, and cardiovascular risks, and somatic effects (fluid retention, bloating, etc.) (Casson 1997).

ESTROGEN THERAPY EFFECTS ON CIRCULATING ANDROGENS

- All androgens and androgen precursors decline with age, a decline that is independent of the menopausal transition
- With surgical ablation of the ovaries, there is a roughly 50% ↓ in T even in menopausal patients, clinical significance remains unclear
- T and E_2 are influenced by SHBG levels while A_4 and E_1 are not
- Study: blinded, randomized >2 mg/day of oral micronized E_2 vs. placebo (Casson et al. 1997). Co-administration of progestin was not studied.
  - ↑ E_2 (8.7 pg/mL → 117 pg/mL)
  - ↓ T by 42%
  - ↑ SHBG by 160%

FUTURE

Selective Androgen Receptor Modulators

- Circulating androgen levels may not reflect intracellular androgen activity which may be critical to clinical conditions: intracellular hormone production and metabolism (i.e., intracrinology) is being investigated for diagnostic and therapeutic purposes
- Androgen receptor cofactors (i.e., coactivators/corepressors) are potential therapeutic targets for androgenic disorders
- Selective androgen receptor modulators (SARMs) are under development for treating androgenic disorders; such agents might permit favorable effects on libido, muscle mass, fat-free mass, and bone maintenance while avoiding undesired androgenic side effects

Tibolone

- Synthetic steroid with estrogenic, androgenic, and progestogenic properties (not available in the United States)
- Tibolone effects (Biglia 2010):
  - ↓ Hot flashes and night sweats: significant reduction (equal to HT)
  - Improves sexual function
  - ↓ Osteoporosis: ↓ bone turnover, significantly improves BMD and reduces fractures
- Uncertainties: possible effects on cardiovascular and breast cancer risks remain incompletely studied.

35

Postmenopausal Hormone Therapy

HORMONE REPLACEMENT THERAPY (1950s–1990s) → HORMONE THERAPY (2002 TO PRESENT)

- Although the Women's Health Initiative (WHI) estradiol (E_2)/progestin and estrogen-only studies (see Hormone Therapy Risks and Benefits section) are not perfect, the indications and duration of hormone therapy (HT) have been revised.
- Many areas are still controversial; the following are general recommendations:
- **Risks** and **benefits** of these interventions for perimenopausal and naturally and surgically postmenopausal women are now more clearly defined.
  - Unopposed estrogen therapy **does not ↑ breast cancer incidence** (see WHI data below); the role of progestins in combined E_2/progestin HT is still controversial.
  - While much data exists on **prevention and treatment of osteoporosis** (with fracture outcomes and bone mineral density [BMD]), estrogen therapy is an option but no longer recommended as first line therapy given the long-term risks associated with treatment (e.g., stroke, VTE). Raloxifene or bisphosphonates are preferred.
  - HT for primary prevention of coronary heart disease (CHD) is no longer recommended; current data suggest that **neither primary nor secondary prevention of CHD is a valid indication** for starting or continuing therapy.
  - Major indications for systemic HT with estrogen ± progestin are relief of **menopausal symptoms** and **prevention of osteoporosis**.

- For **symptom relief,** use the lowest effective dose for the shortest time. Short-term therapy is now recommended (at most 2–3 years, no longer than 5 years).
- **Surgical menopause (MP) (bilateral salpingo-oophorectomy [BSO] ± hysterectomy)** and **prevention/ treatment of osteoporosis** may be indications for **longer-term treatment** (>2–3 years). Use the lowest effective dose; review treatment every few years; and discuss risks, benefits, and alternative treatment options with the patient.
- **Women currently on long-term HT** who are doing well should not automatically stop treatment but should be reevaluated and individually counseled. Stopping HT causes rapid loss of hip fracture protection (within 5 years) (Yates 2004), so women who choose to stop HT need alternative therapy (selective estrogen receptor modulators [SERMs], bisphosphonates) and/or BMD follow-up.

CONTRAINDICATIONS FOR HORMONE THERAPY

- History of breast cancer
- Coronary heart disease or previous stroke
- Previous venous thromboembolic event
- Active liver disease
- Patients at high risk for these complications

COMMON COMPLAINTS AND SYMPTOMS ENCOUNTERED IN THE PERIMENOPAUSE

- Vasomotor symptoms:
  - $\uparrow$ Hot flashes from pre-MP (10%) to MP (approximately 50%), but $\downarrow$ by 4 years after MP (20%).
  - Frequency of hot flashes is associated with $\downarrow E_2$ and $\uparrow$ follicle-stimulating hormone (FSH).
- Irregular bleeding:
  - Must rule out endometrial hyperplasia.
    - → Transvaginal sonography; endometrium >5 mm requires sampling (see page 80).
    - → Hysteroscopy or hysterosonogram (saline or water infusion sonogram) may reveal filling defects (polyps/ submucous myomas) especially when the endometrial stripe is thick but an endometrial biopsy is negative.
- $\downarrow$ BMD:
  - $\uparrow$ Bone loss at all sites, but especially trabecular bone

- ↑ Loss with positive risk factors (smoking, lack of exercise, poor diet, weight)
- Vaginal dryness and urethritis
  - ↑ vaginal dryness from pre-MP (4%) to late peri-MP (21%) and by 3 years after MP (47%).

HORMONE THERAPY IN THE PERIMENOPAUSE

- Standard HT is not an adequate contraceptive.
  - Can use low-dose oral contraceptives (OCs) (20 μg ethinyl E_2) as HT for nonsmokers
  - Change to standard HT (oral, transdermal, etc.) with lower dose estrogen 1–2 years after expected time of MP (mean, 51 years old).

CLASSIC APPROACH TO HORMONE THERAPY (BASED ON OBSERVATIONAL STUDIES ONLY)

- Previously much of the emphasis was on the benefits of estrogen.
- Classically prescribed in the perimenopausal transition.
- Prescribed as long-term therapy.

POST-WHI APPROACH

- Individualize estimates of the benefit to risk ratio for HT.
  - Alleviating menopausal symptoms (no other treatment is as effective, but symptoms were not included in WHI main outcome measures)
  - Bone preservation (annual loss in bone mass after MP: 3–5%).
  - **Risk of breast cancer:** No ↑ risk found with E_2 alone in WHI study; questionable progestin (Provera) effect.
  - Cardioprotection: Observational data (e.g., Nurses' Health Study [NHS]) may well have overstated CHD reduction, *but* younger, healthier patients starting HT closer to MP may still reap benefit vs. older population, smokers, obese patients, and those farther from MP in WHI studies.
  - Memory preservation: weak data; ↓ **cognitive function in WHI studies**

HORMONE THERAPY RISKS AND BENEFITS

Large Observational Studies

Nurses' Health Study

- **NHS:** 48,470 postmenopausal women, 10-year prospective cohort study:

NHS: E2 Users vs. Nonusers	Relative Risk (95% CI)
↑ Breast cancer in current hormone therapy users	1.33 (1.12–1.57)
No significant effect on stroke	0.97 (0.65–1.45)
↓ Rate of CHD events in current E_2 users	0.56 (0.40–0.80)[a]
↓ CHD events in low-CHD-risk women[b]	0.53 (0.31–0.91)[a]
↓ CHD mortality in current/past E_2 users	0.72 (0.55–0.95)[a]

CHD, coronary heart disease; E2, estradiol; CI, confidence interval.
[a]Not supported by large randomized controlled trials (Women's Health Initiative).
[b]Low CHD risk: excludes smoking, diabetes mellitus, hypertension, ↑ cholesterol, or body mass index >90th percentile.
Source: Adapted from Stampfer MJ, Colditz GA, Willett WC, et al. Postmenopausal estrogen therapy and cardiovascular disease. Ten-year follow-up from the nurses' health study. *N Engl J Med* 325(11):756, 1991; and Colditz MJ, Willett WC, et al. Type of postmenopausal hormone use and risk of breast cancer: 12-year follow-up from the Nurses' Health Study. *Cancer Causes Control* 3(5):433, 1992.

- NHS CHD data were based on 10 years' follow-up (337,854 woman-years) and provided a rationale for the widespread use of HT for **primary prevention of CHD** in postmenopausal women.
- The finding of ↑ breast cancer risk in HT users was based on 12 years' follow-up (480,665 woman-years) and was assessed for subgroups as follows:

NHS: Breast Cancer Risks	Relative Risk (95% CI)
↑ Breast cancer in unopposed E_2 users	1.42 (1.19–1.70)[a]
Breast cancer in E_2 + progestin users	1.54 (0.99–2.39)
Breast cancer in progestin-only users	2.52 (0.66–9.63)

E_2, estradiol.
[a]Not supported by large randomized controlled trials (Women's Health Initiative).
Source: Adapted from Stampfer MJ, Colditz GA, Willett WC, et al. Postmenopausal estrogen therapy and cardiovascular disease. Ten-year follow-up from the nurses' health study. *N Engl J Med* 325(11):756, 1991; and Colditz GA, Stampfer MJ, Willett WC, et al. Type of postmenopausal hormone use and risk of breast cancer: 12-year follow-up from the Nurses' Health Study. *Cancer Causes Control* 3(5):433, 1992.

- Neither the strong benefit for primary prevention of CHD nor the ↑ breast cancer risk with unopposed E$_2$ has been supported by later randomized controlled trials (Heart and Estrogen/Progestin Replacement Study [HERS] and the two WHI studies, see below).

Randomized Controlled Trials

Heart and Estrogen/Progestin Replacement Study

- HERS: 2321 women with CHD and a uterus:

HERS: Estradiol + Progestins vs. Placebo	Hazard Ratio (95% CI)
↑ Venous thromboembolism	2.08 (1.28–3.40)
↑ Biliary tract surgery	1.48 (1.12–1.95)
No significant effect on cancers	1.19 (0.95–1.50)
No significant effect on hip, wrist, other fractures	1.04 (0.87–1.25)^a
Similar rate of coronary heart disease events	0.96 (0.77–1.19)

Source: Adapted from Grady D, Herrington D, Bittner V, et al. Cardiovascular Disease outcomes during 6.8 years of hormone therapy: heart and estrogen/progestin replacement study follow-up (HERS II). *JAMA* 288(1):49, 2002; and Hulley S, Furberg C, Barrett-Connor E, et al. Noncardiovascular Disease Outcomes During 6.8 Years of Hormone Therapy: Heart and Estrogen/Progestin Replacement Study Follow-up (HERS II). *JAMA* 288(1):58, 2002.
^{a}Maybe different if ≥10 year estrogen therapy

Kronos Early Estrogen Prevention Study (KEEPS trial) (Pending)

- KEEPS: 728 perimenopausal women aged 42–58 years within 3 years of menopause; primary outcome of carotid intimal-medial thickening did not reveal any less thickening in either of the estrogen treated groups compared to placebo.

The Early vs. Late Intervention Trial with Estradiol (ELITE trial) (Pending)

- ELITE: 643 healthy postmenopausal women < 6 years and > 10 years since menopause; primary outcome carotid artery wall intima-media thickness; secondary outcomes rate of cognitive decline and coronary vessel disease based on CT imaging; results expected in 2013.

Women's Health Initiative

- **WHI E$_2$ + progestin:** 16,608 postmenopausal women without CHD: effect of E$_2$ + progestin in women *without* CHD; results at 5.2 years:

Parameter	Hazard Ratio (95% CI)	Absolute Risk[a]
↑ Invasive breast cancer	1.26 (1.00–1.59)	+8
↑ Coronary heart disease events	1.29 (1.02–1.63)	+7
↑ Stroke	1.41 (1.07–1.85)	+8
↑ Pulmonary embolism	2.13 (1.39–3.25)	+8
Endometrial cancer	0.83 (0.47–1.47)	No difference
↓ Colorectal cancer	0.63 (0.43–0.92)	−6
↓ Hip fracture	0.66 (0.45–0.98)	−5
↓ Vertebral fracture[b]	0.66 (0.44–0.98)	−6
↓ Other osteoporotic fracture[b]	0.77 (0.69–0.86)	−39

[a] Absolute risk: number of excess events per 10,000 woman-years of treatment.
[b] Not included in global index of main outcomes.
Source: Adapted from Rossouw JE, Anderson GL, Prentice RL, et al. Risks and benefits of estrogen plus progestin in healthy postmenopausal women: principal results from the Women's Health Initiative randomized controlled trial. *JAMA* 288(3):321, 2002.

- **WHI E$_2$ alone:** 10,739 postmenopausal women without CHD; halted in February 2004. Results from 6.8 years' mean follow-up:

Parameter	Hazard Ratio (95% CI)	Absolute Risk[a]
↑ Stroke	1.39 (1.10–1.77)	+12
Invasive breast cancer	0.77 (0.59–1.01)	No difference
Coronary heart disease	0.91 (0.75–1.12)	No difference
Pulmonary embolism	1.34 (0.87–2.06)	No difference
Colorectal cancer	1.08 (0.75–1.55)	No difference
↓ Hip fracture	0.61 (0.41–0.91)	−6

[a] Absolute risk: number of excess events per 10,000 woman-years of treatment.
Source: Adapted from Anderson GL, Limacher M, Assaf AR, et al.; Women's Health Initiative Steering Committee. Effects of conjugated equine estrogen in postmenopausal women with hysterectomy: the Women's Health Initiative randomized controlled trial. *JAMA* 291(14):1701, 2004.

o Among postmenopausal women with prior hysterectomy followed up for 10.7 years, CEE use for a median of 5.9 years was not associated with an increased or decreased risk of CHD, DVT, stroke, hip fracture, colorectal cancer or total mortality. A decreased risk of breast cancer persisted (HR 0.77; 95 CI, 0.62–0.95). (LaCroix 2011)

- **Women's Health Initiative Memory Study (WHIMS)** found adverse effects of conjugated equine estrogen (CEE) on cognitive function and ↑ dementia and ↑ mild cognitive impairment in both E_2/medroxyprogesterone acetate (MPA) and E_2-alone studies (Shumaker 2004; Espeland 2004), but these findings are based on a subset of WHI patients, as cognitive performance was not one of the primary outcome measures of the WHI study.

Raloxifene Use for the Heart (RUTH)

- **RUTH:** 10,101 postmenopausal women with CHD or multiple risk factors for CHD: see below

RUTH: Raloxifene vs. Placebo	Hazard Ratio (95% CI)	Absolute Risk[a]
↑ Venous thromboembolic event	1.44 (1.06–1.95)	+1.2
Combined coronary events	0.95 (0.81–1.07)	No difference
Stroke	1.10 (0.92–1.32)	No difference
Clinical nonvertebral fracture	0.96 (0.84–1.10)	No difference
Death, any cause	0.92 (0.82–1.03)	No difference
↓ Invasive breast cancers	0.56 (0.38–0.83)	−1.2
↓ Clinical vertebral fracture	0.65 (0.47–0.89)	−1.3

[a]Absolute risk: number of excess events per 1,000 women-years of treatment.
Source: Adapted from Barrett-Connor E, Mosca L, Collins P et al. Effects of raloxifene on cardiovascular events and breast cancer in postmenopausal women. *N Engl J Med.* 355(2):125, 2006.

Postmenopausal Evaluation and Risk-Reduction with Lasofoxifene (PEARL) Study

- **PEARL:** 8556 postmenopausal women with osteoporosis followed for 5 years

PEARL: Lasofoxifene (0.5mg/d) vs. Placebo	Hazard Ratio (95% CI)	Absolute Risk[a]
↑ Venous thromboembolic event	2.06 (1.17–3.60)	+1.5
Death, any cause	1.12 (0.80–1.56)	No difference
↓ Stroke	0.64 (0.41–0.99)	−1.4
↓ Invasive breast cancers	0.15 (0.04−0.50)	−1.4
↓ Coronary heart disease events	0.68 (0.50–0.93)	−2.4
↓ Nonvertebral fracture	0.76 (0.64–0.91)	−5.8
↓ Vertebral fracture	0.58 (0.47–0.70)	−9.3

[a]Absolute risk: number of excess events per 1,000 women-years of treatment.
Source: Adapted from Cummings SR, Ensrud K, Delmas PD, et al. Lasofoxifene in Postmenopausal Women with Osteoporosis. *N Engl J Med.* 362:686, 2010.

- A comparison study of lasofoxifene and raloxifene (CORAL), 2-year placebo-controlled RCT of 410 women, compared lasofoxifene and raloxifene head to head vs placebo and showed greater effects on lumbar spine BMD and equal effects on total hip BMD.

Why the Discrepancy between Observational and Randomized Controlled Trials?

- Why did large observational studies (NHS) show ↓ CHD and ↑ breast cancer incidence in HT users, but these findings were not substantiated in recent large randomized controlled trials (HERS, two WHI studies)?

In Favor of Hormone Therapy

- Primary vs. secondary prevention
- Differences exist between the NHS population and the WHI subjects (e.g., mean age in NHS, 57 years old vs. WHI E$_2$/progestin study, 63 years old). WHI subjects thus started HT at an average of 12 years post-MP, in contrast with women in the NHS, who commenced hormones in the perimenopausal or early postmenopausal periods consistent with both primary prevention goals and with typical clinical practice ("timing hypothesis").
- WHI studies combine a smaller (<20% of the study) primary prevention group of patients in their early 50s at the

start of the study with a much larger secondary prevention group of patients in their late 50s to late 70s. In the E_2/MPA WHI study, only 33% of subjects and control subjects were 50–59 years old, and only 16–17% were within 5 years of the MP at enrollment (Naftolin 2004).

- Despite their large overall size, the WHI trials are **severely underpowered** to detect a CHD reduction resulting from HT started in 50- to 54-year-olds soon after the MP (Naftolin 2004).

In Favor of the Women's Health Initiative Conclusions

- Observational studies like NHS suffer from the *healthy user effect*, in which nurses using HT were more likely to have confounding positive lifestyle factors, such as being less likely to smoke, leading to apparently ↓ CHD in HT users without a direct causative effect. Also, ↑ breast examinations/↑ mammography use may have ↑ breast cancer diagnosis in HT users for the NHS participants.
- NHS excluded silent myocardial infarction, whereas these were included in WHI data (Col and Pauker 2003). Biases in the classification of deaths by unblinded investigators may have occurred in the NHS study.
- RCT data are less subject to confounding and bias such as the effects listed above.

HORMONE THERAPY ADMINISTRATION, DOSING, AND RECOMMENDED MONITORING

- Recommended Surveillance Monitoring:
  - Women 40 to 50 years old: annual clinical breast exam and mammogram every 1-2 years depending on risk based on personal or family history
  - Women ≥50: annual clinical breast exam and mammogram
  - Traditional estrogens used in HT
  - Bioequivalent formulations:
    - → **0.625 mg conjugated estrogens: CEE (Premarin), plant-derived conjugated estrogens** (Cenestin), **esterified estrogen** (Estratab)
    - → **1 mg micronized E_2** (Estrace)
    - → **0.005 mg (5 µg) oral ethinyl E_2** (OCs)
    - → **0.05 mg/day 17β-E_2** (patches)

- Lower estrogen doses for HT
  - Women's Health, Osteoporosis, Progestin, Estrogen (HOPE) study, a randomized controlled trial (Utian 2001), found that lower daily doses of CEE of 0.3 mg or 0.45 mg produced comparable symptom relief to standard doses (0.625 mg/day).
  - Both CEE doses were effective in increasing spine and hip BMD (Lindsay 2002).
  - 14 µg/day transdermal 17β-E_2 weekly patch (Menostar) preserves BMD without endometrial hyperplasia (Ettinger 2004).

Progestins and Natural Progesterone

- **Progestins greatly reduce the risk of endometrial hyperplasia/endometrial carcinoma associated with estrogen therapy** (but not down to zero).
- **Most data exist for MPA** (WHI E_2/MPA arm). The progestin component may be responsible for some of the adverse effects in the combined HT study that were not found by the E_2-alone arm. However, large studies of other progestins are lacking.
- **Possible disadvantages of adding progestins:**
  - ↑ Breast cancer risk? (suggested by WHI data but not proven)
  - Adverse effect on lipid profiles (↑ low-density lipoprotein, ↓ high-density lipoprotein; may reduce E_2 benefits)
  - Impaired glucose tolerance (rarely clinically significant)
- **Cyclic vs. continuous combined therapy** (for women without hysterectomy):
  - Cyclic therapy usually consists of 10–12 days/month of progestin/progesterone (P_4) followed by a withdrawal bleed.
    → May be better tolerated in the peri-MP than continuous combined therapy (↓ breakthrough bleeding)
  - Continuous combined therapy adds a daily dose of progestin/P_4 to estrogen therapy
    → May be via the same administration route as E_2 (i.e., oral CEE and MPA [Prempro], oral E_2/norethindrone acetate [NETA; Activella], or transdermal E_2/progestin [see below])
    → Some combinations require two routes (e.g., transdermal E2 patches/levonorgestrel intrauterine system [LNG-IUS]).
  - **MPA** (Provera)

→ Standard doses are 5 or 10 mg/day × 10–14 days/
month for cyclic HT; 2.5 or 5.0 mg/day for standard-
dose continuous combined HT. Low-dose MPA (1.5
mg/day) is used with CEE 0.3 or 0.45 mg/day for
continuous combined HT.

○ **NETA (norethindrone acetate):** Aygestin alone, FemHRT
with ethinyl E_2

→ Standard doses are 5 or 10 mg/day × 10–14 days/
month for cyclic HT; 1.0–2.5 mg/day for standard-
dose continuous combined HT.

○ **Micronized P_4** (Prometrium)

→ Identical to natural P_4 (bioequivalent HT). May cause
drowsiness; give q.h.s.

→ Standard doses are 200 or 300 mg/day × 10–14 days/
month for cyclic HT; 100–200 mg/day for standard-
dose continuous combined HT.

○ **LNG-IUS levonorgestrel-intrauterine** (Mirena)

→ Induces endometrial atrophy and amenorrhea; lasts
for 5 years (off-label use)

→ Randomized trial of 200 women receiving E_2 with the
LNG-IUS vs. oral E_2/NETA found equal efficacy for
endometrial protection and higher continuation rates
with the LNG-IUS over 2 years' follow-up (Boon et
al. 2003).

○ **Vaginal progesterone gel (Crinone)**

→ Sustained-release 4% (45 mg) progesterone gel administered daily continuous or cyclic for ten doses q monthly

→ if response inadequate, may increase to 8% gel (90
mg) at same schedule

Transdermal Hormone Therapy Patches

• Doses range from 0.015–0.1 mg/day of E_2. 0.05 and 0.1
mg/day doses are most commonly used; typically, start with
0.05 mg/day.

○ Avoiding first-pass liver metabolism is beneficial for
patients with ↑ triglyceridemia but loses the favorable
effects of E_2 on cholesterol profile (E_2 ↓LDL, ↑ HDL).

• **Once-weekly application:**

○ E_2 alone: Climara, Menostar, generic

○ Combination E2/progestin: E2/LNG patch, 0.045 mg E_2/
day (Climara Pro)

• **Twice-weekly application:**

○ E_2 alone: Alora, Esclim, Estraderm, Vivelle, Vivelle-Dot,
generic

    ○ Combination E_2/progestin: E_2/NETA patch, E_2 0.05 mg/
       day, progestin doses 0.14 or 0.25 mg/day (CombiPatch)

NEWER HORMONE THERAPY FORMULATIONS AND ROUTES

New Transdermal Estrogens: Gels, Emulsions, Sprays

- All of these avoid first pass metabolism by liver
- Indicated for moderate to severe vasomotor menopausal symptoms

Divigel

- Estradiol gel (0.25, 0.5, 1 mg per packet)
  - Apply once daily to 5" × 7" area of dry skin (thigh); alternate thighs

Elestrin

- Estradiol gel pump (0.06%)
  - Pump contains 144 g; 100 metered doses of 0.87grams
  - One pump daily to dry area of upper arm

Estrasorb

- Estradiol hemihydrate 2.5mg/g topical emulsion packaged in foil pouches
  - Supplied as 1.74 g pouches
  - Apply contents of 2 pouches onto legs (1 pouch per leg)

Evamist

- Estradiol transdermal spray
  - Pump contains 8.1 mL (56 metered sprays of 1.53 mg/ spray)
  - Apply to dry area of forearm

Ultra-Low Dose Estradiol Patch

Menostar

- Ultra-low dose estradiol (0.014 mg) transdermal patch; shown to increase BMD by 2.3% after 1 year and 3% after 2 years.
  - Apply patch once weekly

- Indicated for postmenopausal osteoporosis prevention
- Low serum E_2 levels: does not relieve hot flashes; may be prescribed continuously or cyclically (3 weeks on, one week off); clinical trials were performed without the addition of progestins in women with an intact uterus

New Oral Combination Estrogen + Progestin

Angeliq

- Oral estradiol 1 mg + drospirenone 0.5 mg tablets
  - Continuous daily administration
  - May cause hyperkalemia
  - Indicated for moderate to severe vasomotor symptoms of menopause and moderate/severe vulvar and vaginal atrophy in women with an intact uterus

Selective Estrogen Receptor Modulators (SERMs)

- Evista
  - Raloxifene: dose 60 mg PO qdaily
    → Indicated for osteoporosis prevention/treatment and breast cancer prevention
    → Not recommended in premenopausal women because of slight increase in risk of VTE & CHD
    → Common side effects: hot flashes, leg cramps; No concern for endometrial effects

- Ospemifene, arzoxifene, bazedoxifene, lasofoxifene: new SERMs developed and currently being investigated in clinical trials
  - Lasofoxifene Dose: 0.5 mg PO daily indicated for osteoporosis treatment
    → May have more endometrial side effects (consider surveillance of endometrium)
  - Ospemifene Dose: 60 mg PO daily indicated for urogenital atrophy
  - Bazedoxifene: 20 or 40 mg PO daily indicated for osteoporosis prevention/treatment
    → No concern for endometrial effects
    → Combination bazedoxifene/conjugated estrogen is under investigation for treatment of postmenopausal vasomotor symptoms and osteoporosis prevention.

APPENDIX A

Hormone Therapy

Active Ingredients	Drug Name	Company	Typical Daily Dosage Choices
Estrogens			
CEEs	Premarin	Wyeth-Ayerst	0.3, 0.625, 0.9, 1.25, 2.5 mg/ continuous daily dosing or cyclic dosing
17β Estradiol (oral)	Estrace	Warner Chilcott	0.5, 1.0, 2.0 mg/ continuous daily dosing
17β Estradiol (transdermal)	Climara	Bayer	0.025, 0.05, 0.075, 0.1 mg weekly patch
	Alora	Watson	0.05, 0.075, 0.1 mg/change patch 2×/week
	Esclim	Women First	0.025, 0.0375, 0.05, 0.075, 0.1mg/ change patch 2×/week
	Estraderm	Novartis	0.05, 0.1mg/ change patch 2×/ week
	Vivelle	Novartis	0.05, 0.1mg/ change patch 2×/ week
	Vivelle dot	Novartis	0.0375, 0.05, 0.075, 0.1 mg/ change patch 2×/ week
	Divigel	Upsher-Smith	0.25, 0.5, 1 g/pkt 0.1% gel/continuous daily dosing
	Estrogel	Ascend	0.75, 1.25 g/ continuous daily dosing

(Continues on next page)

(Continued from previous page)

	Elestrin	Azur	0.06% gel 0.87g/ pump 1–2 pumps daily dosing
	Estrasorb	Esprit	1.74 g pkt; 2 pkts per use/continuous daily dosing
	Evamist	Ther-Rx	1.53 mg/spray; 1–3 sprays to forearm/continuous daily dosing
	Menostar	Bayer	0.014 mg/change patch 1x/week
Estropipate	Ogen	Pharmacia	0.625, 1.25, 2.5 mg/continuous daily dosing or cyclic dosing
	Ortho-EST	Women First	0.625, 1.25 mg/ continuous daily dosing or cyclic dosing
Esterified estrogens	Estratab	Solvay	0.3, 0.625, 2.5 mg/continuous daily dosing
	Menest	Monarch	0.3, 0.625, 1.25, 2.5 mg/cyclic dosing (3 weeks on therapy, 1 week off)
Synthetic conjugated estrogens	Cenestin	Duramed/ Solvay	0.625, 0.9, 1.25 mg/continuous daily dosing
	Enjuvia	Teva	0.3, 0.45, 0.625, 0.9, 1.25 mg/ continuous daily dosing
Estradiol acetate	Femtrace	Warner Chilcott	0.45, 0.9, 1.8 mg/continuous daily dosing

(Continues on next page)

(Continued from previous page)

Oral Estrogen-Progestin Combination Therapy

CEEs and MPA	PremPro	Wyeth-Ayerst	0.625 mg CEE plus 2.5 mg MPA, 0.625 mg CEE plus 5 mg MPA
	PremPhase	Wyeth-Ayerst	0.625 mg CEE days 1–14, 0.625 mg CEE plus 5 mg MPA days 15–28
EE and NE	Fem HRT	Parke-Davis	5 µg EE plus 1 mg NE; continuous daily dosing
	Jinteli	Teva	5 µg EE plus 1 mg NE; continuous daily dosing
Micronized estradiol and norgestimate	Ortho-Prefest	Ortho-McNeil	1 mg 17β estradiol (continuous) and 0.09 mg norgestimate (pulsed in 3-day cycles)
Micronized estradiol and NE	Activella	Pharmacia	1 mg 17β estradiol and 0.5 mg NE; continuous daily dosing
	Mimvey	Teva	1 mg 17β estradiol and 0.5 mg NE; continuous daily dosing
Micronized estradiol and drospirenone	Angeliq	Bayer	1 mg 17β estradiol and 0.5 mg drospirenone; continuous daily dosing

(Continues on next page)

(Continued from previous page)

Combination Oral Estrogen and Testosterone

CEEs and MT	Estratest	Solvay	1.25 mg CEE plus 2.5 mg MT; cyclic dosing (3 weeks on therapy, 1 week off)
	Estratest-HS	Solvay	0.625 mg CEE plus 1.25 mg MT; cyclic dosing (3 weeks on therapy, 1 week off)

Transdermal Combination Therapy

	CombiPatch	Aventis	0.05 mg 17β estradiol and 0.14 mg NE or 0.05 mg 17β estradiol and 0.25 mg NE; change patch 2×/week
	Climara Pro	Bayer	0.45 mg estradiol and 0.015 mg levonorgestrel/day; change patch 1×/week

Vaginal Estrogen Therapy

CEE	Premarin	Wyeth Ayerst	0.625 mg/g; daily
17β Estradiol	Estrace	Warner-Chilcott	0.1 mg/g; daily then 1–3×/week
Estropipate	Ogen	Pharmacia	1.5 mg/g; daily
Dienestrol	Ortho Dienestrol	Ortho-McNeil	0.1 mg/g; daily then 1–3×/week
Estradiol	Vagifem	Pharmacia	25 μg tablets daily for 2 weeks then 2×/week

(Continues on next page)

(Continued from previous page)

Vaginal Estrogen Ring			
Estradiol	Estring	Pharmacia	7.5 µg/day ring; replace every 90 days
	Femring	Warner Chilcott	0.05–0.1mg/day ring; replace every 90 days

CEE, conjugated equine estrogen; EE, ethinyl estradiol; MPA, medroxyprogesterone acetate; MT, methyltestosterone; NE, norethindrone acetate. (Source: Reproduced with permission from Gordon JD, Rydfors JT, et al., eds. *Obstetrics Gynecology and Infertility* [5th ed]. Arlington, VA: Scrub Hill Press, Inc. 2001.)

36

Postmenopausal Osteoporosis

DEFINITION

- Low bone mass and microarchitectural deterioration with consequent ↑ bone fragility and susceptibility to fracture
- Approximately 10–15% of women who take estrogen lose bone.
- Diagnosis requires bone densitometry

PREVALENCE AND INCIDENCE

- 13–18% in women >50 years of age (Looker 1997)
- >1.3 million osteoporotic fractures/year in the United States

Vertebral	Other	Wrist	Hip
46.3%	20.1%	12.4%	20.1%

Annual incidence of osteoporotic fractures in the United States. (Source: Adapted from Ettinger MP. Aging bone and osteoporosis: strategies for preventing fractures in the elderly. *Arch Intern Med* 163[18]:2237, 2003.)

- Postmenopausal women lose approximately 3% cortical and 8% trabecular bone/year.

Distribution of bone mineral density in healthy women aged 30–40 years.

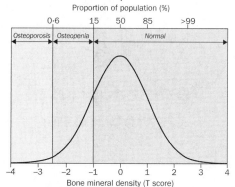

(Source: Reproduced with permission from Kanis JA. Diagnosis of osteoporosis and assessment of fracture risk. *Lancet* 359[9321]:1929, 2002.)

SCREENING

- Controversial but justified for the following reasons:
  - Common disease
  - Associated with high morbidity, mortality, and cost
    - → Estimated cost of osteoporotic fracture in the United States for 1995 was $13.8 billion (Ray 1997).
  - Accurate and safe diagnostic tests are available.
  - Effective treatments are available.
- Check for secondary causes of osteoporosis if (1) a young postmenopausal woman with a fracture or (2) the Z score is below normal for her age group.

FACTORS THAT INCREASE THE LIKELIHOOD OF DEVELOPING OSTEOPOROSIS

- Current low bone mass
- Personal history of fracture after age 50
- History of osteoporotic fracture in a primary relative
- Female gender
- Low body mass index
- Advanced age
- A family history of osteoporosis
- Estrogen deficiency as a result of menopause
  - Especially early or surgically induced
- Abnormal absence of menstrual periods (amenorrhea)
- Anorexia nervosa
- Low lifetime calcium intake

- Vitamin D deficiency
- Use of certain medications, such as corticosteroids and anticonvulsants
- Low testosterone levels in men
- An inactive lifestyle
- Current cigarette smoking
- Excessive use of alcohol
- Race: Caucasian or Asian
- Presence of secondary causes of osteoporosis (see tables below)

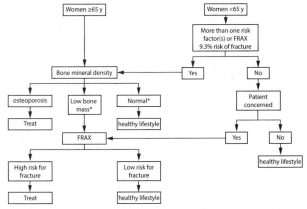

*Fragility fracture is an indication for treatment despite lack of osteoporosis on DXA.

Evaluation of Secondary Causes of Osteoporosis

First Tier

- Complete blood count
- Metabolic profile
- 24-Hour urinary calcium level
- 25-Hydroxyvitamin D level
  - Vit D deficiency is defined as <20 ng/mL (50 nmol/L)
- Thyroid stimulating hormone level

Second Tier

- Celiac panel
- Serum protein electrophoresis

Source: Reproduced from Committee on Practice Bulletins-Gynecology, The American College of Obstetricians and Gynecologists. ACOG Practice Bulletin N. 129. Osteoporosis. *Obstet Gynecol.* Sep;120(3):718-34, 2012.

PATHOGENESIS

- Bone resorption and formation controlled by osteoclasts (resorption) and osteoblasts (formation)
- Follicle stimulating hormone (FSH) stimulates the formation and function of osteoclasts in vitro and in vivo. High circulating FSH may cause hypogonadal bone loss (Sun 2006).
- Mechanism by which hypoestrogenism leads to ↑ bone loss in women is not well understood:
  - Possible direct effect on osteoclast function and changes in the release of certain cytokines (i.e., interleukin [IL]-1, IL-6, tumor necrosis factor [TNF]-α, prostaglandin [PG] E_2)

DIAGNOSIS

- Diagnosis is complicated by the fact that osteoporosis is a silent disease until complicated by a stress fracture
- Vertebral fracture should be suspected in patients with back pain, vertebral deformities by physical examination (kyphosis), or loss of height.
- After a hip fracture, nearly 1 in 6 patients aged 50 to 55 years and more than ½ of those older than 90 years are discharged from the hospital to a nursing home (Walker-Bone 2001).
- Standard x-rays do not detect OP until approximately 40% of bone mass is lost.
- Gold standard of bone mineral density (BMD): **dual energy x-ray absorptiometry (DXA)** of the lumbar spine and hip:
  - Assesses cortical and cancellous bone; BMD ↑ 3–6% in the 1st year of bisphosphonate therapy.
  - DXA can be used to monitor response to treatment.
  - **DXA T score: number of standard deviations (SDs) above or below the average BMD for a healthy 30-year-old woman.**
  - **DXA Z score: number of SDs above or below the average BMD for age- and sex-matched controls;** a Z score below –1 indicates a value in the lowest 25% of the reference range (risk of fractures doubled).
- Note: Z scores rather than T scores should be used for healthy **pre**menopausal women. Z-score may be used to determine if additional screening is necessary for secondary osteoporosis.
- Biochemical markers of bone turnover
  - Assess cancellous bone only.
  - Provide monitoring information; subject to diurnal variation.
  - Change in markers seen as early as 1–3 months into therapy.
  - Some clinicians recommend checking markers at 3 months.

Serum markers of bone **formation**	Alkaline phosphatase, osteocalcin
Serum markers of bone **resorption**	C-telopeptide (CTx)
Urine markers of bone **resorption**	N-telopeptide (NTx), deoxypyridinoline

- **T score:** compares the patient with mean peak bone mass levels as a difference in SD score from a 30-year-old reference point:

T Score	World Health Organization Classification
Greater than or equal to –1	Normal
–1 to –2.5	low bone mass (osteopenia)
Less than –2.5	Osteoporosis

* At any site: femoral neck, total hip, lumbar spine

- −1 SD: twofold ↑ hip fractures
- −2 SD: fourfold ↑ hip fractures
- −3 SD: eightfold ↑ hip fractures

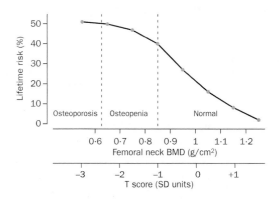

Lifetime risk of hip fractures in women aged 50 years according to bone mineral density (BMD) or T score at the hip. SD, standard deviation. (Source: Reproduced with permission from Kanis JA. Diagnosis of osteoporosis and assessment of fracture risk. *Lancet* 359[9321]:1929, 2002.)

- Obtain DXA if
  - Endocrine diseases (hyperthyroidism, hyperprolactinemia with amenorrhea) (Colao 2000)
  - Secondary amenorrhea (>1 year)
  - Anorexia nervosa ($\downarrow$ follicle-stimulating hormone [FSH], $\downarrow$ luteinizing hormone [LH], $\downarrow$ triiodothyronine [T_3]; $\uparrow$ reverse T_3 [rT_3], $\uparrow$ cortisol)
  - Malabsorption disorders
  - Medications (anticonvulsants, glucocorticoids, excessive levothyroxine sodium [Synthroid], prolonged gonadotropin-releasing hormone [GnRH] agonist)
  - Medical history of a fragility fracture
  - Body weight <127 lb
  - Parental history of hip fracture
  - Current smoker
  - Alcoholism
  - Rheumatoid arthritis
- In response to treatment of OP, markers respond faster and more dramatically than bone density.
  - A 30% or greater reduction in bone turnover is desirable to confirm a response to therapy.

TREATMENT

- WHO Fracture Risk Assessment Tool (FRAX; www .sheffield.ac.uk/FRAX/) can be used to assist treatment decisions.
  - only valid for women >40 years old
  - used for those with T-score –1 to –2.5
  - Treatment considered if there's a 3% risk of hip fracture or a 20% risk of a major osteoporotic fracture (fracture of forearm, hip, shoulder, or clinical spine) in the next 10 years
  - Not valid for women on osteoporosis medicines.
- A medical history of vertebral fracture or fragility fracture is a reason to treat an at risk woman even without a T-score less than –2.5.
- Treatment useful if 10-year probability of hip fracture >3% or 10-year probability of a major osteoporotic fracture >20%.
- All women with a T score less than or equal to –2.0
- Women with risk factors (family history, prior fracture, smokers, <128 lb, high bone turnover) and T scores of –1.5 to –2.0: discuss prevention strategies and treatment

- Combined therapy (e.g., estrogen + alendronate) is synergistic (Greenspan 2003).
- Discontinuing therapy after 5 years is not harmful and may be desirable (Favus 2010).
- Preventive measures for OP:

Drug	Dose
Calcium carbonate, calcium citrate	1,200 mg/day (calcium citrate has fewer side effects)
Vitamin D	800/day. Institute of Medicine recommends supplementation if Vit D level is less than 20 ng/mL.
Exercise[a]	Weight bearing (e.g., walking ≥40 minutes/session, ≥4 sessions/week), resistance exercises and aerobics

[a]Data from Kemmler W, Lauber D, et al. Benefits of 2 years of intense exercise on bone density, physical fitness, and blood lipids in early postmenopausal osteopenic women: results of the Erlangen Fitness Osteoporosis Prevention Study (EFOPS). *Arch Intern Med* 164(10):1084, 2004.

- Estrogen/progestin therapy is no longer a first-line approach for the treatment of OP in postmenopausal women because of increased risk of breast cancer, stroke, venous thromboembolism (VTE), and perhaps coronary disease (Women's Health Initiative [WHI]).
- Atypical fractures of the femoral shaft associated with bisphosphanates: increase in absolute risk was 5 cases per 10,000 patient-years (Schilcher 2011). The benefits of fracture prevention greatly outweigh the risk of atypical femoral fracture (the numbers needed to **treat** would be lower than the numbers needed to harm).
- Bisphosphonates (BPs) reduce bone turnover and increase BMD
  - all BPs decrease vertebral fractures by 35–65%
  - Risedronate also decrease nonvertebral fracture

- o Alendronate and zolendronate significantly decrease hip fractures
- o adverse effects of BPs:
  - → musculoskeletal aches and pains
  - → GI irritation
  - → esophegeal ulceration
  - → osteonecrosis of the jaw
  - → seizures
  - → atypical fracture of the femoral shaft
  - → esophogeal cancer
- o no need to discontinue BPs for dental procedures but, at the same time, no harm in doing so

Drug	Half-Life
Alendronate (Fosamax)	10 years
Risedronate (Actonel)	3 weeks

- Antifracture efficacy of various treatments based on placebo-controlled randomized trials:

Drug	Vertebral Fractures	Hip Fractures
Raloxifene	+++	++
Bisphosphonates	+++	++
Calcitonin (nasal)	+	0
Parathyroid hormone	+++	NA
Vitamin D derivatives	±	0
Estrogen[a]	+	0
Strontium ranelate	++	NA
Fluoride	±	−
Statins[a]	0	0

+++, strong evidence; ++, good evidence; +, some evidence; ±, equivocal; 0, no effects; -, negative effects; NA, none available.
[a]Evidence derived mainly from observational studies.

- Medications:

Generic (Brand Name)	Dose and Route	Indication	Contra indications
Bisphosphonates (oral unless otherwise specified)			
Alendronate (Fosamax)	5 mg/d or 35 mg/week tablet or oral solution	Prevention	• Abnormalities of the esophagus • Inability to stand or sit upright for at least 30 minutes • Hypersensitivity to any component of this product • Hypocalcemia • Patients at increased risk of aspiration should not receive Fosamax oral solution
	10 mg/d or 70 mg/week tablet or oral solution	Treatment	
Alendronate + vitamin D3 (Fosamax Plus D*, Fosavance†)	70 mg + 2,800 IU/week; 70 mg + 5,600 IU/week	Treatment	
Risedronate (Actonel)	5 mg/d p.o.; 35 mg/week; 75 mg in 2 consecutive days/month; 150 mg/month	Prevention + Treatment	
Risedronate (Atelvia)	35 mg/week (delayed release)	Treatment	
Risedronate + calcium carbonate (Actonel with Calcium)	35 mg/week (day 1) + 1,250 mg Ca for no-risedronate days (days 2–7 of 7-d treatment cycle)	Prevention + Treatment	
Ibandronate (Boniva)	150 mg/month; 2.5 mg/day	Prevention + Treatment	
Zoledronic acid (Reclast)	5 mg/2 year I.V.	Prevention	• Hypocalcemia • Creatinine clearance < 35 mL/min/1.73 m^2 and acute renal impairment • Hypersensitivity to Zoledronic acid or any components of this product
	5 mg/year I.V.	Treatment	

(Continues on next page)

(Continued from previous page)

Estrogen Agonist/Antagonist

Raloxifene (Evista)	60 mg/d	Prevention + Treatment	• Venous thromboembolism • Pregnancy, women who may become pregnant, and nursing mothers

Calcitonin

Calcitonin-salmon (Fortical)	200 IU/d nasal spray	Treatment (>5 y postmenopause)	• Allergy to calcitonin-salmon
Calcitonin-salmon (Miacalcin)	200 IU/d nasal spray	Treatment (>5 y postmenopause)	• Allergy to synthetic calcitonin salmon
	100 IU/every other day s.c. or i.m.	Treatment (>5 y postmenopause)	

Parathyroid Hormone

Teriparatide (recombinant human PTH 1–34) (Forteo)	20 μ/d s.c.	Treatment (high Fx risk)	• Hypersensitivity to teriparatide or any of its excipients • Reactions have included angioedema and anaphylaxis

RANK Ligand Inhibitor

Denosumab (Prolia)	60 mg every 6 months s.c.	Treatment	• Hypocalcemia

Estrogen prescription drugs approved for prevention of postmenopausal osteoporosis

Conjugated estrogens (Premarin)	0.3, 0.45, 0.625, 0.9, 1.25 mg/d	Prevention	• Undiagnosed abnormal genital bleeding

(Continues on next page)

(Continued from previous page)

17β-estradiol (Alora*)	0.025, 0.05, 0.075, 0.1 mg/d matrix patch (twice weekly)	Prevention	• Known, suspected, or history of cancer of the breast except in appropriately selected patients being treated for metastatic disease
17β-estradiol (Climara)	0.025, 0.0375, 0.05, 0.075, 0.1 mg/d (0.025 dose not approved in Canada) matrix patch (once weekly)	Prevention	
17β-estradiol (Estrace)	0.5, 1.0, 2.0 mg/d	Prevention	Known or suspected estrogen-dependent neoplasia
17β-estradiol (Menostar*)	0.014 mg/d matrix patch (once weekly)	Prevention	• Active deep vein thrombosis, pulmonary embolism or a history of these conditions
17β-estradiol (Vivelle*)	0.025, 0.0375, 0.05, 0.075, 0.1 mg/d matrix patch (twice weekly)	Prevention	
17β-estradiol (Vivelle-Dot*, Estradot†)	0.025, 0.0375, 0.05, 0.075, 0.1 mg/d matrix patch (twice weekly)	Prevention	• Active or recent (within the past year) arterial thromboembolic disease (for example, stroke, myocardial infarction)
17β-estradiol (Estraderm)	0.05, 0.1 mg/d reservoir patch (twice weekly)	Prevention	• Liver dysfunction or disease • Known thrombophillic disorders (eg. protein C, protein S, or antithrombin deficiency) • Known hypersensitivity to any of the ingredients in this product • Known or suspected pregnancy

(Continues on next page)

(Continued from previous page)

Estrogen-progestin prescription drugs approved
for prevention of postmenopausal osteoporosis

Conjugated estrogens+ medroxyprogesterone acetate (continuous-cyclic) (Premphase*)	0.625 mg E + 5.0 mg P/d (2 tablets: E and E+P)	Prevention Undiagnosed abnonnal genital bleeding	• Undiagnosed abnormal genital bleeding • Known, suspected, or history of breast cancer • Known or suspected estrogen-dependent neoplasia
Conjugated estrogens+ medroxyprogesterone acetate (continuous-combined) (Prempro*)	0.1 or 0.45 mg E + 1.5 mg P/d (1 tablet); 0.625 mg E + 2.5 or 5.0 mg P/d (1 tablet)	Prevention	• Active deep vein thrombosis, pulmonary embolism or a history of these conditions
Ethinyl estradiol + norethindrone acetate (femhrt*, femHRT†)	2.5 µg E + 0.5 mg P/d (1 tablet); 5 µg E + 1 mg P/d (1 tablet)	Prevention	• Active Arterial thromboembolic disease (for example, stroke and myocardial infarction), or a history of these conditions.
17β-estradiol + norethindrone acetate (Activella*)	0.5 mg E + 0.1 mg P/d (1 tablet); 1 mg E + 0.5 mg P/d (1 tablet)	Prevention	• Known liver dysfunction or disease
17β-estradiol + norgestimate (intermittent-combined) (Prefest*)	1 mg E + 0.09 mg P (2 tablets: E and E+P) 1 E tablet/d for 3 d followed by 1 E+P tablet/d for 3 d continuously	Prevention	• Known thromboembolic disorders (e.g., protein C, protein S, or antithrombin deficiency)
17β-estradiol + levonorgestrel (continuous-combined) (Climara Pro*)	0.045 mg E + 0.015 mg P (apply 1 patch once a week)	Prevention	• Known or suspected pregnancy

*Available in the United States but not Canada.
†Available in Canada but not the United States. Products not marked are available in both the United States and Canada
Abbreviations: p.o., by mouth; I.V., intravenous; s.c., subcutaneous; i.m., intramuscular.
Source: Adapted from Modified from North American Menopause Society. Government-approved drugs for postmenopausal osteoporosis in the United States and Canada. Mayfield Heights, OH: NAMS, 2012. Available at http://www.menopause.org/otcharts.pdf. Accessed July 27, 2012.

MONITORING RESPONSE TO THERAPY: SEVERAL APPROACHES

1. Repeat DXA =

- 1st scan normal or mild osteopenia (T −1.5 or higher) → **rDXA in 15 years**

- 1st scan moderate osteopenia (T −1.5 to −1.99) → **rDXA in 5 years**

- 1st scan advanced osteopenia (−2.00 to −2.49) → **rDXA in 1 year**

Source: Adapted from Gourlay ML, Fine JP, Preisser JS, et al; Study of Osteoporotic Fractures Research Group. Bone-density testing interval and transition to osteoporosis in older women. *N Engl J Med.* Jan 19;366(3):225-33, 2012.

2. DXA + biochemical markers of bone turnover
   - Recommended approach
   - Measure at baseline and repeat measurement of markers in 6 months.
   - If marker ↓ significantly (i.e., >50% of urine N-telopeptide [NTx] and >30% for serum C-telopeptide [CTx]) → therapy is having desired effect → repeat DXA after 2 years
- Effective antiresorptive treatments induce a ↓ in bone turnover that reaches plateau within 1–3 months for oral bisphosphonates and usually up to 6 months for various types of estrogen, raloxifene, and nasal calcitonin, depending onthe potency and route of administration of the drug and on the marker (Delmas 2000). Changes in bone turnover markers produced by raloxifene and calcitonin are generally smaller than those produced bythe bisphosphonates and hormone therapy (HT) (Delmas 2000).

Calcium and Vitamin D Supplementation for Postmenopausal Women[a]

Supple-ment	Prepara-tion	Recom-mended Daily Total	Frequency of Doses	Comment
Calcium		1,200–1,500 mg	Two or three times daily	Side effects: nausea and constipation
Calcium carbonate				
	Caltrate	600 mg	Twice daily	With or without vitamin D, at a dose of 200 IU; **food enhances absorption**[b]
	OsCal	250–600 mg	Two or four times daily	With or without vitamin D
	Tums	200–500 mg	Two or three times daily	Available as chew-able antacid tablets and pills
	Viactiv	500 mg	Twice daily	Available as flavored "chews"; with vitamin D[b]
Calcium lactate		42–84 mg	Five or six times daily	Requires taking many tablets very often
Calcium citrate	Citracal	200–500 mg	Two or four times daily	With or without vitamin D at a dose of 200 IU; food enhances absorption[b] proton pump inhibitor allows for better absorption in less acidic environment
Calcium phosphate	Posture	600 mg	Twice daily	Posture is the only calcium phosphate preparation available
Vitamin D		600–800 IU (15–20 μg) daily	Daily	Taken any time of the day

(Continues on next page)

(Continued from previous page)

Multivitamin	400 IU per pill	Daily or twice daily	Good absorption; may contain vitamin D2 or D3
Vitamin D	400 IU per pill	Daily or twice daily	Good absorption
Calcium with vita-min D[b]	125–400 IU per pill	Daily or twice daily	The dose of vitamin D varies in different supplements
Ergocal-ciferol (vitamin D2)	50,000 IU per capsule	Once weekly	For vitamin D defi-ciency, vitamin D3 is preferred
Chole-calciferol (vitamin D3)[c]	50,000 IU per capsule	Once weekly	For vitamin D deficiency

[a]Adequate intake of vitamin D for older postmenopausal women, as established by the Institute of Medicine in 1997, is 600 IU daily; persons living in northern latitudes often have lower serum vitamin D levels and are thought to require 800 IU daily. The recommended daily totals are for elemental calcium and elemental vitamin D.

[b]Often calcium supplements contain vitamin D, but the dose and type of vitamin D vary (e.g., 125 IU to 400 IU per tablet). Similarly, vitamin D supplements often include calcium at various doses (e.g., 125 mg to 500 mg per tablet). Supplements need to be examined carefully by both the patient and the provider, so that proper doses are administered.

[c]Vitamin D3 is preferred for replacement in persons with vitamin D deficiency, because it can be measured more accurately than D2 and is absorbed better. However, high doses (e.g., 50,000 IU) can be difficult to obtain. Vitamin D2 is derived from plant sources. It can be obtained from most formularies and pharmacies. Regardless of the type of vitamin D, treatment with high doses should not continue beyond 3 months and should be followed by a repeated measurement of the serum 25 (OH) vitamin D level. If supplementation is successful in raising the serum level, a dose of 800 IU per day is used for maintenance. If supplementation is unsuccessful and the assay is valid, then consideration should be given to malabsorption, particularly gluten enteropathy.

Source: Modified from Rosen CJ. Postmenopausal osteoporosis. *N Engl J Med.* 2005;353(6):595–603.

37
Hot Flashes

INCIDENCE

- Overall incidence:
  - Premenopausal: 25%
  - Late perimenopausal: 69%
  - Late postmenopause: 39%

BACKGROUND

- Usually a sensation of heat, sweating, flushing, dizziness, palpitations, irritability, anxiety, and/or panic
- Classic hot flash (HF): head-to-toe sensation of heat, culminating in perspiration
- Large cross-cultural variability in prevalence:

%	Culture
0	Mayan women in Mexico
18	Chinese factory workers in Hong Kong
70	North American women (black women > white women)
80	Dutch women

- Despite these vast differences, some trends are seen:
  - HFs usually last 0.5–5.0 years (but may last up to 15 years); one study reported that among women who had experienced moderate to severe HFs, 58% persisted at 5 years, 12% at 8 years, and 10% at 15 years subsequent to reaching menopause.

Onset of HFs	Median duration of HFs (years)
Near entry of menopausal transition	>11.5
Early transition stage	7.4
Late transition stage	3.8

Most common ages at onset of moderate-to-severe HFs = 45-49 years. (Source: Adapted from Freeman EW, Sammel MD, Lin H, et al. Duration of menopausal hot flushes and associated risk factors. *Obstet Gynecol.* May;117(5):1095-104, 2011.

- o Generally more severe in women who undergo surgical menopause; one study reported that 100% of patients undergoing surgical menopause had vasomotor symptoms, and 90% of them had continuing symptoms for 8.5 years. It is postulated that slower, continuous reductions of gonadal steroid levels result in downward regulation of hormone receptors in the hypothalamus in women undergoing natural (vs. surgical) menopause.
- o The lack of correlation between HFs and sleep disturbance seems counterintuitive and challenges the dogma that HFs cause insomnia. (Freedman 2004)
- o HFs have been associated with a diminished sense of well-being (likely as a result of fatigue, irritability, poor concentration, anxiety-type symptoms).
- o Premenopausal/early perimenopausal women with symptoms may be more likely to report a ↓ sense of well-being than late perimenopausal and late postmenopausal women.
- o Some studies estimate that approximately 50% of breast cancer survivors list HF as their most prominent complaint.

ETIOLOGY

- Believed to be related to estrogen withdrawal (not seen in 45,XO patients)
- Estrogen modulates the firing rate of thermosensitive neurons in the preoptic area of the hypothalamus in response to thermal stimulation in the rat.
- Responsiveness of arterioles to catecholamines is greater in women with HFs than in those without HFs. Estrogen enhances α_2-adrenergic activity, and estrogen withdrawal may therefore lead to vasomotor flushes as a result of ↓ α_2-adrenergic activity. Thermogenic changes occurring during a HF may be baroreflex-related since there is **acute hypotension and a brisk increase in heart rate** in both HFs and baroreflex responses to acute hypotensive episodes.
- Women who experience HFs have a significantly smaller thermoneutral zone than women without HF (0.0°C vs.

0.4°C, respectively); small elevations in core body temperature have been shown to precede most HFs.
- Other causes: thyroid disease, epilepsy, infection, insulinoma, pheochromocytoma, carcinoid syndromes, leukemia, pancreatic tumors, autoimmune disorders, and mast-cell disorders

TREATMENT OPTIONS

Estrogens

- Numerous studies have shown the effectiveness of estrogen therapy for HFs. This occurs regardless of route (patch vs. oral) and appears to be dose dependent.
- Overall, estradiol (E_2) treatment is estimated to reduce HFs by 50% in naturally menopausal women and by 70% in surgically menopausal women.

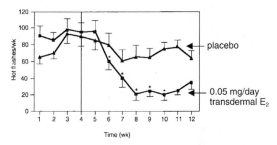

E_2, estradiol. (Source: Reproduced with permission from Bachmann GA. Vasomotor flushes in menopausal women. *Am J Obstet Gynecol* 180[3 Pt 2]:S312, 1999.)

Clonidine

- Clonidine is slightly better for HFs than placebo treatment but comes with some significant toxic effects (mouth dryness, dizziness, drowsiness, and disordered sleeping); this can limit its utility and patient acceptance, which may the reason why only 13 of the intervention patients (39%) continued to use it in one study.

Selective Serotonin Reuptake Inhibitors (SSRIs) or Selective Serotonin Norepinephrine Reuptake Inhibitors (SNRIs)

- The efficacy of SSRIs and SNRIs has been shown in a several randomized trials (see table below for commonly used agents).
- A starting dose of 7.5 mg/day may be preferable for SSRI-naive women

TREATMENT RECOMMENDATIONS *(North American Menopause Society 2004; Grady 2006)*

Lifestyle changes:
  Keep core body temperature as cool as possible.
  Regular exercise
  Paced respiration
  Decrease BMI
  Smoking cessation

Nonprescription treatment (weak supporting evidence):
  Vitamin E (800 IU/day)
  Dietary isoflavones (40–80 mg/day)
  Avoid: progesterone creams, dong quai, black cohosh, evening primrose oil, ginseng, licorice, Chinese herb mixtures, acupuncture, magnet therapy

Preparation	Generic Name	Brand Name	Doses (mg/day)
Estrogen[b]			
Oral	Conjugated estrogens	Premarin	0.3, 0.45, 0.625, 0.9, 1.25
	17-Estradiol	Estrace	0.5, 1.0, 2.0
Spray	17β-Estradiol	Evamist	1.53 mg/spray, 1–3 sprays to forearm daily
Transdermal	17-Estradiol	Alora	0.025, 0.05, 0.075, 0.1 (patch applied twice weekly)
		Climara	0.025, 0.0375, 0.05, 0.075, 0.1 (patch applied weekly)
Vaginal	Estradiol acetate	Femring vaginal ring	0.05, 0.1 (inserted every 90 days)
Progestogen			
Oral	MPA	Provera	10–20
	Micronized progesterone	Prometrium	300 mg qhs
Vaginal	Progesterone	Prochieve 4%	45

(Continues on next page)

((Continued from previous page))

Combination Preparation

Oral sequential[d]	Conjugated estrogens and MPA	Premphase	0.625 conjugated estrogens plus 5.0 MPA
Oral continuous[e]	Conjugated estrogens and MPA	Prempro	0.625 conjugated estrogens plus 2.5 or 5.0 MPA; 0.45 conjugated estrogens plus 2.5 MPA; or 0.3 or 0.45 conjugated estrogens plus 1.5 MPA
Transdermal continuous[e]	17β-Estradiol–norethindrone acetate	Activella	1.0 estradiol plus 0.5 norethindrone
	17β-Estradiol–levonorgestrel	Climara Pro	0.045 estradiol plus 0.015 levonorgestrel (patch applied weekly)
	17β-Estradiol–norethindrone acetate	CombiPatch	0.05 estradiol plus 0.14 or 0.25 norethindrone (patch applied twice weekly)

[a]MPA denotes medroxyprogesterone acetate.

[b]Estrogen should be avoided in women who have a history of or are at high risk for cardiovascular disease, breast cancer, uterine cancer, or venous thromboembolic events and in those with active liver disease. Hormone therapy can cause uterine bleeding, breast tenderness, and headache. Doses of estrogen that are approximately biologically equivalent include the following: 0.625 mg of Premarin, 1.0 mg of Estrace, and 0.05 mg of Alora, Climera, or Femring.

[c]Unlike other vaginal preparations listed in the previous table, Femring delivers a higher systemic level of estrogen and should be opposed by a progestin in women with a uterus.

[d]The first 14 pills contain estrogen and the subsequent pills (15–28) contain estrogen with progestin.

[e]Each pill or patch contains estrogen and progestin.

Source: Adapted from Grady D. Management of menopausal symptoms. *N Engl J Med.* 355(22):2338–2347, 2006.

Preparation	Generic Name	Brand Name	Doses (mg/day)
Progestins			
Oral	Medroxypro-gesterone	Provera	20 mg daily
	Megestrol	Megace ES	20 mg twice daily
Antidepressants			
Oral	Escitalopram	Lexapro	10–20 mg daily
	Citalopram	Celexa	30 mg
	Fluoxetine	Prozac, Sarafem	10–30 mg 10–20 mg
	Paroxetine	Brisdelle	12.5–25 mg
	Desvenlafaxine	Pristiq	75 mg
	Venlafaxine	Effexor XR	75 mg
Gabapentin			
Oral	Gabapentin	Neurontin	300 mg 3 times daily
Alpha-blockers			
Oral	Clonidine	Catapres-TTS	0.1 mg patch daily
	Methyldopa	Aldomet	375-1125 mg daily in divided doses

[a]CR, controlled release; ER, extended release; MPA, medroxyprogesterone acetate; SNRI, serotonin– norepinephrine reuptake inhibitor; SSRI, selective serotonin-reuptake inhibitor.

[b]The hot-flash score was the main outcome of the majority of the clinical trials, measured as the number of hot flashes per day weighted by severity, reported as mild (1), moderate (2), or severe (3).

[c]Side effects were reported in clinical trials of the therapy or on the Epocrates Rx Web site.

[d]Side effects of SSRIs include nausea, vomiting, diarrhea, insomnia, somnolence, anxiety, decreased libido, dry mouth, worsening depression, mania, suicidality, the serotonin syndrome, and the withdrawal syndrome. Paroxetine, and possibly other SSRIs, decrease the activity of cytochrome P-450 enzymes, thereby decreasing the production of active metabolites of tamoxifen, which may interfere with the anti– breast cancer effects of tamoxifen.

Source: Modified from Grady D. Management of menopausal symptoms. *N Engl J Med.* 2006;355(22):2338–2347.

HORMONE THERAPY DECISION-MAKING FLOWCHART

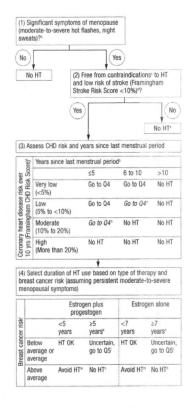

This treatment algorithm is provided only as a guideline for the appropriate use of hormonal therapies in postmenopausal women. The ultimate treatment decisions must be made between a patient and her healthcare professional. As health is unpredictable, the decision whether to start or stay on hormone therapy should be revisited on a regular basis.

[a]Reassess each step at least once every 6–12 months (assuming patient's continued preference for hormone therapy).

[b]Women who have vaginal dryness without moderate-to-severe vasomotor symptoms may be candidates for vaginal estrogen.

^cTraditional contraindications: unexplained vaginal bleeding; active liver disease; history of venous thromboembolism due to pregnancy, oral contraceptive use, or unknown etiology; blood clotting disorder; history of breast or endometrial cancer; history of coronary heart disease, stroke, transient ischemic attack, or diabetes. For other contraindications, including high triglycerides (>400 mg/dL), active gallbladder disease, and history of venous thromboembolism due to past immobility, surgery, or bone fracture, oral hormone therapy should be avoided, but transdermal hormone therapy may be an option (see f below).

^d10-year risk of stroke based on Framingham Stroke Risk Score (D'Agostin 1994;25:40–43).

^eConsider selective serotonin reuptake inhibitor, gabapentin, clonidine, soy, or alternative.

^f10-year risk of coronary heart disease, based on Framingham Coronary Heart Disease Risk Score (Available at www.nhlbi.nih.gov/about/framingham/riskabs.htm)

^gWomen more than 10 years past menopause are not good candidates for starting (first use of) hormone therapy.

^hAvoid oral hormone therapy. Transdermal hormone therapy may be an option because it has a less adverse effect on clotting factors, triglyceride levels, and inflammation factors than oral hormone therapy.

ⁱHormone therapy should be continued only if moderate-to-severe menopausal symptoms persist. The recommended cut points for duration are based on results of the Women's Health Initiative estrogen-progestin and estrogen-alone trials, which lasted 5.6 and 7.1 years, respectively. For longer durations of hormone therapy use, the balance of benefits and risks is not known.

^jAbove-average risk of breast cancer; one or more first-degree relatives with breast cancer; susceptibility genes such as *BRCA1* or *BRCA2*, or a personal history of breast biopsy demonstrating atypia.

^kWomen with premature surgical menopause may take hormone therapy until average age at menopause (age 51 in the United States) and then follow flowchart for subsequent decisionmaking.

^lTry to reduce hormone therapy doses. If progestin is taken daily, avoid extending duration. If progestogen is clinical or infrequent, avoid extending duration more than 1–2 years. For estrogen alone, avoid extending duration more than 2–3 years.

^mIf menopausal symptoms are severe, estrogen plus progestin can be taken for 2–3 years maximum and estrogen alone for 4–5 years maximum.

ⁿIf at high risk of osteoporotic fracture, consider bisphosphonate, raloxifene, or alternative.

^oIncreased risk of osteoporosis; documented osteopenia, personal or family history of nontraumatic fracture, current smoking, or weight less than 125 lbs.

Source: Reproduced with permission from Simon JA, Archer DF, Manson JE et al. Women, hormones, and therapy: new observations from the Women's Health Initiative and the Nurses' Health Study. Trevose, PA: Medical Education Group, 2007:15.

38

Transvaginal Ultrasound in Reproductive Endocrinology and Infertility

BASIC PRINCIPLES OF SCANNING

- Develop a routine to systematically scan all pelvic structures.
- Each structure must be scanned in two planes perpendicular to one another.
- Transducer's position should be monitored during insertion. Once the probe has been properly inserted, the operator should observe the screen at all times, and the position of the probe is determined by optimal visualization of the pelvic viscera. The orientation of the probe is controlled by angulation (accomplished by up and down movement of the transducer handle) and rotation:
  - The probe can be rotated 90 degrees around its axis to obtain sagittal and coronal plane images.
  - The probe can be angled in any plane to direct the plane of image.
  - Deeper insertion or withdrawal can be used to bring the area of interest within the focal zone of the transducer.
- The scan area needs to be thought of as a pie-shaped area emanating from the transducer:

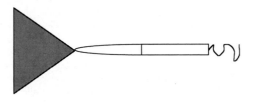

- Rotation of the transducer changes the spatial orientation of that pie between longitudinal and coronal planes:

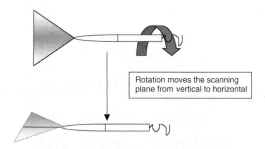

Rotation moves the scanning plane from vertical to horizontal

- Angling the probe (moving the probe up or down) allows for proper orientation of the probe with respect to the pelvic structures, depending on their position (e.g., anteversion, retroversion) within the pelvis:

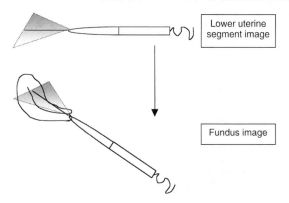

Lower uterine segment image

Fundus image

- The right to left orientation of the image in the coronal plane is controlled in two ways:
  1. Image direction button on the machine itself
  2. Direction of rotation from the sagittal plane
  ○ For example, if the image direction is set on the machine in such a way that the bladder is in the upper left corner while scanning in the sagittal plane, rotation of the probe 90 degrees clockwise will maintain the right to left orientation (patient's left will be displayed on the left of the screen). Rotation of the probe 90 degrees counterclockwise will change that orientation, and now patient's left will be displayed on the right of the screen (Callen 2000).

OVARIAN RESERVE ASSESSMENT

- Ovarian aging is associated with a decline in number of ovarian follicles as well as a possible deterioration of oocyte quality (Toner 2003). Direct measurement of oocyte quantity is not possible at this time; however, ovarian reserve tests reflect the size of the remaining follicular pool:
  - **Antral follicles** 2–8 mm in diameter can be measured on day 2 or 3 of menstrual cycle.
  - **Antral follicle counts** are a reproducible measure of remaining follicle pool and are directly correlated with likelihood of pregnancy after assisted reproductive technology (ART) treatments and inversely correlated with cancellation rates. No antral follicle count, however, can be used as an absolute predictor of pregnancy or cancellation during ART treatments. An antral follicle count of <4 is associated with a high (41–69%) cancellation rate. There is a negative linear correlation between antral follicle counts and gonadotropin dose required to achieve response (Chang 1998; Frattarelli 2000; Frattarelli 2003).
  - **Antral follicle numbers** decrease with advancing chronologic age. The rate of this decline is biphasic, with mean yearly decline of 4.8% in women <37 years of age and increasing to a mean of 11.7% thereafter (Scheffer 1999).

IN-CYCLE MONITORING OF OVARIAN
RESPONSE *(Schwimer and Lebovic 1984)*

- Both size and number of follicles are measured during monitoring for ART treatments; the average growth is 2 mm in diameter per day after stimulation.
- A follicle of ≥18 mm mean diameter is believed to contain a mature oocyte and is used as a marker of when human chorionic gonadotropin (hCG) is to be administered.

Antral Follicle Count and Multiple Pregnancy Rate

- Factors linked to ↑ risk of multiple pregnancies in controlled ovarian hyperstimulation (COH) cycles:
  - Age of the female patient
  - Estradiol levels
  - Total number of follicles developed: The use of ultrasound (US) has been proposed not only to assess follicular

size, but to determine follicle number to reduce multiple pregnancy rates.

ULTRASOUND ASSESSMENT OF THE ENDOMETRIUM IN OVULATION INDUCTION

- Endometrial thickness is best assessed in the longitudinal/ sagittal axis of the uterus, encompassing the thickness of both anterior and posterior endometrial layers. (Note: The figure below is a transverse image to illustrate the layers, although the proper measurement of endometrial thickness should be in the longitudinal/sagittal axis.)

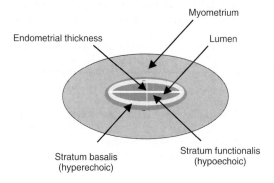

- Endometrial thickness increases slowly in early follicular phase but can thicken by 1–2 mm daily in the late follicular phase. (Note: The figures below are transverse images illustrating the change in endometrial lining, although the proper measurement of endometrial thickness should be in the longitudinal/sagittal axis.)

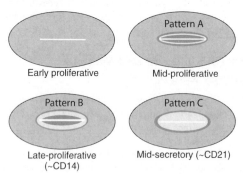

- Thickness of 6 mm appears to represent a critical threshold for achieving pregnancy. No significant improvements in pregnancy rates are seen when endometrial thickness exceeds 6 mm (Dickey 1993).
- A distinct multilayer pattern typically develops within the endometrium in the late follicular phase, commonly referred to as *triple-line* or *trilaminar pattern*. The endometrial patterns are generally divided into three categories:

Pattern A: three hyperechoic lines separated by hypoechoic region
Pattern B: intermediate pattern where three lines are visible, but the intervening endometrium is somewhat hyperechoic.
Pattern C: homogeneous hyperechoic endometrium throughout

  - The uniformly hyperechoic endometrium pattern has been associated with lower implantation rates and poor likelihood of pregnancy (Coulam 1994; Fanchin 2000; Potlog-Nahari 2003).
    - → 447 patients, retrospective analysis, blastocyst transfer (pattern B on day of hCG is associated with ↓ pregnancy rate):

Pattern (no.)	Clinical Pregnancy Rate (%)
A (376)[a]	68
B (66)[a]	47
C (5)	60
B + C (71)	48

[a]P <.001
Source: Adapted from Potlog-Nahari C, Catherino WH, McKeeby JL, et al. A suboptimal endometrial pattern is associated with a reduced likelihood of pregnancy after a day 5 embryo transfer. *Fertil Steril* 83(1):235, 2005.

IMPACT OF ULTRASOUND GUIDANCE AT EMBRYO TRANSFER ON OUTCOME

- Transabdominal US is used during embryo transfers for guidance of the catheter through the cervical canal and to determine the depth of embryo placement within the uterine cavity.
- Many studies have evaluated the impact of this approach with mixed results. The recent meta-analysis of published

studies concluded that US-guided embryo transfer significantly increased implantation rates (Buckett 2003).

- ○ Proposed theories to explain this improvement include:
    - → Confirmation of appropriate placement
    - → Ease of transfer due to guidance through the cervical canal
    - → Placement of embryos in the uterine cavity but away from uterine fundus
- ○ One recent study supported the last theory by demonstrating that clinical pregnancy rates improved with increasing distance between the catheter tip and fundus and by demonstrating US to be superior to clinical touch alone in estimating this distance accurately (Pope 2004).

ULTRASOUND IN ASSESSMENT OF TUBAL PATHOLOGY

- Transvaginal US can be useful in detecting hydrosalpinges with sensitivity as high as 86% confirmedd by large European multicenter study (Sokalska 2009)
- Detection of hydrosalpinx by US during an infertility evaluation is associated with a significant decrease in the expected rates of implantation (OR 0.33%–0.46%, 95% C.I. 0.21–0.96) (de Witt 1998) and proximal occlusion or removal is recommended prior to IVF.

ULTRASOUND ASSESSMENT OF TUBAL PATENCY

- The technique for sonohysterosalpingography (HyCoSy) was first describe in 1984 with the use of Hyscon followed by confirmation of the presence of fluid in cul-de-sac thus confirming patency of at least one fallopian tube. (Richman 1984)
- The use of hyperechoic solution in order to observe flow through fallopian tubes while real time imaging is performed was proposed in 1986 with the use of Echovist-200 (d-galactose microparticle suspension). The technique was utilized in Europe, but was not approved for use in the United States.
- The Femvue Sono Tubal evaluation system approved for use in the United States relies on simultaneous injection of air and saline into the uterus. Intratubal flow can be confirmed by observation of flow extending from tube over the adjacent ovary.
    - ○ A meta-analysis comparing the HyCoSy to HSG and laparoscopic chromopertubation revealed 83% concordance in

detecting tubal pathology between the modalities (Deichert 1989)

- o Another study demonstrated higher prevalence of "uncertain" findings re tubal patency with HyCoSy as compared with HSG (8.8% vs. 0.5%) but the high negative predictive values for both procedures demonstrate their usefulness as screening tests for tubal patency (Strandell 1999)
- o In summary, HyCoSy can be used as a time efficient and well tolerated screening tool for initial evaluation of tubal patency.

SONOHYSTEROGRAPHY

- US technique whereby 10–15 cc of sterile saline is introduced into the uterine cavity via a balloon-tipped catheter. The saline acts as a contrast medium within the uterine cavity and allows for enhanced visualization of endometrial contour.
- Intracervical catheter placement leads to significantly less pain and diminished infused saline necessary for sonohysterography (Spieldoch 2008).
- A meta-analysis examining 2278 procedures compared sonohysterography (SHG) to hysteroscopy as the gold standard for assessment of endometrial lesions (de Kroon 2003):
  - o SHG sensitivity: 95% (confidence interval [CI], 0.83–0.97)
  - o SHG specificity: 88% (CI, 0.85–0.92)
    - → The procedure was more likely to be successfully accomplished in premenopausal vs. postmenopausal women; 93.0% (CI, 92–94) vs. 86.5% (CI, 83.2–89.8).
- When compared to hysterosalpingography (HSG), SHG had greater sensitivity for detecting polypoid lesions (100% vs. 50%) and uterine malformations (77.8% vs. 44.0%). Its sensitivity in detection of intrauterine adhesions was equal to that of an HSG (75%) (Soares 2000).
- The use of SHG significantly enhances the diagnostic capability of transvaginal US alone for both submucosal myomas and endometrial polyps. One study demonstrated that, in 114 patients evaluated for abnormal bleeding, the use of SHG permitted identification of 16 (**14%**) additional lesions in those patients in whom the screening US was **normal** (Laifer-Narin 2002). SHG should therefore be included in a standard protocol for evaluation of abnormal uterine bleeding.

POSTMENOPAUSAL VAGINAL BLEEDING

- Postmenopausal vaginal bleeding (PMB) is a high-risk clini-cal condition for which diagnostic evaluation is indicated. Pelvic US with measurement of midsagittal endometrial thickness (two layers) has been proposed as a screening tool to determine who may benefit from more invasive evalua-tion. Hormone therapy (HT) (sequential and continuous-combined regimens) does influence endometrial thickness (Affinito 1998); however, it is generally recommended that the endometrial thickness cutoff at which invasive testing is recommended is not adjusted even if HT is used.

- The endometrial thickness that should be used as an indica-tion for invasive testing is controversial. When a cutoff level of ≥5 mm is used, the US sensitivity to detect endometrial cancer equals that of nontargeted endometrial biopsy (Gull 2003; Gupta 2002).

39

Hysteroscopy

RESECTOSCOPE HYSTEROSCOPY SETTINGS

Electrode	Current	Watts
VaporTrode (all three types)	Pure cut	200
	Coag	75
Loop	Pure cut	90–120
	Coag	75
Roller ball coag	Pure cut	100–200
	Coag	75

Coag, coagulation.

- Hysteroscopic myomectomy resection: Use VaporTrode cutting and, to clean instrument head, use coagulation setting.

PRESSURE AND POSITIONING

- 40–50 mm Hg to open the uterine cavity (Baker and Adamson 1998)
- 70–75 mm Hg usually adequate for surgery
- Set pump pressure at the patient's mean arterial pressure (MAP); ask anesthesiologists for the patient's MAP; for every foot above the uterus → 10 mm Hg.
- Maximum doses of lidocaine for 60-kg woman: 270 mg (or 27 mL 1% solution) (without epinephrine), 420 mg (with epinephrine) (or 42mL 1% solution)
- Buccal or sublingual misoprostol (200–400 μg) the night before surgery may help dilate the cervix.

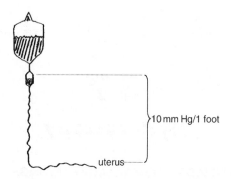

>10 mm Hg/1 foot

uterus

- Avoid Trendelenburg position: By tipping the head down, the heart is below the operative field, and a negative pressure fluids gradient is created, thus predisposing to emboli.
- Fluids:

Solution	Complication
Electrolyte-free solutions, hypotonic (osm) Glycine 1.5% (200) Sorbitol 3% (178) Mannitol 5% (280)	Hypotonic fluid overload Hyponatremia, hyperammonemia and decreased serum osmolality with the potential for seizures, cerebral edema and death.
Electrolyte-containing solutions, isotonic (osm) Normal saline (308) Lactated Ringer solution (273)	Isotonic fluid overload Pulmonary edema and congestive heart failure

- Mechanism to ↓ fluid absorption and to extrude the myoma into the cavity:
  - 5 U vasopressin in 100 mL normal saline (0.05 U/mL): inject 10 mL (20 mL total) into the cervical stroma at 4- and 8-o'clock positions (Phillips 1996)

  - Lactated Ringer (LR) solution for diagnostic hysteroscopy
  - 32% Dextran (Hyskon): nonconductive/immiscible with blood; side effect: anaphylaxis (uncommon)
  - Glycine, sorbitol, or mannitol: Fluid deficit limit of 1,500 mL → stop and promptly conclude procedure; possible use of Lasix (consider sending laboratory tests: electrolytes, renal panel; Na⁺ ↓ 10 mEq/L for every 1 L absorbed)
  - Electrolyte-rich solution: fluid deficit limit of 2,500 mL → stop and promptly conclude procedure.

COMPLICATIONS

- Distinguishing between fluid overload and gas embolus:
  - ↓ CO_2 for both, but the diastolic blood pressure rises with ↑ fluid volume.
- Treatment for gas embolus:
  - Leave the hysteroscope in place (preventing further air access).
  - 100% supplemental oxygen
  - Left lateral decubitus position with the head tilted downward 5 degrees
  - Catheterization of the subclavian vein or right internal jugular vein to aspirate air from the right atrium

- Treatment for acute **hyponatremia** (Na^+ <120): If less than 24 hours, there are few long-term complications from rapid correction
  - O^2
  - Hypocalcemia may accompany; therefore, check Ca_2^+, K^+, Na^+
  - Hypertonic saline, **1.5% NaCl**, to ↑ Na^+ by 1-2 mEq/L/hr but no more than 12 mEq/L in the first 24 hours. Overly rapid correction of severe hyponatremia can lead to osmotic demyelination syndrome (ODS, formerly called central pontine myelinolysis).

ASHERMAN SYNDROME AND INTRAUTERINE ADHESIONS

- Those with normal-appearing endometrium above the level of obstruction on transvaginal ultrasound are likely to have successful hysteroscopic treatment and resumption of menses (Schlaff 1995).
- LR solution pressure may require up to 200 mm Hg to break adhesive disease.
- Postoperative prevention of adhesions (courtesy of Dr. Michael DiMattina, Dominion Fertility, Arlington, Virginia):
  - Intrauterine splint:
    → Place a **No. 14–16 Foley catheter** into the mid- to upper cavity.
    → Inflate with 2–5 mL of sterile water, depending on the size of the cavity.
    → Attach to a leg drainage bag without tension.
    → Maintain for 5–7 days.
  - Medical therapy:

> → **Estradiol valerate, 5 mg IM,** before discharge (lasts for 5–10 days and circumvents nausea with oral estrogen)
> → **Doxycycline, 100 mg PO b.i.d.,** until the catheter is removed
> → **Nonsteroidal anti-inflammatory drug** for the first 48–72 hours postoperative to alleviate pain from catheter and possibly diminish inflammation that can led to adhesion formation
> → Conjugated estrogens (Premarin), 2.5 mg/day, starting 7 days after surgery for 30 days
> → Medroxyprogesterone (Provera), 10 mg/day, starting on day 20 of the Premarin therapy for 10 days

EFFICACY OF HYSTEROSCOPIC SURGERY IN SUBFERTILE WOMEN WITH INTRAUTERINE POLYP *(Bosteels 2010)*

- RCT of polypectomy vs. no polypectomy (Peréz-Medina 2005):
  - Spontaneous pregnancy rate of 29% for polypectomy group vs. 3% in the control group
  - Clinical pregnancy rate of 63% in the polypectomy group compared with 28% in the control group with subsequent FSH/IUI; NNT = 3.
  - No difference with respect to size of polyps

RCT of hysteroscopic polypectomy vs. expected and pregnancy outcome after FSH/IUI (n = 204)

	Polypectomy		P-value
	Study (n = 101)	*Control (n = 103)*	
Pregnant	*Number (%)*	*Number (%)*	*<0.001*
Yes	64 **(63.4)**	29 **(28.2)**	
No	37 (36.6)	74 (71.8)	

RR 2.3 (95% CI 1.6–3.2), NNT=3
Source: Reproduced with permission from Peréz-Medina T, Bajo-Arenas J, Salazar F, et al. Endometrial polyps and their implication in the pregnancy rates of patients undergoing intrauterine insemination: a prospective, randomized study. *Hum Reprod.* Jun;20(6):1632-5, 2005.

40

Laparoscopy

PATIENT PREPARATION AND POSITIONING

Bowel Preparation

- Types: Fleets Phosphosoda, magnesium citrate, GoLYTELY
- Extrapolating from the general surgery literature (Contant 2007), it is reasonable to omit mechanical bowel preparation (which does seem to contradict existing dogma) (Cohen 2011).

Histamine Receptor Blockade

- Recommended for obese patients: ranitidine 50 mg IV 20 minutes prior to surgery.

Positioning

- Modified lithotomy:
  - Hips slightly flexed and thighs parallel to the abdomen; this facilitates access to upper pelvic/abdominal structures and tissue removal.
  - Make sure legs are well positioned and protected (see Positioning Injuries below).
  - Anti-skid material under thorax
  - Sequential compression devices for the lower extremities
- Sacrum: Avoid undue pressure leading to coccydynia.
- Foley catheter for bladder decompression and proper placement of suprapubic port
- Arms adducted and pronated to side and tucked to the patient's side
  - Protect fingers, hands, and elbows with foam cushions.
- Patient supine (0 degrees) for initial Veress needle insertion and primary trocar
- Steep Trendelenburg (20–30 degrees) during the case

POSITIONING INJURIES

Brachial plexus
Caused by outstretched arm or direct compression by shoulder braces during steep Trendelenburg
Result: sensory loss over radial ⅔ of hand, wrist drop if severe

Ulnar nerve
Caused by supination of arm if tucked to the side or pronation if outstretched on arm board
Result: sensory loss of ulnar ⅓ of the hand and parasthesia of the 4th & 5th fingers, claw hand if severe

Peroneal nerve
Compression of the lateral head of the fibula
Result: sensory loss over the lateral aspect of the lower leg, foot drop

Lateral femoral cutaneous nerve
Exaggerated dorsal lithotomy or stretch injury
Result: sensory loss to anterior thigh (lateral femoral cutaneous), inability to raise leg (femoral nerve)

Ergonomics

- Table height at waist level and position yourself so that elbows are comfortably flexed at 90 degrees and shoulders are at resting position
- Locate monitor centrally between the legs or, ideally, two monitors placed at the outside of the patient's knees to minimize neck strain

Anesthesia Considerations

- General anesthesia used for all procedures except perhaps tubal ligation
- Orogastric tube to ↓ possibility of trocar injury to the stomach and ↓ small bowel distention
- CO_2 and Trendelenburg position may lead to splinting of the diaphragm → difficulty maintaining ventilation → hypercapnia

ABDOMINAL ENTRY TECHNIQUE (VERESS NEEDLE)

- Injection of 5 mL 0.25% bupivacaine at the trocar site before incision results in ↓ postoperative pain (Ke 1998).
- Veress needle preparation:
  - Check to ensure the spring-loaded obturator is working before use.

- ○ Stopcock should be open and gas tubing unconnected so that once the negative pressure in the abdomen is encountered, room air enters the abdomen, and bowel and omentum fall away from the tip of the Veress needle.
- Veress needle double-click: puncture of (a) rectus sheath and (b) peritoneum
- Confirmation:
  - ○ First withdraw with a syringe:
    - → **Blood?** Consider vessel injury; need to open immediately if large vessel injury and consult vascular surgery.
    - → **Bile?** Consider small intestine or gallbladder injury.
    - → **Bowel** (feculent)? Do not remove Veress needle; otherwise, difficult to identify bowel perforation; consult general surgery or consider laparoscopic repair after obtaining alternate entry site and accessory trocar placement; simple observation as opposed to suture placement is usually all that is needed for a Veress needle puncture injury.
  - ○ Inject approximately 1 mL normal saline (NS) to remove any possible skin/subcutaneous tissue from Veress tip.
  - ○ Drop test with NS as a sign of intraabdominal negative pressure
  - ○ *Schriock sign*: Initially, intraabdominal pressure reading is a few mm Hg higher to account for a surfactant-like effect requiring some pressure to separate the bowel from the abdominal wall.
  - ○ If entry pressure is >8–10 mm Hg:
    - → Usually incorrect placement in the preperitoneal/subfascial compartment (or a viscus), potentially leading to subcutaneous emphysema
    - → Higher pressures are generally seen in obese patients
- Once intraperitoneal access is obtained:
  - ○ Insufflate with low-flow CO_2 (1 L/min) and percuss over the liver (lose liver dullness—tympanic—after 0.5 L has been insufflated).
  - ○ ↑ CO_2 to high flow (40 L/min though the max flow through a veress needle is 2 L/min) once intraperitoneal placement is assured.
  - ○ Inspect viscera and retroperitoneal structures before requesting Trendelenburg.
  - ○ Operate with CO_2 pressure at 12–15 mm Hg (may need ↑ in obese patients).

ENTRY TECHNIQUES

Umbilical Entry via Modified Alwis Method (*Vellinga 2009*)

- Premise: A surface tension exists from thin layer peritoneal fluid on the peritoneal surface of visceral organs. When the abdominal wall is abruptly lifted and 100–400 cc of gas is insufflated, the negative pressure rises and the air from the positive pressure rushes into the area of negative pressure making an audible sound.
  - If the sound is heard after insufflating 0.1–0.2 L (0.4–0.5 L in obese patients), then the Veress needle is in the intra-peritoneal space.
  - If no sound is heard, the needle is either (a) preperi-toneal, (b) within or against omental or bowel, or (c) there is no blood, fluid, air or excess gas (CO_2) in the pelvis and there is no surface tension to create negative-pressure.
- Technique:
  1. The insufflator is set on high flow and the maximum intraperitoneal pressure is set at 15 mm Hg.
  2. Incision is made with a 15-blade knife in the deepest part of the umbilicus assisted by everting the umbilicus with an Allis clamp and then towel clips laterally. The deepest part of the umbilicus is the thinnest portion of the abdominal wall.
  3. The Veress needle with gas tubing connected is inserted vertically through the incision noting that the normal distance to the peritoneum is only 2 to 3 cm.
  4. Just **when the peritoneum is entered, a negative pressure (<5–6 mm Hg) will appear on the monitor** indicating correct intraperitoneal location.
  5. Turn gas on and isufflate until the intraperitoneal pressure is 15 mm Hg.
  6. Insert 5-mm endoscope into an optical trocar inserted through the umbilical incision under direct vision.

Alternate Access Sites

Left Upper Quadrant (Palmer's Point)

- Midclavicular
- 2 cm below costal margin
- Orogastric tube in place
- **Not recommended** if history of hepatosplenomegaly or gastric surgery

Posterior Vaginal Fornix

- Trendelenburg, long Veress needle, tenaculum on posterior cervix
- Maintain midline entry.
- Remove Veress needle under direct visualization.
- **Not recommended** if cul-de-sac mass, fixed uterine retroversion, rectovaginal endometriosis, or prior vaginal vault surgery

Transfundal

- Approach vaginally, Trendelenburg, long Veress needle, tenaculum on anterior cervix
- Maintain midline entry of uterus.
- Antevert uterus on entry; remove Veress needle under direct visualization.
- **Not recommended** if multiple myomas, fixed retroversion, or high risk for uterine adhesions

Direct Entry (No Veress Needle)

- Advantages: shortened operating time; ↓ incidence of failed entry and ↓ risks associated with the Veress (Ahmad Cochrane 2012)
- Incision large enough to accommodate trocar and avoid skin dystocia
- Elevate abdominal wall; insert trocar directly, aiming toward the sacral hollow.
  - Maintain abdominal elevation until peritoneal confirmation.
- Remove obturator and insert laparoscope to confirm placement.
- If the omentum has been perforated, carefully withdraw laparoscope/trocar in a perpendicular fashion, and omentum should fall off trocar sleeve.

Direct Entry Using Laparoscope

- As above but when a laparoscope is placed within the primary trocar during entry (Visiport, Optiview).

Open Entry (Hasson)

- Skin held up by Allis clamps, incision of skin, reposition of Allis clamps at skin edges, S-retractors placed, dissect to the fascial layer, small Kocher clamps on the fascia, incise fascia carefully, place sutures on lateral edges, enter peritoneum, bluntly enlarge, blunt trocar placed and CO_2 insufflation started, tie sutures to cannula, close fascia with stay sutures, check for fascial defects (may need to place additional suture).

ACCESSORY TROCAR INSERTION

Transillumination

- Helps visualize the superficial epigastric vessels
- If unable to see (obese patients), stay 6–8 cm from the midline (avoids the rectus sheath).
- Make appropriate skin incision along transverse lines of the lower abdominal skin tension (Langer's lines).
- Slow, steady rotational motion with insertion
- Perpendicular to skin and subcutaneous tissue

COMPLICATIONS

Trocar Bleeding

- Abdominal wall: superficial or deep epigastric or deep circumflex vessels
  - Repair under direct visualization.
  - Endoclose device: Place needle and suture on caudad aspect of bleeding vessel, release suture and reenter the needle on the other side of bleeding vessel. Tie suture and repeat on cephalad aspect of bleeding vessel.
  - Keith needle: Same idea but must bring needle back up through trocar (grasp suture instead of needle to facilitate removal)
  - 30-cc Foley balloon: Temporary tamponade
  - Cautery: Only if superficial peritoneal vessels
- Pelvic/aortic vasculature
  - Perform immediate laparotomy, apply pressure, and consult vascular surgery
  - Most common vessel injury: right common iliac

Organ Damage

- Bladder: Repair in layers, may consult urology.
- Bowel: Do not remove trocar! Consult general surgery.

Venous Bleeding

- $\downarrow$ Intraabdominal pressure to 8 mm Hg to help visualize.
- Remember mean venous pressure.
- Visualize under irrigation and low CO_2 pressure.

ELECTROSURGERY

Cut (30–50 W)

- High current, low-voltage (continuous) waveform
- Rapidly elevates tissue temperature, producing vaporization or dissection of tissue with the least effect on coagulation (hemostasis)
- Noncontact means of dissection
  - Activate electrode before touching tissue!
- If energy source left in place, the maximum temperature and width of thermal spread increase with time.

Blend Waveforms

- Interrupts current and increases voltage (noncontinuous)
- Mix between cut and coagulation
- Requires more time to dissect than cut, producing $\uparrow$ thermal spread at the same power setting

Coagulation/Fulguration (30–50 W)

- High-voltage, low-current (noncontinuous) waveform
- Delivers long electrical sparks to tissue
- Superficial eschar produced with minimal depth of necrosis
- Noncontact modality

Monopolar Principles

- Grounding pad
  - Required to help direct the current back to the generator
  - Must be applied correctly to avoid burn at the pad site
- Direct coupling
  - Energy transfer achieved by means of physical contact.
    - → Activated electrode makes unintentional contact with another metal device (e.g., laparoscope and trocar)
- Capacitive coupling
  - Transfer of energy from one circuit to another by means of the mutual capacitance between circuits

→ Induction of stray current to a surrounding conductor through the intact insulation of an active electrode
→ Avoid metal/plastic trocars; use only all metal or all plastic with monopolar electrosurgery.
- Insulation failure
  - Break in insulation provides an alternate pathway for conduction of energy.

Bipolar Principles

- Combines an active electrode with a return electrode in same hand piece
- Eliminates capacitive coupling and alternate current pathways
- Medium-current, low-voltage (continuous) waveform
- Strategies to ↓ thermal injury:
  - Apply current in a pulsatile fashion.
  - Irrigate surrounding tissue.
  - Minimize tissue volume.

Complications

- Thermal injuries to the bowel: incidence of 1.3 in 1,000
  - Usually manifest 2–3 days postoperatively if not identified at the time of laparoscopy
  - Persistent and relatively extreme trocar site pain closest to the bowel injury (local irritation from bowel contents?) (Bishoff 1999)
  - Other possible symptoms: ileus, abdominal pain, abdominal rigidity, leukocytosis with a left shift, fever, and large-volume fluid requirements followed by tachycardia and hypotension
- Residual abdominal gas inducing shoulder pain
  - Intervention to reduce post-op pain:
    → Trendelenburg position (30 degrees), 5 manual pulmonary inflations with a maximum pressure of 60 cm H_2O. Anesthesiologist holds the 5th positive pressure inflation for ~5 seconds. During these maneuvers the trocar sleeve valve ought to be fully open to allow CO_2 gas to escape (Phelps 2008).

Ultrasonic Energy

Harmonic Scalpel/Autosonic Scalpel

- Ultrasound energy converted to mechanical energy by linear oscillation
- 2-mm lateral spread
- Settings:
  - Level 3
    - → Vascular adhesions (shears)
    - → Ovarian cyst (hook)
    - → Oophorectomy (shears)
  - Level 5
    - → Avascular adhesions (hook or shears)
    - → Ablation endometriosis (ball)
    - → Myometrial incisions

LAPAROSCOPIC MYOMECTOMY

- Laparoscopic needle to infiltrate subserosa until blanched with vasopressin
  - Dose: vasopressin (Pitressin): 20 U in 50 cc NS
- Myoma incision
  - Make incision horizontal to ↓ bleeding and facilitate closure.
  - Instruments:
    - → Harmonic scalpel
    - → Monopolar needle: creates ↑ smoke, use suction to clear
- Laparoscopic myoma screw or 5- to 10-mm tenaculum for manipulation of myoma
- Onion-skinning technique
  - Cut on the myoma and not into the myometrial tissue
  - ↓ Blood loss and facilitates closure of the defect
- Specimen removal
  - Electromorcelator (Gynecare: 12 mm; Storz: 12, 15 mm) or
  - Mini-lap incision for removal
- Closure
  - Slow absorbable suture (PDS, Maxon, Vicryl, Polysorb barbed)
  - Intracorporeal needle holders or extracorporeal knot pusher or mini-lap incision

ECTOPIC PREGNANCY

- Large hemoperitoneum may result in increased intraab-dominal pressure on entry
  - Consider using 10-mm suction irrigation (Yankauer) to facilitate faster removal of blood clots.
- Linear salpingotomy
  - Some surgeons inject the mesentery with dilute vasopressin
  - Linear (1–2 cm) incision with monopolar needle or shears on the antimesenteric border
    - → Make incision approximately 0.5 cm from the proximal site of distended tube.
  - Hydrodissection as needed
  - Healing by secondary intention
  - If large incision, consider 5-0 or 6-0 delayed absorbable suture.
  - Specimen removal
    - → Babcock forceps, EndoCatch bag, remove from 10–12 mm port
  - Need to follow serial weekly β-human chorionic gonadotropin(β-hCG) to <5 mIU/mL (rule out persistent ectopic pregnancy)
  - If unable to remove all of ectopic tissue, consider methotrexate.
- Salpingectomy
  - Reserved for severely damaged tube, ruptured tube, or undesired future fertility
  - Electrocoagulate mesosalpinx as close to fallopian tube as possible.
    - → Avoid compromising ovarian blood supply.
  - Follow serial weekly β–hCG to <5 mIU/mL, especially if ovulation induction agents used.
  - Partial salpingectomy best choice if isthmic ectopic

LAPAROSCOPIC CYSTECTOMY

- Sharp shears, curved or straight; lasers used as well
  - Make small incision to separate ovarian cortex from the cyst wall.
  - May use monopolar needle, but ↑ chance of cyst rupture.
- Traction–countertraction
  - Pull tissues apart in a slow motion, holding near the plane of dissection.
  - Hydrodissection with suction irrigator may help.
  - Electrocoagulation of small bleeders, but keep to minimum to preserve maximal ovarian function

- Repair
  - Usually not needed secondary to involution of ovary
  - If large defect, consider suture with 4-0 absorbable suture
- Specimen removal
  - EndoCatch bag: Decompress cyst under direct visualization.
  - Enlarge trocar incision as needed.
  - Posterior colpotomy (Ghezzi 2002)

A. Pelvic Anatomy (Ureters) during Laparoscopy

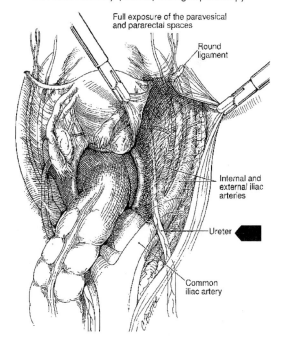

Source: Reproduced with permission from Nezhat CR, Nezhat FR, et al. *Operative Gynecologic Laparoscopy: Principles and Techniques.* New York: McGraw-Hill, 1995.

41
Journal Club Guide

REFERENCE

- Title of article, authors, journal, site(s) of research

BACKGROUND INFORMATION ON THE TOPIC

- Review of the literature suggesting the purpose of the article and how it contributes to the field of knowledge in the specific area

HYPOTHESIS

- Research question (explicitly stated or implied)
- To what population will the findings apply? (relevance of the study)

METHODS/STUDY DESIGN

- Type of study (i.e., descriptive, cross-sectional, cohort, case-control, randomized controlled trial [RCT], meta-analysis, and so forth)
- Selection of study subjects (i.e., How were the subjects chosen? Are there any potential sources of bias? Were the groups similar at the start of the trial? Confounding variables can be controlled for in an RCT [e.g., stratification].)
- Were patients, health workers, and study personnel "blind" to treatment?
- Inclusion/exclusion criteria
- Bias that may have been introduced (ascertainment bias? what was exposure?)
- Control subjects
- IRB approval and clinicaltrials.gov registration (if a clinical trial).

- Adequate randomization: concealed? *SNOSE* (sequentially numbered, opaque, sealed envelopes)? Computer program used? Who holds the code?
- Adequate compliance?
- Outcomes to be measured (are they clearly defined?)
- Types of measurements used
- Were all subjects analyzed in the groups to which they were allocated?
- Was follow-up sufficiently long and complete?

RESULTS

- Statistical analysis used
- Levels of significance used/achieved
- Power analysis
- Findings (review the results in detail)
  - How large was the treatment effect?

CONCLUSIONS

- Stated conclusions
- Do the authors answer the question posed in the hypothesis?
- Are the conclusions justified by the analysis presented?

INTERPRETATION

- Internal validity/external validity (i.e., How does this study apply to the population sampled and to your clinical practice?)
- Clinical vs. statistical significance
- Were all clinically important outcomes considered?
- Are the likely treatment benefits worth the potential harms and costs?
- What alternative treatments are available?
- Is this a significant contribution to the literature?
- Is this study reproducible?

CONSTRUCTION SUGGESTIONS

- How could this study be improved?
- Alternative study design to address this question (make a suggestion about another approach to answering this question)
- Does this study suggest the need for future research in this area?

QUALITY OF EVIDENCE

I. Evidence obtained from at least one properly designed, randomized controlled trial.

II-1. Evidence obtained from well-designed controlled trials without randomization.

II-2. Evidence obtained from well-designed cohort or case-control studies, preferably from more than one center or research group.

II-3. Evidence obtained from multiple time series with or without the intervention. Dramatic results in uncontrolled experiments could also be regarded as this type of evidence.

III. Opinions of respected authorities, based on clinical experience, descriptive studies, or reports of expert committees.

INDICES OF TEST VALIDY:

Sensitivity/Specificity

- Sensitivity denotes those correctly identified by the test
- Specificity denotes the ability of a test to identify those without the condition
- A rule of thumb is that the sensitivity and specificity of a good test should add up to ≥ 1.50, and those of a very good test should add up to ≥ 1.80 (Griffith and Grimes 1990)

Predictive Values

- The predictive value of a diagnostic test is based on both its sensitivity and specificity as well as the prevalence of the target disease in the population being evaluated. Thus, the predictive value of a diagnostic test includes information about both the test itself and the tested population to give a more useful clinical measure.

	Disease		
	+	**—**	
Test **+**	True Positive **a**	False Positive **b**	**PPV = a/a+b**
Test **—**	False Negative **c**	True Negative **d**	**NPV = d/c+d**
	SENS = a/a+c	**SPEC= d/b+d**	

Likelihood Ratio

- A likelihood ratio is the likelihood of a given test result in a person with a disease compared with the likelihood of this result in a person without the disease.
- LR+ greater than 10 means that a positive test is good at ruling in a diagnosis.
- LR- less than 0.1 means that a negative test is good at ruling out a diagnosis.
- Calculation of LRs:
  - LR+ is sensitivity/(1-specificity)
  - LR- is (1-sensitivity)/specificity

Effect Sizes of Interest for Case-Control and Cohort Studies

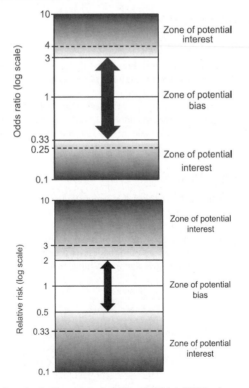

Source: Reproduced with permission from Grimes DA, Schulz KF. False alarms and pseudo-epidemics: the limitations of observational epidemiology. *Obstet Gynecol.* Oct;120(4):920-7, 2012.

STATISTICS

	2 Groups		>2 Groups		
	Related	*Independent*	*Related*	*Independent*	*Measure of Association*
Nominal	McNemar test	Chi², Fisher exact testᵃ	Cochran Q test	Chi²	—
Ordinal	Wilcoxon signed rank test	Mann-Whitney U	Friedman 2-way, ANOVA	Kruskal-Wallis test	Spearman rank correlation
Interval	Paired *t*-test	Unpaired *t*-test	ANOVA	ANOVAᵇ	Pearson correlation, linear regression

ANOVA, analysis of variance.
Note: **nominal** (e.g., surgical complications), **ordinal**: nonparametric (e.g., endometriosis stages), **interval**: normal distribution and continuous variables (e.g., blood pressure), **parametric distribution**: normally distributed and randomly selected.
ᵃUse if there are small numbers (<5 in a cell).
ᵇPost-hoc: Scheffé's or Tukey test.

- o Nominal: surgical complications
- o Ordinal: nonparametric (e.g., endometriosis stages)
- o Interval: normal distribution, continuous variables (e.g., BP)
- o Parametric distribution: normally distributed, randomly selected
- • May run an ANOVA if the data are normally distributed (as determined by Levine's test), then the alpha is chosen at "0.05" and a post-hoc Bonferroni could take into consideration the adjustment (i.e., 3 comparisons would require the Bonferroni alpha to be set at 0.05/3). If the data are not normally distributed then utilize a non-parametric test such as K-W.

SEM vs. SD

- Depends on what question you are trying to answer:
  - SEM, for showing where the means lie
  - SD, for showing where the observations fall

Number Needed to Treat

- Number needed to treat (NNT): the number needed to *obtain* or *avoid* a single additional outcome (http://graphpad.com/quickcalcs/NNT1/)

$$NNT = 1/(EER - CER)$$

  - Where EER = experimental group event rate and CER = control group event rate

For example, if the proportion of getting benefit with **Drug A** was 78% (or 0.78) and 44% (0.44) for **placebo,** the NNT calculation becomes:

$$NNT = 1/(0.78 + 0.44) = 1/0.34 = 3$$

- Using **odds ratios** for calculating NNT:
  - If a systematic review publishes odds ratios but no NNTs you can derive NNTs from the table below:

Odds Ratio (OR)

		Preventive									Treatment								
		0.5	0.55	0.6	0.65	0.7	0.75	0.8	0.85	0.9	1.5	2	2.5	3	3.5	4	4.5	5	10
	0.05	41	46	52	59	69	83	104	139	209	43	22	15	12	9	8	7	6	3
Control	0.1	21	24	27	31	36	43	54	73	110	23	12	9	7	6	5	4	4	2
Event	0.2	11	13	14	17	20	24	30	40	61	14	8	5	4	4	3	3	3	2
Rate	0.3	8	9	10	12	14	18	22	30	46	11	6	5	4	3	3	3	3	2
(CER)	0.4	7	8	9	10	12	15	19	26	40	10	6	4	4	3	3	3	3	2
	0.5	6	7	8	9	11	14	18	25	38	10	6	5	4	4	3	3	3	2
	0.7	6	7	9	10	13	16	20	28	44	13	8	7	6	5	5	5	5	4
	0.9	12	15	18	22	27	34	46	64	101	32	21	17	16	14	14	13	13	11

Odds ratios are on the top line and control event rates: CER down the left hand side and NNTs are in the boxes. So if you have an odds ratio of 0.6 and a CER of 0.5, then NNT will be found where they cross: NNT = 8.

TIPS TO WRITE AN ORIGINAL
RESEARCH ARTICLE: *(Vintzileos 2010)*

Specific Reporting Guidelines: Necessary for Manuscript Submissions

RCT	CONSORT
Meta-analyses and systematic reviews of RCT	QUORUM
Meta-analyses and systematic reviews of observational studies	MOOSE
Studies of diagnostic accuracy	STARD
Observational studies	STROBE
Genetic association studies	STREGA

Source: Adapted from Vintzileos AM, Ananth CV. How to write and publish an original research article. *Am J Obstet Gynecol.* Apr;202(4):344.e1-6, 2010.

Introduction

1. Summarize background information:
   - Leading to a **rationale** for the study
   - Justifying the **need** for the study
   - Clarifying the **new information** that the study aims to offer
2. State study objective/hypothesis

Materials and Methods

1. Study design
2. IRB approval and type of consent obtained
3. Demographics
4. Inclusion and exclusion criteria
5. Description of procedures and tests
6. Definition of exposures and outcomes (primary and secondary)
7. Sample size calculation; power (http://homepage.cs.uiowa.edu/~rlenth/Power/)
8. Types of measurements
9. Statistical methods and level of significance

Data	Report Data as
Continuous data with normal distribution	Mean ± SD
Continuous data without normal distribution, or Ordinal data	Median ± interquartiles or ranges
Categorical data	Proportions (%)

Source: Adapted from Vintzileos AM, Ananth CV. How to write and publish an original research article. *Am J Obstet Gynecol.* Apr;202(4):344.e1-6, 2010.

Results

- Give results for all outcome measures described in M&M
- Use raw numbers WITH percentages
- Confidence intervals provide more accurate indication of the strength of association than P values
- Important findings should be noted

Discussion

- Principal findings
- New knowledge from study
- Strengths and weaknesses of study
- Comparison with prior studies (discuss similarities and differences)
- Explanation of differences
- Succinct conclusion as to how the findings impact clinical practice or future research
- Proposal for future research

References

- Note that within the references lie the potential manuscript reviewers

APPENDIX A

Succinct Expressions for Conclusions of Primary Endpoints Based on P Values

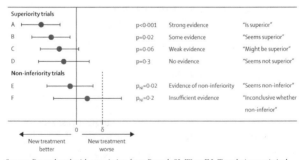

Source: Reproduced with permission from Pocock SJ, Ware JH. Translating statistical findings into plain English. *Lancet*. Jun 6;373(9679):1926-8, 2009.

APPENDIX B

Nomogram for Sample Size Calculation with a Two-Sample Comparison of a Continuous Variable (Normally Distributed) and the Same Number of Patients in Each Arm

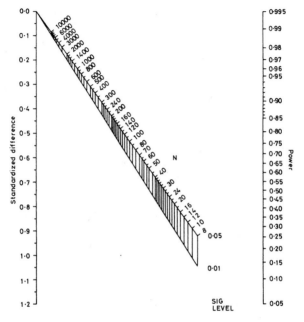

Altman DG. Statistics and ethics in medical research: III How large a sample? *BMJ*. Nov 15;281(6251):1336-8, 1980.

Chapter Key Points

SEXUAL DIFFERENTIATION

- Imperforate hymen and transverse vaginal septum can be difficult to differentiate and are associated with other GU and bony abnormalities. MRI can be useful in the pre-operative evaluation.
- Patients with Congenital Adrenal Hyperplasia require corticosteroids. During childhood, growth curves are one of the most sensitive ways to follow them—if they are over-replaced, the growth curve will taper.
- Timing of gonadectomy in CAIS is controversial, with some recommendations favoring post pubertal gonadectomy to permit normal breast development and pubertal growth, and others cautioning against the age-related risk of gonadoblastoma.
- Male reproductive development requires an active process. The 'default' reproductive phenotype is female (although not necessarily a gonadally competent female). A testis determining factor must be produced and female reproductive organ development must be suppressed.
- Y chromosome containing gonadal tissue should NOT reside in the abdominal cavity!—gonadectomy should be performed—timing depends upon exact defect, always before age 30.
- Genitoplasty guidelines are evolving, trend is to wait until adolescence if parents and child can tolerate ambiguity.
- Most common primary amenorrhea genetic disorders are Turner Syndrome (1/2500) and Mullerian Agenesis (1/4000–1/10,000).

PUBERTY

- Although the median age at onset of puberty and menarche has grown earlier over the past century, the median age at menopause has remained the same.

- Physiologic or 'constitutional' delay of puberty is more common in boys than girls and is usually psychogenic.
- Because of their precocious growth, children with central precocious puberty are often held to behaviors that are inappropriately advanced for their chronological age. This behavioral stress can lead to poor performance at school and further social problems that affect the entire family.
- The largest contribution to female delayed puberty is hypergonadotropic hypogonadism. Early diagnosis might allow for egg harvesting, as is currently offered to girls with Turner Syndrome in the Netherlands.
- Premature adrenarche is associated with later-life hyperandrogenic anovulation

PEDIATRIC AND ADOLESCENT GYNECOLOGY

- Although a biopsy is almost always recommended to diagnose lichen sclerosis et atrophicus, in children and adolescents, a course of high potency topical corticosteroids is a reasonable course of action.

MULLERIAN AGENESIS

- With Mullerian agenesis, creation of an adequate vagina can often be accomplished with manual dilation. Given the amount of effort required to use standard dilators, it is best to introduce their use when the patient has decided to become sexually active. Her partner can often be brought into the therapeutic relationship.

SEPTATE UTERUS

- When a complete septum is present, it can sometimes be quite challenging to incise it. If you do not have a favorable angle, a curved uterine sound can be inserted into the contralateral cavity and pointed toward the operative site to allow you to visualize where you need to make an incision.

TURNER SYNDROME

- Girls with Turner Syndrome may be candidates for fertility preservation, should they have oocytes. Spontaneous menses and mosiacism were the best predictors of follicles on ovarian biopsy. (Borgstrom B, et al Fertiltiy preservation in girls with Turner Syndrome: prognostic signs of the presence of ovarian follicles. *J Clin Endocrinol Metab* 94:74–80, 2009.

MENSTRUAL CYCLE

- Long follicular phases are usually associated with shorter luteal phases when a woman's cycle length exceeds 35 days. This is believed to be a consequence of less efficient folliculogenesis—and thus a less robust corpus luteum. Correcting the follicular phase deficit with ovulation induction treatments will usually correct this problem.
- The midluteal phase appears to be the easiest point at which to disrupt a cycle, either intentionally (when using GnRH agonist to initiate an IVF cycle) or spontaneously (as when women acquire hypothalamic amenorrhea).

ABNORMAL UTERINE BLEEDING

- Although much older literature suggests that women are not accurate about the quantity of their menstrual blood loss, more recent data indicate that self-reported menstrual blood loss is adequate for clinical determination of menorrhagia.
- Most menopausal women present for a work-up of abnormal bleeding concerned that they have uterine cancer; however, atrophy is the most likely diagnosis.
- When treating acute menorrhagia with exogenous estrogens, expect nausea and treat prophylactically with anti-emetics.
- Using the ultrasound-based algorithm for post-menopausal bleeding will avoid the need for many endometrial biopsies.

ORAL CONTRACEPTIVES

- Waiting until Sunday to initiate oral contraceptives OR waiting until the beginning of a menstrual is not clinically helpful in avoiding breakthrough bleeding and may delay initiation of the pill, thereby unnecessarily exposing a woman to a risk of unwanted pregnancy. Patients should initiate therapy as soon as they have the prescribed medication in hand.
- The large reduction in ovarian cancer and protection against endometrial cancer from taking oral contraceptives are particularly beneficial for perimenopausal women, as

the incidence of these conditions is relatively high in women in this age group. This benefit can help offset the increased risk of thromboembolism and MI in women in the 5th decade of life.

- Conception in the first month after discontinuing oral contraceptives has been associated with a greater risk of miscarriage in some studies.

AMENORRHEA

- When administering a progestin withdrawal test to assess the 'depth' of amenorrhea, it is very important to ask specifically about the bleeding pattern. Do not ask the patient if she 'got her period'. Many women will experience spotting or staining after a progestin challenge—which is a positive test to a doctor, but your patient expects a period that resembles 'full flow.'

EXERCISE-INDUCED AMENORRHEA

- In women with eating disorder-related amenorrhea, the FSH: LH ratio is usually elevated, even though both hormones are very low.
- In women with exercise-induced amenorrhea, frequent small feedings may prevent hypoglycemia and negative energy balance and improve the condition.
- In women with functional hypothalamic amenorrhea, cognitive behavioral therapy (CBT) may be superior to other forms of treatment and should be tried before, or in conjunction with, hormone treatment.

ECTOPIC PREGNANCY

- Given that the outcomes of laparoscopic salpingectomy/ salpingostomy and MTX treatment are so similar (see page 125), the treatment choice more often rests on patient preference and other less tangible factors, such as likelihood of adequate follow-up, distance from the patient's home to the treatment site, and out of pocket costs of care to the patient.
- When the clinical picture is not consistent with a positive hCG—get a urine test! It's the quickest first step in ruling out 'phantom' hCG.

SHEEHAN SYNDROME

- Although there is a 'classic' progression of pituitary damage associated with Sheehan Syndrome, it does not always present in this typical fashion. If the diagnosis is suspected, do a complete endocrine investigation including dynamic testing, if necessary, to exclude the diagnosis.

PREMENSTRUAL SYNDROME

- Remember for billing purposes that PMDD is the more severe condition and without this level of severity, many of the possible off-label treatments will be denied to your patient.
- In using the DSM-V criteria, note that PMDD cannot be associated with another primary disorder that is exacerbated premenstrualy. This latter phenomenon is called 'menstrual magnification' and is present in many conditions: migraine, asthma, atopy of various types, and many psychiatric disorders (primarily major depression). This does not mean that the patient should not be treated, rather it helps the clinician disentangle the symptoms and directs him or her to a collaborative approach with the medical provider treating the primary disorder.

CHRONIC PELVIC PAIN

- Lichen sclerosus et atrophicus can sometimes cause chronic dyspareunia and vulvodynia symptoms and may not always present with a classic vulvar appearance (attenuated labia, smooth skin, whitish coloration of the external genitalia). Consider obtaining a vulvar biopsy.

ENDOMETRIOSIS

- Endometriomas greater than 4 cm rarely regress with medical treatment. However, for perimenopausal women who are not having significant pain, observation, progestin therapy or a course of GnRH agonist may allow the patient to reach menopause without surgical intervention.

FIBROIDS

- Even though there is no overall benefit to GnRH agonist pre-operative treatment, in selected cases it may provide a surgical advantage (e.g., allow the surgeon to use a Pfannensteil incision rather than a vertical incision, or allow a laparotomy case to be done laparoscopically or robotically).

- As with endometriosis, women with relatively large fibroids may be able to be managed medically through menopause, avoiding surgical intervention. In this case, progestins are not as useful and will often result in fibroid growth.

POLYCYSTIC OVARY SYNDROME

- Polycystic appearing ovaries have a typical ovarian appearance: >12 follicles 2–9mm in size that line the periphery of the ovary ('black pearl necklace' sign) with an increased ovarian volume. The ovarian stroma can appear hyperechoic, and look bright white next to the darker follicular cysts. Some systems of identification of a PCOS like appearance include ratios of stroma to follicles. This takes into account the stromal hyperplasia that is seen in true PCOS. Don't just focus on the follicles when you are scanning a woman to look for PCOS.
- Mass spectrometry based testosterone assays are becoming more widely available and will improve the ability to diagnose hyperandrogenemia in women.
- A PCOS work-up need only be performed ONCE. The condition does not reverse in adulthood.
- Glucose challenge with insulin levels is a more sensitive test for insulin resistance than a HgbA1c or a fasting glucose/insulin ratio. Provocation of insulin secretion in individuals with insulin resistance yields a greatly exaggerated response compared to insulin sensitive individuals. However, this is an expensive test that is not practical to perform in many clinical settings.
- When suspicious for a tumor in PCOS women, DHEA-S may not be elevated because some tumors lack sulfotransferase activity. If the clinical presentation is consistent with a tumor but the lab tests are normal, consider a DHEA level.
- Women with PCOS who have elevated prolactin may benefit from dopamine agonist treatment even in the absence of a prolactinoma.
- It is prudent to recheck a potassium level within 6–8 weeks of initiating spironolactone therapy to assure that hyperkalemia has not occurred.

FEMALE SUBFERTILITY

- Supposedly 'normal' cycles in fertile women are sometimes anovulatory despite a positive LH surge by OPK. This was seen in 7% of women in a Reproductive Medicine Network trial.
- Aromatase inhibitors are pregnancy category X but their short half life (2 days) suggests that they are not significantly bioavailable to an early gestation if they are given solely in the follicular phase. This is in constrast to clomiphene, also pregnancy category X, which remains in the enterohepatic circulation for up to 6 weeks.
- In cases where surgical removal or clipping of the hydrosalpinx is not practical or not feasible, extended treatment with doxycycline may be an effective alternative.

MALE SUBFERTILITY

- In obtaining a history for male infertility, be aware that cryptorchidism corrected in infancy is sometimes described in families as 'hernia surgery'.
- In couples with barriers to surgery for correction of a varicocoele, IUI may be an alternative, if an acceptable total motile sperm count can be achieved.
- Regional differences and temporal trends in male reproductive health disorders: semen quality may be a sensitive marker of environmental exposures.
- Endocrine disruptors have been shown to affect male sexual development and fertility in animal species. Possible effects on human spermatogenesis remain to be elucidated, should they exist.

DIMINISHED OVARIAN RESERVE

- While many women with DOR will go on to have an earlier menopause than the average woman without DOR, this is not always the case. Be cautious when providing a prognosis about age at menopause!
- Based on data from perimenopausal women, the window for a 'day 3' FSH can be as wide as Day 2–5 after a menstrual period.
- A patient's prognosis is only as good as her HIGHEST day 3 FSH or LOWEST AMH suggest.

ASSISTED REPRODUCTIVE TECHNOLOGIES

- There are many covariates that influence the success of ART. Race-ethnicity and BMI are now known to have a large effect on the likelihood of successful pregnancy with IVF. Both high and low BMI are negative predictors for pregnancy. African-American women are less likely to conceive with IVF, as are Asian women. Hispanic women have a worse prognosis, much of which is attributable to language barriers.

FINANCIALLY EFFICIENT FERTILITY CARE

- Most cost effective formulas for fertility treatments do not take into account downstream costs of multiple pregnancies, resulting poor perinatal outcomes, and long term care of handicapped offspring. This is mostly because these costs are almost impossible to assess in our current medical care system.

OVARIAN HYPERSTIMULATION SYNDROME

- Patients with late-onset OHSS can be reassured that their difficult course is NOT having a negative impact on the pregnancy.
- A report from the emergency room about a hypotensive woman with abdominal pain and a positive pregnancy test can trigger reflexes that will lead to immediate concern for ectopic pregnancy. Ask about any treatments that led to the pregnancy and stop and assess (if the patient is sufficiently stable) before you race to the OR! It might be OHSS.

HYPEREMESIS IN PREGNANCY

- Poor perinatal outcomes occur in women who are subjected to prolonged hypoglycemia in pregnancy. It is important to get an accurate history about intake from pregnant patients.

GAMETE PRESERVATION

- iSaveFertility is an app that provides patient information and also much information that is useful for physicians in counseling. It reviews chemotherapy doses and probabilities of infertility. Fertile Hope has a similar chemotherapy calculator.

- It is not clear how high the utilization of cryopreserved eggs will be. In two studies of men who have cryopreserved sperm, one series revealed utilization of only 3% while the other series showed 27% of men utilized their sperm for reproductive purposes within 10 years of cryopreservation.

LUTEAL PHASE DEFICIENCY

- The 'luteal phase deficiency' phenotype is similar to what is seen in obesity associated subfertility
- The luteal phase deficiency seems to be a reproductive endocrine 'way station' between normal cycling and anovulation. Women who have been observed recovering from secondary hypothalamic amenorrhea demonstrate cycles of this type, with long follicular phases, low FSH, and short or inadequate luteal phases.

HYPERPROLACTINEMIA AND GALACTORRHEA

- Hyperprolactinemia due to pharmacologic agents can present a clinical dilemma. If a patient is on antipsychotic medication, it is often not practical to simply stop the medication to see if the elevated prolactin becomes normal. Yet, an MRI performed in this setting has a low yield. If the clinician has a relationship with the treating psychiatrist, it is sometimes possible to obtain a prolactin level prior to initiating a treatment that is associated with elevated prolactin. If it is normal, that makes it possible to avoid performing the low-yield workup for elevated prolactin in this setting.

RECURRENT PREGNANCY LOSS

- Given the overall good prognosis of couples with RPL who have a negative workup, there is little that the clinician can or need do. Careful surveillance of hCG may present an opportunity to engage in 'watchful waiting' with the couple—which can, in and of itself, have a therapeutic benefit.

MANAGEMENT OF EARLY PREGNANCY FAILURE

- Terms such as 'blighted ovum' and 'missed abortion' are best avoided in the patient's presence. They are non-specific, sound derogatory and can be very confusing to patients.

Women with infertility and early pregnancy loss are typically bereft and very vulnerable to blaming themselves. Do not provide them with fodder for negative delusions.

PRIMARY OVARIAN INSUFFICIENCY/ PREMATURE OVARIAN FAILURE

- If mosaicism is suspected, it can be helpful to increase detection by requesting that the cytogenetics laboratory count 50 cells, not the usual 20 cells.
- To screen out the very rare associations with POI/POF such as autoimmune liver disease, it is relatively inexpensive to check a complete metabolic panel, which will also include calcium and phosphorus (to rule out hypoparathyroidism), serum protein, and potentially pick up Addison disease (if hyperkalemia is detected).
- It is helpful to explain to women with a diagnosis of POI/POF that their chances of natural conception are NOT zero! Many patients faced with this diagnosis are not immediately amenable to egg donation.
- Reactive depressive symptoms are nearly universal in women who are diagnosed with POI/POF. Patients should be made aware and queried frequently about adverse mood, as sometimes medical treatment may be necessary.
- ALWAYS deliver this diagnosis in person at a follow-up visit. The diagnosis is often a devastating surprise for a young woman, and the news should be delivered in a supportive environment with ample time for the patient to express her shock and grief.

GENETIC TESTING

- Overall, the costs in obtaining a pre-emptive diagnosis of a severe genetic defect far outweigh the costs of screening. However, the societal 'price' that we pay for the estimation of risk poses many difficulties for pregnant women and their partners. It is important to provide emotional support for the downstream anxiety that screening engenders.

ANDROGEN REPLACEMENT THERAPY

- When considering treating sexual complaints in menopausal women with testosterone, it is important to identify the locus of the problem. Hypoactive sexual desire disorder is the clearest reason to initiate treatment. If testosterone does not work within a matter of weeks, it should be discontinued. There are essentially no long term safety data on testosterone therapy for menopausal women.

POSTMENOPAUSAL HORMONE THERAPY

- It is important to remember that the WHI results indicated less risk for estrogen alone therapy for women who had had a hysterectomy than estrogen plus progestin therapy for women who did not. However, women who have had a hysterectomy had different health risks than women who did not and thus this clinical trial did not isolate the variable of progestin exposure. For example, women who had hysterectomies were more likely to be hypertensive, and had more overall breast cancer and cardiovascular events even when they took placebo.
- The KEEPS trial did not demonstrate less carotid intimal-medial thickening in either of the estrogen treated groups compared to placebo (primary outcome). Coronary calcium, measured by CT, was low in all groups at baseline, and no between group differences were detected (secondary endpoint). A detailed cognitive battery performed in conjunction with KEEPS did not find any major cognitive differences between groups over the 4 year follow up period. A longer-term follow up study is planned.

POSTMENOPAUSAL OSTEOPOROSIS

- Unfortunately, the FRAX model, which is a guideline, has been applied across the board to all bone density test requests by many insurance companies. It can be challenging to get an earlier screening test on a woman who is younger than age 65!
- The National Osteoporosis Foundation (www.nof.org) website has useful information about the calcium content of many commonly consumed foods. It is preferable for patients to get their daily calcium through the diet, as supplements have been associated with an increased risk of cardiovascular disease in several large series. This may be because supplemental calcium causes transient spikes in circulating calcium and can lead to soft tissue deposition. Patients should be advised to supplement up to the RDA and not beyond.

- There are concerns that the IOM recommendations on vitamin D supplementation are too conservative. Many endocrinologists prefer to supplement to achieve levels over 30 ng/mL. More is not necessarily better.
- Remember it takes BOTH low bone density AND a fall to have a fracture! Patients with low BMD can mitigate their chances for a fracture by working on balance and strength training.

HOT FLASHES

- In one clinical trial from Canada, 300 mg micronized progesterone nightly significantly reduced hot flashes.
- When initiating gabapentin, it is important to start with a low dose (100–300 mg) and increase as needed to obtain relief, as significant side effects of drowsiness occur frequently.
- The Hormone Health Network website (http://www.hormone.org) has a Menopause calculator that helps a woman determine, based on the best available evidence, whether hormone therapy makes sense for her.

TRANSVAGINAL ULTRASOUND IN REPRODUCTIVE ENDOCRINOLOGY AND INFERTILITY

- When performing transvaginal ultrasound to examine the uterine lining in postmenopausal women, the endometrial tissue should contribute to the measurement, and not the fluid, if any.

HYSTEROSCOPY

- Patients undergoing hysteroscopic lysis of adhesions who have secondary amenorrhea SHOULD maintain estrogen therapy postoperatively to assure a good outcome.
- Women with underlying hypoestrogenic amenorrhea (hypogonadotropic or hypergonadotropic) who undergo a pregnancy loss are at very high risk for postoperative Asherman Syndrome.

LAPAROSCOPY

- Get the insufflating gas out! Post-laparoscopy shoulder pain is an avoidable complication.

- To avoid any thermal damage with a laparoscopic cystectomy, the cyst can be shelled out intact and a topical hemostatic agent can be used.

JOURNAL CLUB GUIDE

- When evaluating clinical trials, always keep in mind that a good randomization can make up for a lot of other potential problems with the trail. It is important to peruse 'Table 1'—which is usually the table that describes the baseline characteristics in the overall cohort and in each randomization group.
- Look for sensitivity analyses. This level of effort in reporting results helps let the reader understand the robustness of the study findings. Studies that seem to only be statistically significant when the groups are broken down by a single variable or when only certain cutoffs are used are suspect for validity, because it is possible that the authors chose those key values retrospectively and not prospectively.
- When examining bivariate versus multivariate analyses, look for stability in the point estimate of relative risk or odds ratio. Stability of these numbers indicates that the variable(s) of interest are, indeed, predictive of the outcome.
- Studies that are 'exempt' from IRB approval still require notification of one's local IRB.

References

Abdalla H, Thum MY. Repeated testing of basal FSH levels has no predictive value for IVF outcome in women with elevated basal FSH. *Hum Reprod* 21(1):171–174, 2006.

Abdulmaaboud M, Shokeir A, Farage Y, et al. Treatment of varicocele: a comparative study of conventional open surgery, percutaneous retrograde sclerotherapy, and laparoscopy. *Urology* 1998; 52:294–300.

Abdel Gadir A, Alnaser HMI, et al. The response of patients with polycystic ovarian disease to human menopausal gonadotropin therapy after ovarian electrocautery or a luteinizing hormone-releasing hormone agonist. *Fertil Steril* 57:309, 1992.

Abdel Gadir A, Mowafi RS, et al. Ovarian electrocautery versus human menopausal gonadotrophins and pure follicle stimulating hormone therapy in the treatment of patients with polycystic ovarian disease. *Clin Endocrinol (Oxf)* 33(5):585, 1990.

Abdel-Meguid T, Al-Sayyad A, et al. Does varicocele repair improve male infertility? An evidence-based perspective from a randomized, controlled trial. *Europ Assoc Urology* 59(3):455–61, 2010.

Abdulmaaboud MR, Shokeir AA, et al. Treatment of varicocele: a comparative study of conventionalopen surgery, percutaneous retrograde sclerotherapy, and laparoscopy. *Urology* 52(2):294–300, 1998.

Abrao M, Podgaec S, et al. Deeply infiltrating endometriosis affecting the rectum and lymph nodes.*Fertil Steril* 86(3):543–7, 2006.

Adam Z, Poulin F, et al. Increased risk of neural tube defects after recurrent pregnancy losses. *Am J Med Genet* 55(4):512, 1995.

Affinito P, Palomba S, et al. Ultrasonographic measurement of endometrial thickness during hormonal replacement therapy in postmenopausal women. *Ultrasound Obstet Gynecol* 11(5):343, 1998.

Ahmad G, O'Flynn H, et al. Laparoscopic entry techniques. *Cochrane Summaries* 15;2:CD006583, 2012.

Ailawadi M, Lorch SA, et al. Cost-effectiveness of presumptively medically treating women at risk for ectopic pregnancy compared with first performing a dilatation and curettage. *Fertil Steril* 83(2):376, 2005.

Ailawadi RK, Jobanputra S, et al. Treatment of endometriosis and chronic pelvic pain with letrozole and norethindrone acetate: a pilot study. *Fertil Steril* 81(2):290, 2004.

Aitken RJ, Clarkson JS, et al. Analysis of the relationship between defective sperm function and the generation of reactive oxygen species in cases of oligozoospermia. *J Androl* 10(3):214, 1989.

REFERENCES

Akande VA, Hunt LP, et al. Differences in time to natural conception between women with unexplained infertility and infertile women with minor endometriosis. *Hum Reprod* 19(1):96, 2004.

Alberman E. The epidemiology of repeated abortion. In Beard RW, Sharp F. *Early Pregnancy Loss: Mechanisms and Treatment.* New York: Springer-Verlag, 1988:9.

Álvarez C, Martí-Bonmatí L, et al. Dopamine agonist cabergonline reduces hemoconcentration andascites in hyperstimulated women undergoing assisted reproduction. *J Clinic Endocrinol Metab*92(8)2931–2937, 2007.

Amar AP, Couldwell WT, et al. Predictive value of serum prolactin levels measured immediately after transsphenoidal surgery. *J Neurosurg* 97(2):307, 2002.

Amer SA, Li TC, et al. Ovulation induction using laparoscopic ovarian drilling in women with polycystic ovarian syndrome: predictors of success. *Hum Reprod* 19(8):1719, 2004.

American College of Obstetricians and Gynecologists. ACOG Committee Opinion No. 469: Carrier screening for fragile X syndrome. *American College of Obstetricians and Gynecologists* 116(4):1008–10, 2010.

American College of Obstetricians and Gynecologists. Practice Bulletin no. 73. Clinical management guidelines for obstetrician-gynecologists. 2006.

American College of Obstetricians and Gynecologists. Practice Bulletin no. 94. Washington, DC: American College of Obstetricians and Gynecologists, 2008.

The American Fertility Society. The American Fertility Society classifications of adnexal adhesions, distal tubal occlusion, tubal occlusion secondary to tubal ligation, tubal pregnancies, müllerian anomalies and intrauterine adhesions. *Fertil Steril* 49(6):944, 1988.

American Society for Reproductive Medicine. Diagnostic evaluation of the infertile male: a committee opinion. *Fertil Steril* 98(2):294–301.

American Society for Reproductive Medicine. Increased maternal cardiovascular mortality associatedwith pregnancy in women with turner syndrome. *Fertil Steril* 97(2):282–4, 2012.

American Society for Reproductive Medicine. Prevalence of chronic endometritis in recurrent miscarriages. *American Society for Reproductive Medicine* 95(3):1156–8, 2011.

American Society for Reproductive Medicine. Revised American Society for Reproductive Medicine classification of endometriosis: 1996. *Fertil Steril* 67(5):817, 1997.

Amita M, Takahashi T, et al. Molecular mechanism of the inhibition of estradiol-induced endometrial epithelial cell proliferation by clomiphene citrate. *Reprod Develop* 151(1):394–405, 2010.

Anasti JN. Premature ovarian failure: an update. *Fertil Steril* 70(1):1, 1998.

Andersen AG, Als-Nielsen B, et al. Time interval from human chorionic gonadotrophin (HCG) injection to follicular rupture. *Hum Reprod* 10(12):3202, 1995.

Anderson GL, Limacher M, et al.; Women's Health Initiative Steering Committee. Effects of conjugated equine estrogen in postmenopausal women with hysterectomy: the Women's Health Initiative randomized controlled trial. *JAMA* 291(14):1701, 2004.

Anderson GM, Kieser DC, et al. Hypothalamic prolactin receptor messenger ribonucleic acid levels,prolactin signaling, and hyperprolactinemic inhibition of pulsatile luteinizing hormone secretionare dependent on estradiol. *Endocrinology* 149(4):1562–70, 2008.

Arici A, Byrd W, et al. Evaluation of clomiphene citrate and human chorionic gonadotropin treatment: a prospective, randomized, crossover study during intrauterine insemination cycles. *Fertil Steril* 61(2):314, 1994.

Asante A, Leonard PH, et al. Fertility drug use and the risk of ovarian tumors in infertile women: a case-control study. *Fertil Steril.* 2013 Jun;99(7):2031–6.

Ayvaliotis B, Bronson R, et al. Conception rates in couples where autoimmunity to sperm is detected. *Fertil Steril* 43(5):739, 1985.

Aziz A, Bergquist C, et al. Prophylactic oophorectomy at elective hysterectomy. Effects on psychologicalwell-being at 1-year follow-up and its correlations to sexuality. *Maturitas* 51(4):349–57, 2005.

Bach F, Glanville J, et al. An observational study of women with müllerian agenesis and their need for vaginal dilator therapy. *Fertil Steril* 96:438–6, 2011.

Bachmann GA. Vasomotor flushes in menopausal women. *Am J Obstet Gynecol* 180(3 Pt 2):S312, 1999.

Bachmann GA, Kemmann E. Prevalence of oligomenorrhea and amenorrhea in a college population. *Am J Obstet Gynecol* 144(1):98, 1982.

Backer LC, Rubin CS et al. Serum follicle-stimulating hormone and luteinizing hormone levels in womenaged 35–60 in the us population: the third national health and nutrition examination survey(NHANES III, 1988–1994). *Menopause* 6(1):29–35, 1999.

Bagratee JS, Khullar V, et al. A randomized controlled trial comparing medical and expectant management of first trimester miscarriage. *Hum Reprod* 19(2):266, 2004.

Badaway A, Elnashar A, et al. Gonadotropin-releasing hormone agonists for prevention ofchemotherapy-induced ovarian damage: prospective randomized study. *Fertil Steril* 91(3):694–7, 2009.

Badaway A, Mosbah A, et al. Extended letrozole therapy for ovulation induction in clomiphene-resistant women with polycystic ovary syndrome: a novel protocol. *Fertil Steril* 92(1):236–9, 2009.

Baerwald AR, Olatunbosun OA, et al. Effects of oral contraceptives administered at defined stages ofovarian follicular development. *Fertil Steril* 86(1):27–35, 2006.

Baird DD, Dunson DB, et al. High cumulative incidence of uterine leiomyoma in black and white women. *AJOG* 188:100, 2003

Bajekal N, Li TC. Fibroids, infertility and pregnancy wastage. *Hum Reprod Update* 6(6):614, 2000.

Bakalov VK, Vanderhoof VH, et al. Adrenal antibodies detect asymptomatic auto-immune adrenal insufficiency in young women with spontaneous premature ovarian failure. *Hum Reprod* 17(8):2096, 2002.

Baker VL, Adamson GD. Minimum intrauterine pressure required for uterine distention. *J Am Assoc Gynecol Laparosc* 5(1):51, 1998.

Balasch J, Creus M, et al. Lack of endometriosis in patients with repeated abortion. *Hum Reprod* 3(2):263, 1988.

Balasch J, Creus M, et al. Visible and non-visible endometriosis at laparoscopy in fertile and infertile women and in patients with chronic pelvic pain: a prospective study. *Hum Reprod* 11(2):1163, 1996.

Barbieri RL. Hormone treatment of endometriosis: the estrogen threshold hypothesis. *Am J Obstet Gynecol* 166:740, 1992.

Barnhart K, Dunsmoor-Su R, et al. Effect of endometriosis on in vitro fertilization. *Fertil Steril* 77(6):1148, 2002.

Barnhart K, Hummel A, et al. Use of "2-dose" regimen of methotrexate to treat ectopic pregnancy. *Fertil Steril* 87(2):250–6, 2007.

Barnhart K, Osheroff J. Follicle stimulating hormone as a predictor of fertility. *Curr Opin Obstet Gynecol* 10(3):227, 1998.

Barnhart KT, Sammel MD, et al. Decline of serum human chorionic gonadotropin and spontaneous complete abortion: defining the normal curve. *Obstet Gynecol* 104(5):975, 2004a.

Barnhart KT, Sammel MD, et al. Symptomatic patients with an early viable intrauterine pregnancy: HCG curves redefined. *Obstet Gynecol* 104(1):50, 2004b.

Barnhart K, Schreiber C. Return to fertility following discontinuation of oral contraceptives. *Fertil Steril* 91(3)659–63, 2009.

Bateman BG, Taylor PT, Jr. Reproductive considerations during abdominal surgical procedures in young women. *Surg Clin North Am* 71(5):1053, 1991.

Bates GW, Jr., Hill JA. Autoimmune ovarian failure. *Infertil Reprod Med Clinics NA* 13(1):65, 2002.

Bayrak A, Saadat P, et al. Pituitary imaging is indicated for the evaluation of hyperprolactinemia. *Fertil Steril* 84(1):181–5, 2005.

Bayram N, Van Wely M, et al. Using an electrocautery strategy or recombinant follicle stimulating hormone to induce ovulation in polycystic ovary syndrome: randomised controlled trial. *BMJ* 328(7433):192, 2004.

Beck LE, Gevirtz R, et al. The predictive role of psychosocial stress on symptom severity in premenstrual syndrome. *Psychosom Med* 52(5):536, 1990.

Beerendonk CC, Van Dop PA, et al. Ovarian hyperstimulation syndrome: facts and fallacies. *Obstet Gynecol Surv* 53(7):439, 1998.

Belker AM, Thomas AJ, Jr., et al. Results of 1,469 microsurgical vasectomy reversals by the Vasovasostomy Study Group. *J Urol* 145(3):505, 1991.

Belsey EM, Pinol AP. Menstrual bleeding patterns in untreated women. Task force on long-acting systemic agents for fertility regulation. *Contraception* 55(2):57–65, 1997.

Benaglia L, Bermejo A, et al. In vitro fertilization outcome in women with unoperated bilateral endometriomas. *Fertil Steril.* 99(6):1714–9, 2013.

Beretta P, Franchi M, et al. Randomized clinical trial of two laparoscopic treatments of endometriomas: cystectomy versus drainage and coagulation. *Fertil Steril* 70(6):1176, 1998.

Berkkanoglu M, Isikoglu M, et al. What is the best time to perform intracytoplasmic sperm injection/embryo transfer cycle after hysteroscopic surgery for incomplete uterine septum? *Fertil Steril* 90(6):2112–5, 2008.

Berube S, Marcoux S, et al. Fecundity of infertile women with minimal or mild endometriosis and women with unexplained infertility. The Canadian Collaborative Group on Endometriosis. *Fertil Steril* 69(6):1034, 1998.

Bhattacharya S, Harris K, et al. Clomifene citrate or unstimulated intrauterine insemination comparedwith expectant management for unexplained infertility: pragmatic randomized controlled trial.*BMJ* 337:a716

Bidet M, Bachelot A, et al. Resumption of ovarian function and pregnancies in 358 patients with premature ovarian failure. *J Clin Endocrinol Metab* 96(12):3864–3872, 2011.

Biglia N, Maffei S, et al. Tibolone in postmenopausal women: a review based on recent randomizedcontrolled clinical trials. *Gynecol Endocrinol* 26(11):804–14, 2010.

Bishoff JT, Allaf ME, et al. Laparoscopic bowel injury: incidence and clinical presentation. *J Urol* 161(3):887, 1999.

Bishry G, Tselos V, et al. Correlation between laparoscopic and histological diagnosis in patients with endometriosis. *J Obstet Gynecol* 28(5):511–515, 2008.

Bissonnette F, Lapensee L, et al. Outpatient laparoscopic tubal anastomosis and subsequent fertility. *Fertil Steril* 72(3):549, 1999.

Blumenfeld Z, Avivi I, et al. Prevention of irreversible chemotherapy-induced ovarian damage in young women with lymphoma by a gonadotrophin-releasing hormone agonist in parallel to chemotherapy. *Hum Reprod* 11(8):1620, 1996.

Boer-Meisel ME, te Velde ER, et al. Predicting the pregnancy outcome in patients treated for hydrosalpinx: a prospective study. *Fertil Steril* 45(1):23, 1986.

Boivin J, Griffiths E, et al. Emotional distress in infertile women and failure of assisted reproductive technologies: meta-analysis of prospective psychosocial studies. *BMJ* 342:d223, 2011.

Boivin J, Schmidt L. Use of complementary and alternative medicines associated with a 30% lower ongoing pregnancy/live birth rate during 12 months of fertility treatment. *Hum Reprod*24(7):1626–1631, 2009.

Bonduelle M, Aytoz A, et al. Incidence of chromosomal aberrations in children born after assisted reproduction through intracytoplasmic sperm injection. *Hum Reprod* 13(4):781, 1998a.

Bonduelle M, Wilikens A, et al. A follow-up study of children born after intracytoplasmic sperm injection (ICSI) with epididymal and testicular spermatozoa and after replacement of cryopreserved embryos obtained after ICSI. *Hum Reprod* 13[Suppl 1]:196, 1998b.

Bosch E, Labarta E, et al. Circulating progesterone levels and ongoing pregnancy rates in controlledovarian stimulation cycles for in vitro fertilization: analysis of over 4000 cycles. *Hum Reprod* 25(8):2092–2100, 2010.

Bosdou JK, Venetis CA, et al. The use of androgens or androgen-modulating agents in poor responders undergoing in vitro fertilization: a systematic review and meta-analysis. *Hum Reprod Update.* 2012 Mar-Apr;18(2):127–45.

Bosteels J, Weyers S, et al. The effectiveness of hysteroscopy in improving pregnancy rates in subfertilewomen without other hynaecological symptoms: a systematic review. *Hum Reprod* 16(1):1–11, 2010.

Boue A, Boue J, et al. Cytogenetics of pregnancy wastage. *Adv Hum Genet* 14:1, 1985.

Breitkopf DM, Frederickson RA, et al. Detection of benign endometrial masses by endometrial stripe measurement in premenopausal women. *Obstet Gynecol* 104(1):120, 2004.

Brahma P, Martel K, et al. Future directions in myoma research. *Obstet Gynecol Clin N Am* 33(1):199–224, 2006.

Branch DW, Gibson M, et al. Recurrent Miscarriage. *N Engl J Med* 363(18):1740–747, 2010.

Branch W. Report of the obstetric APS task force: 13th international congress on antiphospholipid antibodies, 13th April 2010. *Lupus* 20(2):158–64, 2011.

Braunstein GD, Grodin JM, et al. Secretory rates of human chorionic gonadotropin by normal trophoblast. *Am J Obstet Gynecol* 15;115(4):447, 1973.

REFERENCES

Breast cancer and hormonal contraceptives: collaborative reanalysis of individual data on 53 297 women with breast cancer and 100 239 women without breast cancer from 54 epidemiological studies. Collaborative Group on Hormonal Factors in Breast Cancer. *Lancet.* Jun 22;347(9017):1713–27, 1996.

Brinton LA, Trabert B, et al. In vitro fertilization and risk of breast and gynecologic cancers: a retrospective cohort study within the Israeli Maccabi Healthcare Services. *Fertil Steril.* 2013–99(5):1189-96.

Broekmans F, Ziegler D, et al. The antral follicle count: practicle recommendations for better standardization. *Fertil Steril* 94(3):1044–51, 2010.

Brodin T, Hadziosmanovic N, et al. Antimüllerian hormone levels are strongly associated with live birth rates after assisted reproduction. *J Clin Endocrinol Metab.* Mar;98(3):1107–14, 2013.

Bromer JG, Aldad TS, et al. Defining the proliferative phase endometrial defect. *Fertil Steril* 91(1):698–704, 2009.

Brown DL, Felker RE, et al. Serial endovaginal sonography of ectopic pregnancies treated with methotrexate. *Obstet Gynecol* 77:406, 1991.

Brugers JA, Fong SL, et al. Oligoovulatory and anovulatory cycles in women with polycystic ovary syndrome (PCOS): what's the difference? *J Clin Endocrinol Metab* 95(12):485–489, 2010.

Brzezinski AA, Wurtman JJ, et al. d-Fenfluramine suppresses the increased calorie and carbohydrate intakes and improves the mood of women with premenstrual depression. *Obstet Gynecol* 76(2):296, 1990.

Buchholz T, Lohse P, et al. Polymorphisms in the ACE and PAI-1 genes are associated with recurrent spontaneous miscarriages. *Hum Reprod* 18(11):2473–2477, 2003.

Buckett WM. A meta-analysis of ultrasound-guided versus clinical touch embryo transfer. *Fertil Steril* 80(4):1037, 2003.

Burrow GN, Wortzman G, et al. Microadenomas of the pituitary and abnormal sellar tomograms in an unselected autopsy series. *N Engl J Med* 304(3):156, 1981.

Buster JE, Pisarska MD. Medical management of ectopic pregnancy. *Clinical Obstet Gynecol* 42(1):23, 1999.

Buttram VC, Jr. Mullerian anomalies and their management. *Fertil Steril* 40(2):159, 1983.

Buttram VC, Jr., Reiter RC. Abdominal myomectomy and subsequent fertility. *Fertil Steril* 36:433, 1981.

Buyalos RP, Ghosh K, et al. Infertile women of advanced reproductive age. Variability of day 3 FSH and E_2 levels. *J Reprod Med* 43(12):1023, 1998.

Callen PW. *Ultrasonography in Obstetrics and Gynecology.* San Francisco: WB Saunders, 2000.

Camus E, Poncelet C, et al. Pregnancy rates after in vitro fertilization in cases of tubal infertility with and without hydrosalpinx: a meta-analysis of published comparative studies. *Hum Reprod* 14(5):1243, 1999.

Carli C, Leclerc P, et al. Direct effect of macrophage migration inhibitory factor on sperm function: possible involvement in endometriosis-associated infertility. *Fertil Steril* 88(4):1240–47, 2007.

Carr B, Breslau N, et al. Oral contraceptive pill, GnRH agonists, or use in combination for treatment of hirsutism. *J Clin Endocrinol Metab* 60(4): 1169, 1995.

Carrell DT, Liu L, et al. Sperm DNA fragmentation is increased in couples with unexplained recurrent pregnancy loss. *Archives Andrology* 49(1):49–55, 2003.

Carrington BM, Hricak H, et al. Mullerian duct anomalies: MR imaging evaluation. *Radiology* 176(3):715, 1990.

Casper RF. Treatment of premenstrual dysphoric disorder. UpToDate Patient Information Web site: http://www.utdol.com. Accessed February 2005.

Casson PR, Elkind-Hirsch KE, et al. Effect of postmenopausal estrogen replacement on circulating androgens. *Obstet Gynecol* 90(6):995, 1997.

Castellano JM, Gaytan M. Expression of kiss-1 in rat ovary: putative local regulator of ovulation? *Endocrinology* 147(10):4852–62, 2006.

Catarci T, Fiacco F, et al. Empty sella and headache. *Headache* 34(10):583, 1994.

Centers for Disease Control and Prevention. *2001 Assisted Reproductive Technology Success Rates*, December 2003.

Chan AF, Mortola JF, et al. Persistence of premenstrual syndrome during low-dose administration of the progesterone antagonist RU 486. *Obstet Gynecol* 84(6):1001, 1994.

Chan YY, Jayaprakasan K, et al. The prevalence of congenital uterine anomalies in unselected and high-risk populations: a systematic review. *Hum Repod Update* 17(6):761–771, 2011.

Chang MY, Chiang CH, et al. Use of the antral follicle count to predict the outcome of assisted reproductive technologies. *Fertil Steril* 69(3):505, 1998.

Charny CW. The spermatogenic potential of the undescended testies before and after treatment. *J Urol* 83(1):697–705, 1960.

Chatellier G, Zapletal E, et al. The number needed to treat: a clinically useful nomogram in its proper context. *BMJ* 312(7028):426, 1996.

Chen C. Pregnancy after human oocyte cryopreservation. *Lancet* 1(8486):884–6, 1986.

Chevalier N, Letur H, et al. Materno-fetal cardiovascular complications in turner syndrome after oocytedonation: insufficient prepregnancy screening and pregnancy follow-up are associated with poor outcome. *JCEM* 96(2):0000, 2011.

Cheung AP. Ultrasound and menstrual history in predicting endometrial hyperplasia in polycystic ovary syndrome. *Obstet Gynecol* 98(2):325, 2001.

Chillon M, Casals T, et al. Mutations in the cystic fibrosis gene in patients with congenital absence of the vas deferens. *N Engl J Med* 332(22):1475, 1995.

Chipchase J, James D. Randomised trial of expectant versus surgical management of spontaneous miscarriage. *Br J Obstet Gynaecol* 104(7):840, 1997.

Choudhury SR, Knapp LA. Human reproductive failure II: immunogenetic and interacting factors. *Hum Reprod Update* 7(2):135, 2001.

Christiansen OB, Mathiesen O, et al. Idiopathic recurrent spontaneous abortion. Evidence of a familial predisposition. *Acta Obstet Gynecol Scand* 69(7–8):597–601, 1990.

Christiansen OB, Pedersen B, et al. A randomized, double-blind, placebo-controlled trial of intravenous immunoglobulin in the prevention of recurrent miscarriage: evidence for a therapeutic effect in women with secondary recurrent miscarriage. *Hum Reprod* 17(3):809, 2002.

Chuong CJ, Dawson EB, et al. Vitamin A levels in premenstrual syndrome. *Fertil Steril* 54(4):643, 1990a.

Chuong CJ, Dawson EB, et al. Vitamin E levels in premenstrual syndrome. *Am J Obstet Gynecol* 163(5 Pt 1):1591, 1990b.

Chung K, Sammel M, et al. Defining the curve when initial levels of human chorionic gonadotropin in patients with spontaneous abortions are low. *Fertil Steril* 85(2):508–10, 2006.

REFERENCES

Cibula D, Zikan M, et al. Oral contraceptives and risk of ovarian and breast cancers in BRCA mutation carriers: a meta-analysis. *Expert Rev Anticancer Ther.* Aug;11(8):1197–207, 2011.

Ciccarelli E, Camanni F. Diagnosis and drug therapy of prolactinoma. *Drugs* 51(6):954, 1996.

Ciotta L, Cianci A, et al. Clinical and endocrine effects of finasteride, a 5 α-reductase inhibitor, in women with idiopathic hirsutism. *Fertil Steril* 64(2): 299, 1995.

Cicinelli E, Resta L. et al. Endometrial micropolyps at fluid hysteroscopy suggest the existence of chronic endometrits. *Hum Reprod* 5(1):1386–9, 2005.

Clarke GN, Elliott PJ, et al. Detection of sperm antibodies in semen using the immunobead test: a survey of 813 consecutive patients. *Am J Reprod Immunol Microbiol* 7(3):118, 1985.

Cnattingius S, Signorello LB, et al. Caffeine intake and the risk of first-trimester spontaneous abortion. *N Engl J Med* 343(25):1839, 2000.

Cobo A, Meseguer M, et al. Use of cryo-banked oocytes in an ovum donation programme: a prospective, randomized, controlled, clinical trial. *Hum Reprod* 25(9):2239–2246, 2010.

Coccia E, Rizello F, et al. Endometriosis and infertility surgery and ART: an integrated approach for successful management. *Euro J Obstet Gynecol* 138(1):54–59, 2008.

Cocksedge KA, Li TC, et al. A reappraisal of the role of polycystic ovary syndrome in recurrentmiscarriage. *Reprod Biomed Online* 17(1):151–60, 2008.

Cohen S, Einarsson J. The role of mechanical bowel preparation in gynecologic laparoscopy. *Obstest Gynecol* 4(1):28–31, 2011.

Cohen L, Valle R. Role of vaginal sonography and hysterosonography in the endoscopic treatment of uterine myomas. *Fertil Steril* 73(2):197–204, 2000.

Col NF, Pauker SG. The discrepancy between observational studies and randomized trials of menopausal hormone therapy: did expectations shape experience? *Ann Intern Med* 139(11):923, 2003.

Colao A, Di Sarno A, et al. Withdrawal of long-term cabergoline therapy for tumoral and nontumoral hyperprolactinemia. *N Engl J Med* 349(21):2023, 2003.

Colao A, Di Somma C, et al. Prolactinomas in adolescents: persistent bone loss after 2 years of prolactin normalization. *Clin Endocrinol (Oxf)* 52(3):319, 2000.

Colditz GA, Stampfer MJ, et al. Type of postmenopausal hormone use and risk of breast cancer: 12-year follow-up from the Nurses' Health Study. *Cancer Causes Control* 3(5):433, 1992.

Cole LA. Phantom hCG and phantom choriocarcinoma. *Gynecol Oncol* 71(2): 325, 1998.

Cole LA, Khanlian SA, et al. Accuracy of home pregnancy tests at the time of missed menses. *Am J Obstet Gynecol* 190(1):100, 2004.

Conde-Agudelo A, Rosas-Bermúdez A, et al. Birth spacing and risk of adverse perinatal outcomes: a meta-analysis. *JAMA* 295(15):1809–23, 2006.

Condon JT. The premenstrual syndrome: a twin study. *Br J Psychiatry* 162:481, 1993.

Contant C, Hop W, et al. Mechanical bowel preparation for elective colorectal surgery: a multicentre randomized trial. *Lancet* 370(1):2112–17,2007.

Cooper DS. Subclinical hypothyroidism. *New Engl J Med* 345(4):260, 2001.

Cooper T, Noonan E, et al. World health organization reference values for human semen characteristics. *Hum Reprod* 0(0):1–15, 2009.

Copperman AB, Wells V, et al. Presence of hydrosalpinx correlated to endometrial inflammatory response in vivo. *Fertil Steril* 86(4):972–6, 2006.

Corenblum B, Donovan L. The safety of physiological estrogen plus progestin replacement therapy and with oral contraceptive therapy in women with pathological hyperprolactinemia. *Fertil Steril* 59(3):671, 1993.

Coric M, Barisic D, et al. Electrocoagulation versus suture after laparoscopic stripping of ovarian endometriomas assessed by antral follicle count: preliminary results of randomized clinical trial. *Arch Gynecol Obstet* 283:373–378, 2011.

Coulam CB, Adamson SC, et al. Incidence of premature ovarian failure. *Obstet Gynecol* 67:604, 1986.

Coulam CB, Bustillo M, et al. Ultrasonographic predictors of implantation after assisted reproduction. *Fertil Steril* 62(5):1004, 1994.

Courbiere B, Oborski V, et al. Obstetric outcome of women with in vitro fertilization pregnancieshospitalized for ovarian hyperstimulation syndrome: a case-control study. *Fertil Steril* 95(5):1629–32, 2011.

Coutifaris C, Myers ER, et al. Histological dating of timed endometrial biopsy tissue is not related to fertility status. *Fertil Steril* 82(5):1264, 2004.

Coutinho EM, Mascarenhas I, et al. Comparative study on the efficacy, acceptability, and side effects of a contraceptive pill administered by the oral and the vaginal route: an international multicenter clinical trial. *Clin Pharmacol Ther* 54(5):540, 1993.

Couzinet B, Meduri G, et al. The postmenopausal ovary is not a major androgen-producing gland. *J Clin Endocrinol Metab* 86(10):5060, 2001.

Craig LB, Ke RW, et al. Increased prevalence of insulin resistance in women with a history of recurrent pregnancy loss. *Fertil Steril* 78(3):487, 2002.

Creinin MD. Laboratory criteria for menopause in women using oral contraceptives. *Fertil Steril* 66(1):101, 1996.

Creinin MD, Schwartz JL, et al. Early pregnancy failure—current management concepts. *Obstet Gynecol Surv* 56(2):105, 2001.

Creus M, Penarrubia J, et al. Day 3 serum inhibin B and FSH and age as predictors of assisted reproduction treatment outcome. *Hum Reprod* 15(11):2341, 2000.

Crosignani P. Current treatment issues in female hyperprolactinaemia. *Euro J Obstet Gynecol* 125(2):152–64, 2006.

Cruz Lee S, Kaunitz A, et al. The oncogenic potential of endometrial polyps. *Obstet Gynecol* 116(5):1197–1205, 2010

Csapo AI, Pulkkinen M. Indispensability of the human corpus luteum in the maintenance of early pregnancy. Luteectomy evidence. *Obstet Gynecol Surv* 33(2):69, 1978.

Csokmay JM, Frattarelli JL. Basal ovarian cysts and clomiphene citrate ovulation induction cycles. *Obstet Gynecol* 107(6):1292–96, 2006.

Curtis KM, Chrisman CE, et al. Contraception for women in selected circumstances. *Obstet Gynecol* 99(6):1100, 2002.

Cutting R, Morroll D, et al. Elective single embryo transfer: guidelines for practice british fertility societyand association of clinical embryologists. *Hum Fertility* 11(3):131–146, 2008.

D'Agostino RB, Wolf PA, et al. Stroke risk profile: adjustment for antihypertensive medication. The Framingham study. *Stroke* 25(1):40–43, 1994.

D'Ercole M, Della Pepa G, et al. Two diagnostic pitfalls mimicking a prolactin-secreting microdenoma. *J Clin Endocrinol Metab* 95(12):5171, 2010.

REFERENCES

Dabirashrafi H, Bahadori M, et al. Septate uterus: new idea on the histologic features of the septum in this abnormal uterus. *Am J Obstet Gynecol* 172(1 Pt 1):105, 1995.

Dabirashrafi H, Mohammad K, et al. Is estrogen necessary after hysteroscopic incision of the uterine septum? *J Am Assoc Gynecol Laparosc.* 3(4):623-5, 1996.

Daftary G, Kayisli U, et al. Salpingectomy increases peri-implantation endometrial HOXA10 expression in women with hydrosalpinx. *Fertil Steril* 87(2):367–72, 2007.

Daly DC, Walters CA, et al. A randomized study of dexamethasone in ovulation induction with clomiphene citrate. *Fertil Steril* 41(6):844, 1984.

Damewood MD, Shen W, et al. Disappearance of exogenously administered human chronic gonadotropin. *Fertil Steril* 52(3):398–400, 1989.

Daniell JF, Miller W. Polycystic ovaries treated by laparoscopic laser vaporization. *Fertil Steril* 51(2):232, 1989.

Davies MJ, Moore VM, et al. Reproductive technologies and the risk of birth defects. N Engl J Med. 10;366(19):1803–13, 2012.

Davis AR, Kroll R, et al. Occurance of menses or pregnancy after cessation of a continuous oral contraceptive. *Fertil Steril* 89(5):1059–63, 2008.

Davis AR, Moreau M, et al. Testosterone for low libido in postmenopausal women not taking estrogen. *N Engl Med* 19(1):359, 2008.

Davis OK, Berkeley AS, et al. The incidence of luteal phase defect in normal, fertile women, determined by serial endometrial biopsies. *Fertil Steril* 51(4):582, 1989.

Davis SR, Burger HG. Androgens and the postmenopausal woman. *J Clin Endorinol Metab* 81(8):2759–63, 2007.

Davis SR, Davison SL, et al. Circulating androgen levels and self-reported sexual function in women. *JAMA* 294(1):91–96, 2005.

Davison SL, Bell R, et al. Androgen levels in adult females: changes with age, menopause, andoophorectomy. *J of Clin Endocrinol Metab* 90(7):3847–3853, 2005.

Davenport M. Approach to the patient with turner syndrome. *JCEM* 95(4):1487–1495, 2010.

Davis RO, Katz DF. Computer-aided sperm analysis: technology at a crossroads. *Fertil Steril* 59(5):953, 1993.

Daya S, Ward S, et al. Progesterone profiles in luteal phase defect cycles and outcome of progesterone treatment in patients with recurrent spontaneous abortion. *Am J Obstet Gynecol* 158(2):225, 1988.

De Cherney AH, Boyer SP. Isthmic ectopic pregnancy: segmental resection as the treatment choice. *Fertil Steril* 44(3):307–12, 1985.

de Kroon CD, de Bock GH, et al. Saline contrast hysterosonography in abnormal uterine bleeding: a systematic review and meta-analysis. *BJOG* 110(10):938, 2003.

De Placido G, Alviggi C, et al. Serum concentrations of soluble human leukocyte class I antigens and of the soluble intercellular adhesion molecule-1 in endometriosis: relationship with stage and non-pigmented peritoneal lesions. *Hum Reprod* 13(11):3206, 1998.

De Souza MJ, Miller BE, et al. High frequency of luteal phase deficiency and anovulation in recreational women runners: blunted elevation in follicle-stimulating hormone observed during luteal-follicular transition. *J Clin Endocrinol Metab* 83(12):4220, 1998.

De Witt, W., Gowrising, CJ., Kuik, DJ. et al. (1997) Only hydrosalpinges visible on ultrasound are associated with reduced implantation and pregnancy rates after IVF. (Abstr.) *Hum.Reprod.*, 12 (Abstract book 1), 170, P-105.

de Ziegler D, Borghese B, Chapron C. Endometriosis and infertility: pathophysiology and management. *Lancet.* 2010 Aug 28;376(9742):730–8.

Deaton JL, Gibson M, et al. A randomized, controlled trial of clomiphene citrate and intrauterine insemination in couples with unexplained infertility or surgically corrected endometriosis. *Fertil Steril* 54(6):1083, 1990.

Deaton JL, Honore GM, et al. Early transvaginal ultrasound following an accurately dated pregnancy: the importance of finding a yolk sac or fetal heart motion. *Hum Reprod* 12(12):2820, 1997.

Deichert U, Schleif R, et al. Transvaginal hysterosalpingo-contrast-sonography (Hy-Co-Sy) compared with conventional tubal diagnostics. *Hum Reprod* 4(4):418–24, 1989.

Dekkers OM, Pereira AM, et al. Treatment and follow-up of clinically nonfunctioning pituitary macroadenomas. *J Clin Endocrinol Metab* 93(10):3717–3726, 2008.

Delemarre-van de Waal HA. Regulation of puberty. *Best Pract Res Clin Endocrinol Metab* 16(1):1, 2002.

Delmas PD. Markers of bone turnover for monitoring treatment of osteoporosis with antiresorptive drugs. *Osteoporos Int* 11[Suppl 6]:S66, 2000.

Del Mastro L, Boni L, et al. Effect of the gonadotropin-releasing hormone analogue triptorelin on the occurrence of chemotherapy-induced early menopause in premenopausal women with breast cancer: a randomized trial. *JAMA.* 306(3):269–76, 2011.

Dennerstein L, Randolph J, et al. Hormones, mood, sexuality, and the menopausal transition. *Fertil Steril* 77[Suppl 4]:S42, 2002.

DeWaay DJ, Syrop CH, et al. Natural history of uterine polyps and leiomyomata. *American College of Obstetricians and Gynecologists* 100(1):3–7, 2002.

D'Hooghe TM, Debrock S, et al. Endometriosis and subfertility: is the relationship resolved? *Semin Reprod Med* 21(2):243, 2003.

D'Hooghe TM, Hill JA. Killer cell activity, statistics, and endometriosis. *Fertil Steril* 64(1):226, 1995.

Dias Pereira G, Hajenius PJ, et al. Fertility outcome after systemic methotrexate and laparoscopic salpingostomy for tubal pregnancy. *Lancet* 353(9154):724, 1999.

Diaz I, Navarro J, et al. Impact of stage III-IV endometriosis on recipients of sibling oocytes: matched case-control study. *Fertil Steril* 74(1):31–34, 2000.

Dickey RP, Olar TT, et al. Relationship of endometrial thickness and pattern to fecundity in ovulation induction cycles: effect of clomiphene citrate alone and with human menopausal gonadotropin. *Fertil Steril* 59(4):756, 1993.

DiSaia PJ, Creasman WT. Epithelial ovarian cancer. In *Clinical Gynecologic Oncology.* St. Louis: Mosby Year Book, 1997:529.

Dizerega GS, Barber DL, et al. Endometriosis: role of ovarian steroids in initiation, maintenance, and suppression. *Fertil Steril* 33(6):649, 1980.

Djahanbakhch O, McNeily AS, et al. Changes in plasma levels of prolactin, in relation to those of FSH, oestradiol, androstenedione and progesterone around the preovulatory surge of LH in women. *Clin Endocrinol (Oxf)* 20:463, 1984.

Dohle GR, Halley DJ, et al. Genetic risk factors in infertile men with severe oligozoospermia and azoospermia. *Hum Reprod* 17(1):13, 2002.

REFERENCES

Dokras, A, Baredziak L, et al. Obstetric outcomes after in vitro fertilization in obese and morbidly obese women. *American College of Obstetricians and Gynecologists* 108(1):61–69, 2006.

Dolmans MM, Luyckx V, et al. Risk of transferring malignant cells with transplanted frozen-thawed ovarian tissue. *Fertil Steril.* 99(6):1514–22, 2013.

Donnez J, Dolmans MM, et al. Livebirth after orthotopic transplantation of cryopreserved ovarian tissue. *Lancet* 364(9443):1405, 2004.

Donnez J, Dolmans MM, et al. Restoration of ovarian activity and pregnancy after transplantation of cryopreserved ovarian tissue: a review of 60 cases of reimplantation. *Fertil Steril.* 99(6):1503–13, 2013

Donnez J, Nisolle M, et al. Peritoneal endometriosis and "endometriotic" nodules of the rectovaginal septum are two different entities. *Fertil Steril* 66:362, 1996.

Dorn C, Mouillet JF, et al. Insulin enhances the transcription of luteinizing hormone-beta gene. *Am J Obstet Gynecol* 191(1):132, 2004.

Duffy JM, Ahmad G, et al. Growth hormone for in vitro fertilization. *Cochrane Database Syst Rev.* 2010 Jan 20;(1):CD000099.

Dunaif A. Insulin resistance and the polycystic ovary syndrome: mechanism and implications for pathogenesis. *Endocr Rev* 18(6):774, 1997.

Dunaif A, Zia J, et al. Excessive insulin receptor serine phosphorylation in cultured fibroblasts and in skeletal muscle. A potential mechanism for insulin resistance in the polycystic ovary syndrome. *J Clin Invest* 96(2):801, 1995.

Dunn JF, Nisula BC, et al. Transport of steroid hormones: binding of 21 endogenous steroids to both testosterone-binding globulin and corticosteroid-binding globulin in human plasma. *J Clin Endocrinol Metab* 53(1):58, 1981.

Dunson DB, Colombo B, et al. Changes with age in the level and duration of fertility in the menstrual cycle. *Hum Reprod* 17(5):1399, 2002.

Ecochard R, Gougeon A. Side of ovulation and cycle characteristics in normally fertile women. *Hum Reprod* 15(4):752, 2000.

Edmonds DK, Lindsay KS, et al. Early embryonic mortality in women. *Fertil Steril* 38(4):447, 1982.

Elias KA, Weiner RI. Direct arterial vascularization of estrogen-induced prolactin-secreting anterior pituitary tumors. *Proc Natl Acad Sci USA* 81(14):4549, 1984.

Elnashar A, Abdelmageed E, et al. Clomiphene citrate and dexamethazone in treatment of clomiphene citrate-resistant polycystic ovary syndrome: a prospective placebo-controlled study. *Hum Reprod.* 2006 Jul;21(7):1805–8.

Elting MW, Korsen TJ, et al. Women with polycystic ovary syndrome gain regular menstrual cycles when ageing. *Hum Reprod* 15(1):24, 2000.

Empson M, Lassere M, et al. Recurrent pregnancy loss with antiphospholipid antibody: a systematic review of therapeutic trials. *Obstet Gynecol* 99(1):135, 2002.

Erdem M, Erdem M, et al. Impact of luteal phase support on pregnancy rates in intrauterine insemination cycles: a prospective randomized study. *Fertil Steril* 91(6):2508–13, 2009.

Erickson GF, Magoffin DA, et al. The ovarian androgen producing cells: a review of structure/function relationships. *Endocr Rev* 6(3):371, 1985.

Eskenazi B, Wyrobek AJ, et al. The association of age and semen quality in healthy men. *Hum Reprod* 18(2):447, 2003.

Espeland MA, Rapp SR, et al. Conjugated equine estrogens and global cognitive function in postmenopausal women: Women's Health Initiative Memory study. *JAMA* 291(24):2959, 2004.

Ettinger B, Ensrud KE, et al. Effects of ultralow-dose transdermal estradiol on bone mineral density: a randomized clinical trial. *Obstet Gynecol* 104(3):443, 2004.

Ettinger MP. Aging bone and osteoporosis: strategies for preventing fractures in the elderly. *Arch Intern Med* 163(18):2237, 2003.

Facchinetti F, Borella P, et al. Oral magnesium successfully relieves premenstrual mood changes. *Obstet Gynecol* 78(2):177, 1991.

Fanchin R, Righini C, et al. New look at endometrial echogenicity: objective computer-assisted measurements predict endometrial receptivity in in vitro fertilization-embryo transfer. *Fertil Steril* 74(2):274, 2000.

Farhi J, Ashkenazi J, et al. Effect of uterine leiomyomata on the results of in vitro fertilization treatment. *Hum Reprod* 10(10):2576, 1995.

Farley TM, Meirik O, et al. Cardiovascular disease and combined oral contraceptives: reviewing the evidence and balancing the risks. *Hum Reprod Update* 5(6):721, 1999.

Farquhar C. Eptopic Pregnancy. *Lancet.* 366:583–91, 2005.

Farquhar CM, Harvey SA, et al. A prospective study of 3 years of outcomes after hysterectomy with and without oophorectomy. *Am J Obstet Gynecol* 194(3):711–7, 2006.

Farquhar CM, Lethaby A, et al. An evaluation of risk factors for endometrial hyperplasia in premenopausal women with abnormal menstrual bleeding. *Am J Obstet Gynecol* 181(3):525, 1999.

Fassnacht M, Schlenz N, et al. Beyond adrenal and ovarian androgen generation: increased peripheral 5 alpha-reductase activity in women with polycystic ovary syndrome. *J Clin Endocrinol Metab* 88(6):2760, 2003.

Fatemi HM. The luteal phase and ovarian stimulation. *Erupean Obstet Gynecol* 4(1):26–29, 2009.

Fatemi HM, Kasius JC, et al. Prevalence of unsuspected uterine cavity abnormalities diagnosed by office hysteroscopy prior to in vitro fertilization. *Hum Reprod.* 25(8):1959–65, 2010.

Favus, MJ. Bisphosphonates for osteoporosis. *N Engl J Med* 363(21):2027–35, 2010.

Fechner P, Davenport M, et al. Differences in follicle-stimulating hormone secretion between 45,X monosomy turner syndrome and 45,X/46,XX mosaicism are evident at an early age. *JCEM* 91(12):4896–4902, 2006.

Fedele L, Bianchi S, et al. Superovulation with human menopausal gonadotropins in the treatment of infertility associated with minimal or mild endometriosis: a controlled randomized study. *Fertil Steril* 58(1):28, 1992.

Fedele L, Bianchi S, et al. Residual uterine septum of less than 1 cm after hysteroscopic metroplasty does not impair reproductive outcome. *Hum Reprod* 11(4):727, 1996a.

Fedele L, Bianchi S, et al. Ultrastructural aspects of endometrium in infertile women with septate uterus. *Fertil Steril* 65(4):750, 1996b.

Fedele L, Bianchi S, et al. Transrectal ultrasonography in the assessment of rectovaginal endometriosis. *Obstet Gynecol* 91:444, 1998.

Feicht CB, Johnson TS, et al. Secondary amenorrhoea in athletes. *Lancet* 2(8100):1145, 1978.

Feigenbaum SL, Downey DE, et al. Transsphenoidal pituitary resection for preoperative diagnosis of prolactin-secreting pituitary adenoma in women: long term follow-up. *J Clin Endocrinol Metab* 81(5):1711, 1996.

Feinberg EC, Molitch ME, et al. The incidence of sheehan's syndrome after obstetric hemorrhage. *Fertil Steril* 84(4):975–9, 2005.

REFERENCES

Felemban A, Tan SL, et al. Laparoscopic treatment of polycystic ovaries with insulated needle cautery: a reappraisal. *Fertil Steril* 73(2):266, 2000.

Ferrero S, Gillott DJ, et al. Use of aromatase inhibitors to treat endometriosis-related pain symptoms: a systematic review. *Reprod Biol Endo* 9:89, 2011.

Fernandez E, La Vecchia C, et al. Oral contraceptives and colorectal cancer risk: a meta-analysis. *Br J Cancer* 84(5):722, 2001.

Ferriman D, Gallwey JD. Clinical assessment of body hair growth in women. *J Clin Endocrinol Metab* 21:1440, 1961.

Fertility Plus. http://www.fertilityplus.org. Accessed February 2005.

Feuillan P, Calis K, et al. Letrozole treatment of precocious puberty in girls with the McCune-Albright Syndrome: A pilot study. *J Clin Endocrinol Metab* 92(6):2100–2106, 2007.

Filicori M, Cognigni GE. Roles and novel regimens of luteinizing hormone and follicle-stimulating hormone in ovulation induction. *J Clin Endocrinol Metab* 86(4):1437, 2001.

Fishel SB, Edwards RG, et al. Human chorionic gonadotropin secreted by preimplantation embryos cultured in vitro. *Science* 223(4638):816, 1984.

Foma F, Gulmezoglu AM. Surgical procedures to evacuate incomplete abortion (Cochrane Review). In *The Cochrane Library*. Chichester, UK: John Wiley and Sons, 2003.

Fordney Settlage DS, Motoshima M, et al. Sperm transport from the external cervical os to the fallopian tubes in women: a time and quantitation study. *Fertil Steril* 24(9):655–61, 1973.

Foresta C, Moro E, et al. Prognostic value of Y deletion analysis. The role of current methods. *Hum Reprod* 16(8):1543, 2001.

Forman EJ, Upham KM, et al. Comprehensive chromosome screening alters traditional morphology-based embryo selection: a prospective study of 100 consecutive cycles of planned fresh euploid blastocyst transfer. *Fertil Steril*. 2013 [Epub ahead of print]

Forman EJ, Hong KH, et al. In vitro fertilization with single euploid blastocyst transfer: a randomized controlled trial. *Fertil Steril*. 2013 [Epub 2013]

Foulk RA, Martin MC, et al. Hyperreactio luteinalis differentiated from severe ovarian hyperstimulation syndrome in a spontaneously conceived pregnancy. *Am J Obstet Gynecol* 176(6):1300; discussion, 1302, 1997.

Frank RT. The hormonal causes of premenstrual tension. *Arch Neurol Psychiatr* 26:1052, 1931.

Frank RT. Formation of artificial vagina without operation. *Am J Obstet Gynecol* 35:1053, 1938.

Franssen MT, Musters AM, et al. Reproductive outcome after PGD in couples with recurrent miscarriagecarrying a structural chromosome abnormality: a systematic review. *Hum Reprod Update* 17(4):467–75, 2011.

Frattarelli JL, Lauria-Costab DF, et al. Basal antral follicle number and mean ovarian diameter predict cycle cancellation and ovarian responsiveness in assisted reproductive technology cycles. *Fertil Steril* 74(3):512, 2000.

Frattarelli JL, Levi AJ, et al. A prospective assessment of the predictive value of basal antral follicles in in vitro fertilization cycles. *Fertil Steril* 80(2):350, 2003.

Freedman RR, Roehrs TA. Lack of sleep disturbance from menopausal hot flashes. *Fertil Steril* 82(1):138, 2004.

Freeman EW, Kroll R, et al.; PMS/PMDD Research Group. Evaluation of a unique oral contraceptive in the treatment of premenstrual dysphoric disorder. *J Womens Health Gend Based Med* 10(6):561, 2001.

Freeman EW, Sammel MD, et al. Duration of menopausal hot flushes and associated risk factors. *Obstet Gynecol* 117(5):1095–104, 2011.

Freiesleben N, Lossl K, et al. Predictors of ovarian response in intrauterine insemination patients and development of a dosage nomogram. *Reprod BioMed Online* 17(5):632–641, 2008.

Friedler S, Margalioth EJ, et al. Incidence of post-abortion intra-uterine adhesions evaluated by hysteroscopy—a prospective study. *Hum Reprod* 8(3):442, 1993.

Friedman AJ, Daly M, et al. Recurrence of myomas after myomectomy in women pretreated with leuprolide acetate depot or placebo. *Fertil Steril* 58(1):205, 1992.

Fritz B, Hallermann C, et al. Cytogenetic analyses of culture failures by comparative genomic hybridisation (CGH)-Re-evaluation of chromosome aberration rates in early spontaneous abortions. *Eur J Hum Genet* 9(7):539, 2001.

Fruzzetti F, Bersi C, et al. Treatment of hirsutism: comparisons between different antiandrogens with central and peripheral effects. *Fertil Steril* 71:445, 1999.

Fujimoto VY, Clifton DK, et al. Variability of serum prolactin and progesterone levels in normal women: the relevance of single hormone measurements in the clinical setting. *Obstet Gynecol* 76(1):71, 1990.

Fulghesu AM, Romualdi D, et al. Is there a dose-response relationship of metformin treatment in patients with polycystic ovary syndrome? Results from a multicentric study. *Hum Reprod.* 10:3057, 2012

Garcia-Enguidanos A. Long-term use of oral contraceptives increases the risk of miscarriage. *Fertil Steril* 83:1864–66, 2005.

Garcia-Velasco JA, Arici A, et al. Macrophage derived growth factors modulate Fas ligand expression in cultured endometrial stromal cells: a role in endometriosis. *Mol Hum Reprod* 5(7):642, 1999.

Garcia-Velasco JA, Mahutte NG, et al. Removal of endometriomas before in vitro fertilization does not improve fertility outcomes: a matched, case-control study. *Fertil Steril* 81(5):1194, 2004.

Gebbie AE, Glasier A, et al. Incidence of ovulation in perimenopausal women before and during hormone replacement therapy. *Contraception* 52(4):221–22, 1995.

George L, Mills JL, et al. Plasma folate levels and risk of spontaneous abortion. *JAMA* 288(15):1867, 2002.

Ghanem M, Bakre N, et al. The effects of timing of intrauterine insemination in relation to ovulation and the number of inseminations on cycle pregnancy rate in common infertility etiologies. *Hum Reprod* 26(3):576–583, 2011.

Ghezzi F, Beretta P, et al. Recurrence of ovarian endometriosis and anatomical location of the primary lesion. *Fertil Steril* 75(1):136, 2001.

Ghezzi F, Raio L, et al. Vaginal extraction of pelvic masses following operative laparoscopy. *Surg Endosc* 16(12):1691, 2002.

Gillam MP, Midder S, et al. The novel use of very high doses of cabergoline and a combination of testosterone and a aromatase inhibitor in the treatment of a giant prolactinoma. *J Clin Endocrinol Metab* 87(10):4447–451, 2002.

Givens JR. Polycystic ovaries—a sign, not a diagnosis. *Semin Reprod Endocrinol* 34:67, 1984.

Gjønnæss H. Polycystic ovarian syndrome treated by ovarian electrocautery through the laparoscope. *Fertil Steril* 41(1):20, 1984.

Gjønnæss H. Late endocrine effects of ovarian electrocautery in women with polycystic ovary syndrome. *Fertil Steril* 69(4):697, 1998.

Glasow A, Breidert M, et al. Functional aspects of the effect of prolactin (PRL) on adrenal steroidogenesis and distribution of the PRL receptor in the human adrenal gland. *J Clin Endocrinol Metab* 81(8):3103, 1996.

Glatstein IZ, Pang SC, McShane PM. Successful pregnancies with the use of laminaria tents before embryo transfer for refractory cervical stenosis. *Fertil Steril*. 1997 Jun;67(6):1172–4.

Glick H, Endicott J, et al. Premenstrual changes: are they familial? *Acta Psychiatr Scand* 88(3):149, 1993.

Glueck CJ, Wang P, et al. Metformin therapy throughout pregnancy reduces the development of gestational diabetes in women with polycystic ovary syndrome. *Fertil Steril* 77(3):520, 2002a.

Gnoth C, Godehardt D, et al. Time to pregnancy: results of the German prospective study and impact on the management of infertility. *Hum Reprod* 18(9):1959, 2003.

Golan A, Ron-El R, et al. Ovarian hyperstimulation syndrome: an update review. *Obstet Gynecol Surv* 44:430, 1989.

Golbus MJ. Chromosome aberrations and mammalian reproduction. In Mastroianni L, Biggers JD, eds. *Fertilization and Embryonic Development In Vitro*. New York: Plenum Press, 1981.

Goldstein SR. Modern evaluation of the endometrium. *Obstet Gynecol*. 116(1):168–76, 2010.

Gordon C. Functional hypothalamic amenorrhea. *N Engl J Med* 363:365–71, 2010.

Gordon JD, Rydfors JT, et al., eds. *Obstetrics Gynecology and Infertility* (5th ed). Arlington, VA: Scrub Hill Press, Inc., 2001.

Gordts S, Campo R, et al. Clinical factors determining pregnancy outcome after microsurgical tubal reanastomsis. *Fertil Steril* 92(4):1198–202, 2009.

Gougeon A. Dynamics of follicular growth in the human: a model from preliminary results. *Hum Reprod* 1(2):81, 1986.

Gosden RG, Wade JC, et al. Impact of congenital or experimental hypogonadotrophism on the radiation sensitivity of the mouse ovary. *Hum Reprod* 12(11):2483–88, 1997.

Gnoth C, Schuring AN, et al. Relevance of anti-müllerian hormone measurement in a routine IVF program. *Hum Reprod* 23(6):1359–1365, 2008.

Gnoth C, Godehardt E, et al. Definition and nprevalence of subfertility and infertility. *Hum Reprod* 20(5):1144–47, 2005.

Grady D. Management of menopausal symptoms. *N Engl J Med* 355(1):2338–47, 2006.

Grady D, Herrington D, et al. Cardiovascular disease outcomes during 6.8 years of hormone therapy: Heart and Estrogen/Progestin Replacement Study Follow-up (HERS II). *JAMA* 288(1):49, 2002.

Gravholt CH, Fedder J, et al. Occurrence of gonadoblastoma in females with Turner syndrome and Y chromosome material: a population study. *J Clin Endocrinol Metab* 85(9):3199, 2000.

Green J, Berrington G, et al. Risk factors for adenocarcinoma and squamous cell carcinoma of the cervix in women aged 20–44 years: the UK national case-control study of cervical cancer. *Cancer* 89(1):2078–86, 2003.

Greene R, Dalton K. The premenstrual syndrome. *Br Med J* i:1007, 1953.

Greenspan SL, Resnick NM, et al. Combination therapy with hormone replacement and alendronate for prevention of bone loss in elderly women: a randomized controlled trial. *JAMA* 289(19):2525, 2003.

Greer IA. Exploring the role of low-molecular-weight heparins in pregnancy. *Semin Thromb Hemost* 28[Suppl 3]:25, 2002.

Griffin JE, Edwards C, et al. Congenital absence of the vagina. *Ann Intern Med* 85:224, 1976.

Griffith CS, Grimes DA. The validity of the postcoital test. *Am J Obstet Gynecol* 162(3):615, 1990.

Grimes DA, Jones LB, et al. Oral contraceptives for functional ovarian cysts. *Cochrane Database Syst Rev* 7(9):6134, 2011.

Grimes DA, Schulz KF. False alarms and pseudo-epidemics: the limitations of observational epidemiology. *Obstet Gynecol.* 2012 Oct;120(4):920–7.

Groeneveld E, Broeze KA, et al. Is asprin effective in women undergoing in vitro fertilization (IVF)?Results from an individual patient data meta-analysis (IPD MA). *Hum Reprod* 17(4):501–509, 2011.

Gull B, Karlsson B, et al. Can ultrasound replace dilation and curettage? A longitudinal evaluation of postmenopausal bleeding and transvaginal sonographic measurement of the endometrium as predictors of endometrial cancer. *Am J Obstet Gynecol* 188(2):401, 2003.

Gupta JK, Chien PF, et al. Ultrasonographic endometrial thickness for diagnosing endometrial pathology in women with postmenopausal bleeding: a meta-analysis. *Acta Obstet Gynecol Scand* 81(9):799, 2002.

Gupta S. Weight gain on the combined pill—is it real? *Hum Reprod Update* 6(5):427, 2000.

Guzick D, Huang L, et al. Randomized trial of leuprolide versus continuous oral contraceptives in the treatment of endometriosis-associated pelvic pain. *Fertil Steril* 95(5):1568–73, 2011.

Guzick D, Wing R, et al. Endocrine consequences of weight loss in obese, hyperandrogenic, anovulatory women. *Fertil Steril* 61(4):598, 1994.

Guzick DS, Carson SA, et al. Efficacy of superovulation and intrauterine insemination in the treatment of infertility. National Cooperative Reproductive Medicine Network. *N Engl J Med* 340(3):177, 1999.

Guzick DS, Overstreet JW, et al. Sperm morphology, motility, and concentration in fertile and infertile men. *N Engl J Med* 345(19):1388, 2001.

Guzick DS, Sullivan MW, et al. Efficacy of treatment for unexplained infertility. *Fertil Steril* 70(2):207, 1998.

Gyang A, Hartman M, Lamvu G. Muskuloskeletal causes of chronic pelvic pain: What a gynecologist should know. *Obstetrics and Gynecology* 121:645,2013

Gysler M, March CM, et al. A decade's experience with an individualized clomiphene treatment regimen including its effect on the postcoital test. *Fertil Steril* 37(2):161, 1982.

Hagman A, Källén K, et al. Obstetric outcomes in women with turner karyotype. *JCEM* 96(11):3475–3482, 2011.

Haimov-Kochman R et al. Spontaneous ovarian hyperstimulation syndrome and hyperreactio luteinalis are entities in continuum. *Ultrasound Obstet Gynecol* 24:675, 2004.

Halbreich U, Smoller JW. Intermittent luteal phase sertraline treatment of dysphoric premenstrual syndrome. *J Clin Psychiatry* 58(9):399, 1997.

Halbreich U, Tworek H. Altered serotonergic activity in women with dysphoric premenstrual syndromes. *Int J Psychiatry Med* 23(1):1, 1993.

Hallberg L, Högdahl AM, et al. Menstrual blood loss—a population study. Variation at different ages and attempts to define normality. *Acta Obstet Gynecol Scand* 45(3):320–51, 1966.

Halme J, Becker S, et al. Altered maturation and function of peritoneal macrophages: possible role in pathogenesis of endometriosis. *Am J Obstet Gynecol* 156(4):783, 1987.

Hammadieh N, Coomarasamy A, et al. Ultrasound-guided hydrosalpinx aspiration during oocytecollection improves pregnancy outcome in IVF: a randomized controlled trial. *Hum Reprod* 23(5):1113–1117, 2008

Hammond MG, Jordan S, et al. Factors affecting pregnancy rates in a donor insemination program using frozen semen. *Am J Obstet Gynecol* 155(3): 480, 1986.

Hanafi M. Predictors of leiomyoma recurrence after myomectomy. *Am J Obstet Gynecol* 105(4):877–81, 2005.

Hankinson SE, Willett WC, et al. Plasma prolactin levels and subsequent risk of breast cancer in postmenopausal women. *J Natl Cancer Inst* 91(7):629, 1999.

Hansen LM, Batzer FR, et al. Evaluating ovarian reserve: follicle stimulating hormone and oestradiol variability during cycle days 2–5. *Hum Reprod* 11(3):486, 1996.

Harada T, Momoeda M, et al. Low-dose oral contraceptive pill for dysmenorrheal associated withendometriosis: a placebo-controlled double-blind, randomized trial. *Fertil Steril* 90(5):1583–8, 2007.

Harada M, Osuga Y, et al. Concentration of osteoprotegerin (OPG) in peritoneal fluid is increased in women with endometriosis. *Hum Reprod* 19(10):2188, 2004.

Hardiman P, Pillay OC, et al. Polycystic ovary syndrome and endometrial carcinoma. *Lancet* 361(9371):1810, 2003.

Harris SE, Chand AL, et al. INHA promoter polymorphisms are associate with premature ovarian failure. *Mol Hum Reprod* 11(11):779–84, 2005.

Harrison RF, Barry-Kinsella C. Efficacy of medroxyprogesterone treatment in infertile women with endometriosis: a prospective, randomized, placebo-controlled study. *Fertil Steril* 74(1):24, 2000.

Haynes PJ, Hodgson H, et al. Measurement of menstrual blood loss in patients complaining of menorrhagia. *Br J Obstet Gynaecol* 84(10):763, 1977.

Hecht BR, Bardawil WA, et al. Luteal insufficiency: correlation between endometrial dating and integrated progesterone output in clomiphene citrate-induced cycles. *Am J Obstet Gynecol* 163(6 Pt 1):1986, 1990.

Heck KE, Schoendorf KC, et al. Delayed childbearing by education level in the United States, 1969–1994. *Matern Child Health J* 1(2):81, 1997.

Hellmuth E, Damm P, et al. Oral hypoglycaemic agents in 118 diabetic pregnancies. *Diabet Med* 17(7):507, 2000.

Hickman TN, Namnoum AB, et al. Timing of estrogen replacement therapy following hysterectomy with oophorectomy for endometriosis. *Obstet Gynecol* 91(5 Pt 1):673, 1998.

Hill JA. Recurrent pregnancy loss: male and female factor, etiology and treatment. Frontiers in Reproductive Endocrinology, Washington, DC, Serono Symposia USA, Inc., 2001.

Hill JA, Polgar K, et al. T-helper 1-type immunity to trophoblast in women with recurrent spontaneous abortion. *JAMA* 273(24):1933, 1995.

Hinckley MD, Milki AA. 1000 office-based hysteroscopies prior to in vitro fertilization: feasibility and findings. *JSLS.* 8(2):103–7, 2004.

Hirata J, Kikuchi Y, et al. Endometriotic tissues produce immunosuppressive factors. *Gynecol Obstet Invest* 37(1):43, 1994.

Hobbs L, Ort R, et al. Synopsis of laser assisted hair removal systems. *Skin Therapy Lett* 5(3):1, 2000.

Hock DL, Sharafi K, et al. Contribution of diminished ovarian reserve to hypofertility associated with endometriosis. *J Reprod Med* 46(1):7, 2001.

Höfle G, Gasser R, et al. Surgery combined with dopamine agonists versus dopamine agonists alone inlong-term treatment of macroprolactinoma: a retrospective study. *Exp Clin Endocrinol Diabetes* 106(3):211–16, 1998.

Hoff JD, Quigley ME, et al. Hormonal dynamics at midcycle: a reevaluation. *J Clin Endocrinol Metab* 57(4):792, 1983.

Hofmann GE, Khoury J, et al. Recurrent pregnancy loss and diminished ovarian reserve. *Fertil Steril* 74(6):1192, 2000.

Hollowell JG, Staehling NW, et al. Serum TSH, T(4), and thyroid antibodies in the United States population (1988 to 1994): national health and nutrition examination survey (NHANES III). *J Clin Endocrinol Metab* 87(2):489–99, 2002.

Holoch P, Wald M. Current options for preservation of fertility in the male. *Fertil Steril* 96(2):286–90, 2011.

Homer HA, Li TC, et al. The septate uterus: a review of management and reproductive outcome. *Fertil Steril* 73(1):1, 2000.

Honda I, Sato T, et al. [Uterine artery embolization for leiomyoma: complications and effects on fertility]. *Nippon Igaku Hoshasen Gakkai Zasshi* 63(6):294, 2003.

Horcajadas J, Goyri E, et al. Endometrial receptivity and implantation are not affected by the presence of uterine intramural leiomyomas: a clinical and functional genomics analysis. *J Clin Endocrinol Metab* 93(9):3490–3498, 2008.

Hornstein MD, Hemmings R, et al. Use of nafarelin versus placebo after reductive laparoscopic surgery for endometriosis. *Fertil Steril* 68(5):860, 1997.

Hornstein MD, Yuzpe AA, et al. Prospective randomized double-blind trial of 3 versus 6 months of nafarelin therapy for endometriosis associated pelvic pain. *Fertil Steril* 63(5):955, 1995.

Howard FM. The role of laparoscopy in chronic pelvic pain: promise and pitfalls. *Obstet Gynecol Surv* 48(6):357, 1993.

Howards SS. Treatment of male infertility. *N Engl J Med* 332(5):312, 1995.

Howell S, Shalet S. Gonadal damage from chemotherapy and radiotherapy. *Endocrinol Metab Clin North Am* 27(4):927–43, 1998.

Huang KE. The primary treatment of luteal phase inadequacy: progesterone versus clomiphene citrate. *Am J Obstet Gynecol* 155(4):824, 1986.

Hubacher D, Lara-Ricalde R, et al. Use of copper intrauterine devices and the risk of tubal infertility among nulligravid women. *N Engl J Med* 345(8):561, 2001.

Hughes E, Collins J, et al. Clomiphene citrate for unexplained subfertility in women. *Cochrane Database Syst Rev* (3):CD000057, 2000.

Hull MG, Savage PE, et al. The value of a single serum progesterone measurement in the midluteal phase as a criterion of a potentially fertile cycle ("ovulation") derived form treated and untreated conception cycles. *Fertil Steril* 37(3):355, 1982.

REFERENCES

Hulley S, Furberg C, et al. Noncardiovascular disease outcomes during 6.8 years of hormone therapy: Heart and Estrogen/Progestin Replacement Study Follow-up (HERS II). *JAMA* 288(1):58, 2002.

Hurd WW, Whitfield RR, et al. Expectant management versus elective curettage for the treatment of spontaneous abortion. *Fertil Steril* 68(4):601, 1997.

Hurst BS, Hickman JM, et al. Novel clomiphene "stair-step" protocol reduces time to ovulation in women with polycystic ovarian syndrome. *Am J Obstet Gynecol* 200(5):510.e1–4, 2009.

Hussein A, Ozgok Y, Ross L, Niederberger C. Clomiphene administration for cases of nonobstructive azoospermia: a multicenter study. *J Androl.* 2005 Nov-Dec;26(6):787–91.

Hussein A, Ozgok Y, et al. Optimization of spermatogenesis-regulating hormones in patients with non-obstructive azoospermia and its impact on sperm retrieval: a multicentre study. *BJU Int.* 2013 [Epub 2012]

Imani B, Eijkemans MJ, et al. Predictors of patients remaining anovulatory during clomiphene citrate induction of ovulation in normogonadotropic oligoamenorrheic infertility. *J Clin Endocrinol Metab* 83(7):2361, 1998.

Imani B, Eijkemans MJ, et al. Predictors of chances to conceive in ovulatory patients during clomiphene citrate induction of ovulation in normogonadotropic oligoamenorrheic infertility. *J Clin Endocrinol Metab* 84(5):1617, 1999.

Imudia AN, Awonuga AO, et al. Peak serum estradiol level during controlled ovarian hyperstimulation is associated with increased risk of small for gestational age and preeclampsia in singleton pregnancies after in vitro fertilization. *Fertil Steril.* 2012 Jun;97(6):1374–9.

Imudia AN, Awonuga AO, et al. Elective cryopreservation of all embryos with subsequent cryothaw embryo transfer in patients at risk for ovarian hyperstimulation syndrome reduces the risk of adverse obstetric outcomes: a preliminary study. *Fertil Steril.* 2013 Jan;99(1):168–73.

Isik AZ, Gulekli B, et al. Endocrinological and clinical analysis of hyperprolactinemic patients with and without ultrasonically diagnosed polycystic ovarian changes. *Gynecol Obstet Invest* 43(3):183, 1997.

Jaffe R, Jauniaux E, et al. Maternal circulation in the first-trimester human placenta—myth or reality? *Am J Obstet Gynecol* 176(3):695, 1997.

Jakubowicz DJ, Iuorno MJ, et al. Effects of metformin on early pregnancy loss in the polycystic ovary syndrome. *J Clin Endocrinol Metab* 87(2):524, 2002.

Jansen R, Elliott P. Angular and interstitial pregnancies should not be called 'cornual'. *Aust NZJ Obstet Gynaecol* 23(2):123, 1983.

Jarow JP, Ogle SR, et al. Seminal improvement following repair of ultrasound detected subclinical varicoceles. *J Urol* 155(4):1287, 1996.

Jaslow CR, Carney JL, Kutteh WH. Diagnostic factors identified in 1020 women with two versus three or more recurrent pregnancy losses. *Fertil Steril.* 1;93(4):1234–43, 2010.

Jasonni VM, Raffelli R, et al. Vaginal bromocriptine in hyperprolactinemic patients and puerperal women. *Acta Obstet Gynecol Scand* 70(6):493, 1991.

Jauniaux E, Johns J, et al. The role of ultrasound imaging in diagnosing and investigating early pregnancy failure. *Ultrasound Obstet Gynecol* 25(6):613–24, 2005.

Jeng GT, Scott JR, et al. A comparison of meta-analytic results using literature vs individual patient data. Paternal cell immunization for recurrent miscarriage. *JAMA* 274(10):830, 1995.

Jenkins S, Olive DL, et al. Endometriosis: pathogenic implications of the anatomic distribution. *Obstet Gynecol* 67:335, 1986.

Jensen I, Rinaldo CH, et al. Human umbilical vein endothelial cells lack expression of the estrogen receptor. *Endothelium* 6(1):9, 1998.

Joffe H, Cohen LS, Harlow BL. Impact of oral contraceptive pill use on premenstrual mood: predictors of improvement and deterioration. *Am J Obstet Gynecol* 189(6):1523, 2003.

Johnson J, Canning J, et al. Germline stem cells and follicular renewal in the postnatal mammalian ovary. *Nature* 428(6979):145, 2004a.

Johnson NP, Farquhar CM, et al. A double-blind randomised controlled trial of laparoscopic uterine nerve ablation for women with chronic pelvic pain. *BJOG* 111(9):950, 2004b.

Johnson NP, Mak W, et al. Laparoscopic salpingectomy for women with hydrosalpinges enhances the success of IVF: a Cochrane review. *Hum Reprod* 17(3):543, 2002.

Juliano M, Dabulis S, et al. Characteristics of women with fetal loss in symptomatic first trimester pregnancies with documented fetal cardiac activity. *Ann Emerg Med* 52(2):143–47, 2008.

Jordan J, Craig K, et al. Luteal phase defect: the sensitivity and specificity of diagnostic methods in common clinical use. *Fertil Steril* 62(1):54, 1994.

Jordan RM, Kendall JW, et al. The primary empty sella syndrome: analysis of the clinical characteristics, radiographic features, pituitary function and cerebrospinal fluid adenohypophysial hormone concentrations. *Am J Med* 62(4):569, 1977.

Jurema M, Vieira A, et al. Effect of ejaculatory abstinence period on the pregnancy rate after intrauterine insemination. *Fertil Steril* 84(3):678–81, 2005.

Jurkovic D, Ross JA, et al. Expectant management of missed miscarriage. *Br J Obstet Gynaecol* 105(6):670, 1998.

Kalsi J, Thum MY, et al. Analysis of the outcome of intracytoplasmic sperm injection using fresh or frozen sperm. *BJU Int.* 2011 Apr;107(7):1124–8.

Kahnlian SA, Cole LA. Management of gestational trophoblastic disease and other cases with low serum levels of human chronic gonadotropin. *J Reprod Med* 51(10):812–8, 2006.

Kahraman K, Berker B, et al. Microdose gonadotropin-releasing hormone agonist flare-up protocol versus multiple dose gonadotropin-releasing hormone antagonist protocol in poor responders undergoing intracytoplasmic sperm injection-embryo transfer cycle. *Fertil Steril.* 2009 Jun;91(6):2437–44.

Kahsar-Miller MD, Nixon C, et al. Prevalence of polycystic ovary syndrome (PCOS) in first-degree relatives of patients with PCOS. *Fertil Steril* 75(1):53, 2001.

Källén B, Lindam A, et al. Cancer risk in children and young adults conceived by in vitro fertilization. *Pediatrics* 126(2):270–76, 2010.

Kallio S, Puurunen J, et al. Antimullerian hormone levels decrease in women using combined contraception independently of administration route. *Fertil Steril* 99:1305, 2013

Kalra SK, Ratcliffe SJ, et al. Ovarian stimulation and low birth weight in newborns conceived through in vitro fertilization. *Obstet Gynecol.* 2011 Oct;118(4):863–71.

Kalsi J, Thum MY, et al. In the era of micro-dissection sperm retrieval (m-TESE) is an isolated testicular biopsy necessary in the management of men with non-obstructive azoospermia? *BJU Int.* 2012 Feb;109(3):418–24.

REFERENCES

Kalsi J, Thum MY, et al. Analysis of the outcome of intracytoplasmic sperm injection using fresh or frozen sperm. *BJU Int.* 2011 Apr;107(7):1124–8.

Kamel HS, Darwish AM, et al. Comparison of transvaginal ultrasonography and vaginal sonohysterography in the detection of endometrial polyps. *Acta Obstet Gynecol Scand* 79(1):60, 2000.

Kanis JA. Diagnosis of osteoporosis and assessment of fracture risk. *Lancet* 359(9321):1929, 2002.

Kaplowitz P. Clinical characteristics of 104 children referred for evaluation of precocious puberty. *J Clin Endocrinol Metab* 89(8):3644, 2004.

Kaplowitz PB, Oberfield SE. Reexamination of the age limit for defining when puberty is precocious in girls in the United States: implications for evaluation and treatment. Drug and Therapeutics and Executive Committees of the Lawson Wilkins Pediatric Endocrine Society. *Pediatrics* 104(4 Pt 1):936, 1999.

Kalra SK, Barnhart KT. In vitro fertilization and adverse childhood outcomes: what we know, where we are going, and how we will get there. A glimpse into what lies behind and beckons ahead. *Fertil Steril.* 2011 May;95(6):1887–9.

Katsuragawa H, Kanzaki H, et al. Monoclonal antibody against phosphatidylserine inhibits in vitro human trophoblastic hormone production and invasion. *Biol Reprod* 56(1):50, 1997.

Kaufman RH, Adam E, et al. Continued follow-up of pregnancy outcomes in diethylstilbestrol-exposed offspring. *Obstet Gynecol* 96(4):483, 2000.

Kaunitz A. Hormonal contraception in women of older reproductive age. *N Engl J Med* 358:1262–70, 2008.

Ke RW, Portera SG, et al. A randomized, double-blinded trial of preemptive analgesia in laparoscopy. *Obstet Gynecol* 92(6):972, 1998.

Kennedy S, Berggvist A, et al. ESHRE guideline for the diagnosis and treatment of endometriosis. *Hum Reprod* 20(10):2698–704, 2005.

Khalaf Y, Ross C, et al. The effect of small intramural uterine fibroids on the cumulative outcome of assisted conception. *Hum Reprod* 21(10):2640–644, 2006.

Khalifa E, Toner JP, et al. Significance of basal follicle-stimulating hormone levels in women with one ovary in a program of in vitro fertilization. *Fertil Steril* 57(4):835, 1992.

Khalil MR et al. Homologous intrauterine insemination. An evaluation of prognostic factors based on a review of 2473 cycles. *Acta Obstet Gynecol Scand* 80:74, 2001.

Khorram O, Lessey B. Alterations in expression of endometrial endothelial nitric oxide synthase and $\alpha_v\beta_3$ integrin in women with endometriosis. *Fertil Steril* 78(4):860–64, 2002.

Kiddy DS, Hamilton-Fairley D, et al. Improvement in endocrine and ovarian function during dietary treatment of obese women with polycystic ovary syndrome. *Clin Endocrinol (Oxf)* 36:105, 1992.

Kim S, Klemp J, et al. Breast cancer and fertility preservation. *Fertil Steril* 95(5):1535–43, 2011.

Klatsky PC, Lane DE, et al. The effect of fibroids without cavity involvement on ART outcomes independent of ovarian age. *Hum Reprod.* 2007 Feb;22(2):521–6.

Klein JR, Litt IF. Epidemiology of adolescent dysmenorrhea. *Pediatrics* 68(5):661, 1981.

Kleinhaus K, Perrin M, et al. Paternal age and spontaneous abortion. *Obstet Gynecol* 108(2):369–77, 2006.

Klinkert ER, Broekmans FJ, et al. A poor response in the first in vitro fertilization cycle is not necessarily related to a poor prognosis in subsequent cycles. *Fertil Steril* 81(5):1247–53, 2004.

Kodama H, Fukuda J, et al. Characteristics of blood hemostatic markers in a patient with ovarian hyperstimulation syndrome who actually developed thromboembolism. *Fertil Steril* 64:1207, 1995.

Koga K, Osuga Y, et al. A case of giant cystic adenomyosis. *Fertil Steril* 85(3)748–9, 2006.

Koga K, Osuga Y, et al. Increased concentrations of soluble tumour necrosis factor receptor (sTNFR) I and II in peritoneal fluid from women with endometriosis. *Mol Hum Reprod* 6(10):929, 2000.

Kokay IC, Petersen SL, et al. Identification of prolactin-sensitive GABA and kisspeptin neuron in regionsof the rat hypothalamus involved in the control of fertility. *Neuroendocrinology* 152(2):526–535, 2011.

Kolibanakis EM, Schultze-Mosgau A, et al. A lower ongoing pregnancy rate can be expected when GnRH agonist is used for triggering final ooctye maturation instead of HCG in patients undergoing IVF with GnHR antagonists. *Hum Reprod* 20(10):2887–2892, 2005.

Kongnyuy EJ, Wiysonge CS. Interventions to reduce haemorrhage during myomectomy for fibroids. *Cochrane Database Syst Rev* 3:CD005355, 2009.

Koninckx PR, Mueleman C, et al. Suggestive evidence that pelvic endometriosis is a progressive disease, whereas deeply infiltrating endometriosis is associated with pelvic pain. *Fertil Steril* 55(4):759, 1991.

Kontoravids A, Makrakis E, et al. Proximal tubal occlusion and salpingectomy result in similar improvement in in vitro fertilization outcome in patients with hydrosalpinx. *Fertil Steril* 86(6):1642–49, 2006.

Kouides PA, Phatak PD, et al. Gynaecological and obstetrical morbidity in women with type I von Willebrand disease: results of a patient survey. *Haemophilia* 6(6):643, 2000.

Kruger TF, Acosta AA, et al. New method of evaluating sperm morphology with predictive value for human in vitro fertilization. *Urology* 30(3):248, 1987.

Kundsin RB, Driscoll SG, et al. Ureaplasma urealyticum incriminated in perinatal morbidity and mortality. *Science* 213(4506):474, 1981.

Kupfer MC, Schwimer SR, et al. Transvaginal sonographic appearance of endometrioma: spectrum of findings. *J Ultrasound Med* 11:129, 1992.

Kurman RJ, Kaminski PF, et al. The behavior of endometrial hyperplasia. A long-term study of "untreated" hyperplasia in 170 patients. *Cancer* 56(2): 403, 1985.

Kutteh WH. Antiphospholipid antibody-associated recurrent pregnancy loss: treatment with heparin and low-dose aspirin is superior to low-dose aspirin alone. *Am J Obstet Gynecol* 174(5):1584, 1996.

Kyrou D, Fatemi HM, et al. Luteal phase support in normo-ovulatory women stimulated with clomiphene citrate for intrauterine insemination: need or habit? *Hum Reprod* 25(10):2501–2506, 2010.

La Marca A, Giulini S, et al. Anti-Müllerian hormone measurement on any day of the menstrual cycle strongly predicts ovarian response in assisted reproductive technology. *Hum Reprod.* Mar;22(3):766–71, 2007.

La Marca A, Nelson SM, et al. Anti-Müllerian hormone–based prediction model for a live birth in assisted reproduction. *Reprod Biomed Online.* 2011 Apr;22(4):341–49.

LaCroix AZ, Chlebowski RT, et al. Health outcomes after stopping conjugated equine estrogens among postmenopausal women with prior hysterectomy. *JAMA* 305(13):1305–14, 2011.

Laifer-Narin S, Ragavendra N, et al. False-normal appearance of the endometrium on conventional transvaginal sonography: comparison with saline hysterosonography. *AJR Am J Roentgenol* 178(1):129, 2002.

Lamvu G. Role of hysterectomy in treatment of chronic pelvic pain. *Obstet Gynecol* 117(5):1175–78, 2011.

Lanigan SW. Incidence of side effects after laser hair removal. *J Am Acad Dermatol* 49(5):882, 2003.

Lashen H, Fear K, et al. Obesity is associated with increased risk of first trimester and recurrent miscarriage: matched case-control study. *Hum Reprod* 19(7):1644, 2004.

Lara-Torre E, Schroeder B. Adolescent compliance and side effects with quick start initiation of oral contraceptive pills. *Contraception* 66(2):81–85, 2002.

Laughlin GA, Barrett-Connor E, et al. Hysterectomy, oophorectomy, and endogenous sex hormone levels in older women: the Rancho Bernardo Study. *J Clin Endocrinol Metab* 85(2):645, 2000.

Laughlin GA, Yen SS. Nutritional and endocrine-metabolic aberrations in amenorrheic athletes. *J Clin Endocrinol Metab* 81(12):4301, 1996.

Laughlin GA, Yen SS. Hypoleptinemia in women athletes: absence of a diurnal rhythm with amenorrhea. *J Clin Endocrinol Metab* 82(1):318, 1997.

Laughlin S, Baird D, et al. Prevalence of uterine leiomyomas in the first trimester of pregnancy. *Obstet Gynecol* 113(3):630–35, 2009.

Lazovic G, Milacic D, et al. Medicaments or surgical therapy of PCOS. *Fertil Steril* 70(3):472 (abst), 1998.

Lebovic DI, Mueller MD, et al. Immunobiology of endometriosis. *Fertil Steril* 75(1):1, 2001.

Legro R, Barnhart H, et al. Clomphene, metformin, or both for infertility in the polycystic ovary syndrome. *N Engl J Med* 356(6):551–66, 2007.

Lethaby A, Hickey M. Endometrial destruction techniques for heavy menstrual bleeding: a Cochrane review. *Hum Reprod* 17(11):2795, 2002.

Lethaby A, Vollenhoven B, et al. Efficacy of pre-operative gonadotrophin hormone releasing analogues for women with uterine fibroids undergoing hysterectomy or myomectomy: a systematic review. *BJOG* 109(10):1097, 2002.

Lev-Toaff AS, Coleman BG, et al. Leiomyomas in pregnancy: sonographic study. *Radiology* 164:375, 1987.

Levi AJ, Raynault MF, et al. Reproductive outcome in patients with diminished ovarian reserve. *Fertil Steril* 76(4):666, 2001.

Levitas E, Lunenfel E, et al. Relationship between the duration of sexual abstinence and semen quality: analysis of 9,489 semen samples. *Fertil Steril* 83(6):1680–86, 2005.

Lewis V, Queenan Jr J, et al. Clomiphene citrate monitoring for intrauterine insemination timing: a randomized trial. *Fertil Steril* 85(2):401–16, 2006.

Li DK, Liu L, et al. Exposure to non-steroidal anti-inflammatory drugs during pregnancy and risk of miscarriage: population based cohort study. *BMJ* 327(7411):368, 2003.

Li S, Qayyum A, et al. Association of renal agenesis and müllerian duct anomalies. *J Comput Assist Tomogr* 24(6):829, 2000.

Liewan H, Santoro N. Premature ovarian failure: a modern approach to diagnosis and treatment. *Endocrinologist* 7:314, 1997.

Lincoln SR, Ke RW, et al. Screening for hypothyroidism in infertile women. *J Reprod Med* 44(5):455, 1999.

Linden MG, Bender BG, et al. Intrauterine diagnosis of sex chromosome aneuploidy. *Obstet Gynecol* 87(3):468, 1996.

Lindsay R, Gallagher JC, et al. Effect of lower doses of conjugated equine estrogens with and without medroxyprogesterone acetate on bone in early postmenopausal women. *JAMA* 287(20):2668, 2002.

Lippman SA, Warner M, et al. Uterine fibroids and gynecologic pain symptoms in a population-based study. *Fertil Steril* 80(6):1488, 2003.

Lipscomb GH, Bran D, et al. Analysis of three hundred fifteen ectopic pregnancies treated with single-dose methotrexate. *Am J Obstet Gynecol* 178:1354, 1998.

Lipscomb GH, Givens VM, et al. Comparison of multidose and single-dose methotrexate protocols forthe treatment of ectopic pregnancy. *Am J Obstet Gynecol* 192(2):1844–47, 2005.

Lipscomb GH, Givens VA, et al. Previous ectopic pregnancy as a predictor of failure of systemic methotrexate therapy. *Fertil Steril* 81(5):1221, 2004.

Lipscomb GH, McCord ML, et al. Predictors of success of methotrexate treatment in women with tubal ectopic pregnancies. *N Engl J Med* 341:1974, 1999a.

Lipscomb GH, Stovall TG, et al. Nonsurgical treatment of ectopic pregnancy. *N Engl J Med* 343(18):1325, 2000.

Liu HC, Kreiner D, et al. Beta-human chorionic gonadotropin as a monitor of pregnancy outcome in in vitro fertilization-embryo transfer patients. *Fertil Steril* 50(1):89, 1988.

Liu J, Rebar RW, et al. Neuroendocrine control of the postpartum period. *Clin Perinatol* 10(3):723, 1983.

Liu JH, Yen SS. Induction of midcycle gonadotropin surge by ovarian steroids in women: a critical evaluation. *J Clin Endocrinol Metab* 57(4):797, 1983.

Lo JC, Schwitzgebel VM, et al. Normal female infants born of mothers with classic congenital adrenal hyperplasia due to 21-hydroxylase deficiency. *J Clin Endocrinol Metab* 84(3):930, 1999.

Lobo R, Shoupe D, et al. The effects of two doses of spironolactone on serum androgens and anagen hair in hirsute women. *Fertil Steril* 43(2):200, 1985.

Lockhat FB, Emembolu JO, et al. The evaluation of the effectiveness of an intrauterine-administered progestogen (levonorgestrel) in the symptomatic treatment of endometriosis and in the staging of the disease. *Hum Reprod* 19(1):179, 2004.

Lockwood C, Bauer K, et al. Inherited thrombophilias in pregnancy. *Obstet Gynecol* 118(3):730–40, 2011.

Looker AC, Orwoll ES, et al. Prevalence of low femoral bone density in older U.S. adults from NHANES III. *J Bone Miner Res* 12(11):1761, 1997.

Luborsky JL, Meyer P, et al. Premature menopause in a multi-ethnic population study of the menopause transition. *Hum Reprod* 18(1):199, 2003.

Luk J, Arici A. Does the ovarian reserve decrease from repeated ovulation stimulations? *Curr Opin Obstest Gynecol* 22(3):177–182, 2010.

Luke B, Brown M, et al. Female obesity adversely affects assisted reproductive technology (ART) pregnancy and live birth rates. *Hum Reprod* 26(1):245–52, 2011.

Lutfallah C, Wang W, et al. Newly proposed hormonal criteria via genotypic proof for type II 3beta-hydroxysteroid dehydrogenase deficiency. *J Clin Endocrinol Metab* 87(6):2611, 2002.

Lutfey KE, Link CL, et al. Prevalence and correlates of sexual activity and function in women: results fromthe Boston area community health (BACH) survey. *Arch Sex Behav* 38(4):514–27, 2009.

Lyons RA, Saridogan E, et al. The reproductive significance of human fallopian tube cilia. *Hum Reprod Update* 12(4):363–372, 2006.

Mahabeer S, Naidoo C, et al. Metabolic profiles and lipoprotein lipid concentrations in non-obese patients with polycystic ovarian disease. *Horm Metab Res* 22(10):537, 1990.

Maheshwari A, Bhattacharya S. Elective frozen replacement cycles for all: ready for prime time? *Hum Reprod.* Jan;28(1):6–9, 2013.

Mains L, Van Voorhis BJ. Optimizing the technique of embryo transfer. Fertil Steril. 2010 Aug;94(3):785–90.

Manners CV. Endometrial assessment in a group of infertile women on stimulated cycles for IVF: immunohistochemical findings. *Hum Reprod* 5(2):128, 1990.

Manning AP, Thompson WG, et al. Towards positive diagnosis of the irritable bowel. *Br Med J* 2(6138):653, 1978.

Mannix L, Martin V, et al. Combination treatment for menstrual migraine and dysmenorrhea using sumatriptan-naproxen. *ACOG* 114(1):106–113, 2009.

Marchbanks PA, McDonald JA, et al. Oral contraceptives and the risk of breast cancer. *N Engl J Med* 346(26):2025, 2002.

Marcoux S, Maheux R, et al. Laparoscopic surgery in infertile women with minimal or mild endometriosis. *N Engl J Med* 337:217, 1997.

Markee JE. Menstruation in intraocular endometrial transplants in the rhesus monkey. *Contrib Embryol* 177:221, 1940.

Marshall WA, Tanner JM. Variations in pattern of pubertal changes in girls. *Arch Dis Child* 44(235):291, 1969.

Maruo T, Laoag-Fernandez JB, et al. Effects of the levonorgestrel-releasing intrauterine system on proliferation and apoptosis in the endometrium. *Hum Reprod* 16(10):2103, 2001.

Massie J, Shahine L, et al. Ovarian stimulation and the risk of aneuploid conceptions. *Fertil Steril* 95(3):970–72, 2011.

Matorras R, Corcóstegui B, et al. Fertility in women with minimal endometriosis compared with normal women was assessed by means of a doctor insemination program in unstimulated cycles. *Am J Obstet Gynecol* 203(4):345 e1–6, 2010.

Matsuzaki S, Houlle C, et al. Analysis of risk factors for the removal of normal ovarian tissue during laparoscopic cystectomy for ovarian endometriosis. *Hum Reprod* 24(6):1402–1406, 2009.

Mavrelos D, Ben-Nagi J, et al. The value of pre-operative treatment with GnRH analogues in women with submucous fibroids: a double-blind, placebo-controlled randomized trial. *Hum Reprod* 25(9):2264–2269, 2010.

Mayani A, Barel S, et al. Dioxin concentrations. *Hum Reprod* 12(2):373, 1997.

McCord ML, Muram D, et al. Single serum progesterone as a screen for ectopic pregnancy: exchanging specificity and sensitivity to obtain optimal test performance. *Fertil Steril* 66(4):513, 1996.

McDonough PG. Puberty. In *Precis, Reproductive Endocrinology: An Update in Obstetrics and Gynecology.* Washington, DC: American College of Obstetricians and Gynecologists, 1998:32.

McElreavey K, Krausz C, et al. The human Y chromosome and male infertility. *Results Probl Cell Differ* 28:211, 2000.

McGovern PG, Legro RS, et al. Utility of screening for other causes of infertility in women with "known" polycystic ovary syndrome. *Fertil Steril* 87(2):442–44, 2007.

McLachlan R, O'Bryan M. State of the art for genetic testing of infertile men. *J Clin Endocrinol Metab* 95(3):1013–1024, 2010.

McNatty KP, Makris A, et al. Metabolism of androstenedione by human ovarian tissues in vitro with particular reference to reductase and aromatase activity. *Ster-oids* 34(4):429, 1979.

Meldrum DR, Fisher AR, et al. Acupuncture–help, harm, or placebo? *Fertil Steril.* 2013 Jun;99(7):1821–4.

Melin A, Spafen P, et al. Endometriosis and the risk of cancer with special emphasis on ovarian cancer. *Hum Reprod* 21(5):1237–1242, 2006.

Melo M, Busso CE, et al. GnRH agonist versus recombinant HCG in an oocyte donation programme: a randomized, prospective, controlled, assessor-blind study. *Reprod Biomed Online.* 2009 Oct;19(4):486–92.

Messinis IE, Templeton AA. Endocrine and follicle characteristics of cycles with and without endogenous luteinizing hormone surges during superovulation induction with pulsatile follicle-stimulating hormone. *Hum Repod* 2(1):11–16, 1987.

Meyer WR, Castelbaum AJ, et al. Hydrosalpinges adversely affect markers of endometrial receptivity. *Hum Reprod* 12(7):1393, 1997.

Michaëlsson K, Baron JA, et al. Oral-contraceptive use and risk of hip fracture: a case-control study. *Lancet* 353(9163):1481, 1999.

Migeon CJ, Wisniewski AB. Human sex differentiation and its abnormalities. *Best Pract Res Clin Obstet Gynaecol* 17(1):1, 2003.

Miller L, Hughes JP. Continuous combination oral contraceptive pills to eliminate withdrawal bleeding: a randomized trial. *Obstet Gynecol* 101(4):653, 2003.

Miller JD, Shaw RW, et al. Historical prospective cohort study of the recurrence of pain after discontinuation of treatment with danazol or a gonadotropin-releasing hormone agonistt. *Fertil Steril* 70(2):293, 1998.

Mishell DR, Darney PD, et al. Practice guidelines for OC selection: update. *Dialogues Contracept* 5(4):7, 1997.

Mitwally MF, Casper RF. Aromatase inhibition reduces gonadotrophin dose required for controlled ovarian stimulation in women with unexplained infertility. *Hum Reprod* 18(8):1588, 2003.

Mitwally MF, Casper RF. Single-dose administration of an aromatase inhibitor for ovarian stimulation. *Fertil Steril* 83(1):229, 2005.

Moawad N, Mahajan S, et al. Current diagnosis and treatment of interstitial pregnancy. *Am J Obstet Gynecol* 2010.

Modan B, Hartge P, et al. Parity, oral contraceptives, and the risk of ovarian cancer among carriers and noncarriers of a BRCA1 or BRCA2 mutation. *N Engl J Med* 345(4):235, 2001.

Moen MH and Magnus P. The familial risk of endometriosis. Acta Obstet Gynecol Scand, 72:560, 1993.

Molitch ME. Pregnancy and the hyperprolactinemic woman. *N Engl J Med* 312(21):1364, 1985.

Molitch ME, Reichlin S. Hyperprolactinemic disorders. *Dis Mon* 28(9):1, 1982.

Monajatur Rahman S, Karmakar D, et al. Timing of intrauterine insemination: an attempt to unravel the enigma. *Arch Gynecol Obstet* 284(4):1023–27, 2011.

REFERENCES

Morris RS, Paulson R. Ovarian hyperstimulation syndrome: classification and management. *Contemporary Ob/Gyn*, Sept:43, 1994.

Morris SN, Missmer SA, et al. Effects of lifetime exercise on the outcome of in vitro fertilization. *American College of Obstetricians and Gynecologists* 108(4):935–45, 2006.

Mortola JF, Girton L, et al. Diagnosis of premenstrual syndrome by a simple, prospective, and reliable instrument: the calendar of premenstrual experiences. *Obstet Gynecol* 76(2):302, 1990.

Moy I, Milad M, et al. Randomized controlled trial: effects of acupuncture on pregnancy rates in women undergoing in vitro fertilization. *Fertil Steril* 95(2):583–87, 2011.

Muller P, Musset R, et al. [State of the upper urinary tract in patients with uterine malformations. Study of 133 cases]. *Presse Med* 75(26):1331, 1967.

Murphy AA, Green WR, et al. Unsuspected endometriosis documented by scanning electron microscopy in visually normal peritoneum. *Fertil Steril* 46(3): 522, 1986.

Murray DL, Reich L, et al. Oral clomiphene citrate and vaginal progesterone suppositories in the treatment of luteal phase dysfunction: a comparative study. *Fertil Steril* 51(1):35, 1989.

Murray MJ, Meyer WR, et al. A critical analysis of the accuracy, reproducibility, and clinical utility of histologic endometrial dating in fertile women. *Fertil Steril* 81(5):1333, 2004.

Muse KN, Cetel NS, et al. The premenstrual syndrome. Effects of "medical ovariectomy." *N Engl J Med* 311(21):1345, 1984.

Naftolin F, Taylor HS, et al. The Women's Health Initiative could not have detected cardioprotective effects of starting hormone therapy during the menopausal transition. *Fertil Steril* 81(6):1498, 2004.

Nakai Y, Plant TM, et al. On the sites of the negative and positive feedback actions of estradiol in the control of gonadotropin secretion in the rhesus monkey. *Endocrinology* 102(4):1008, 1978.

Nakashima A, Araki R, et al. Implications of assisted reproductive technologies on term singleton birth weight: an analysis of 25,777 children in the national assisted reproduction registry of Japan. *Fertil Steril.* 2013 Feb;99(2):450–5.

Nakamura S, Douchi T, et al. Relationship between sonographic endometrial thickness and progestin-induced withdrawal bleeding. *Obstet Gynecol* 87(5 Pt 1):722, 1996.

Nappi RG et al. Natural pregnancy in hypothyroid woman complicated by spontaneous ovarian hyperstimulation syndrome. *Am J Obstet Gynecol* 178:610, 1998.

Narod SA, Risch H, et al. Oral contraceptives and the risk of hereditary ovarian cancer. Hereditary Ovarian Cancer Clinical Study Group. *N Engl J Med* 339(7):424, 1998.

Nawroth F, Gohar R, et al. Is there an association between septate uterus and endometriosis? *Hum Repod* 21(2):542–544, 2006.

Nestler JE. Metformin and the polycystic ovary syndrome. *J Clin Endocrinol Metab* 86(3):1430, 2001.

Negro R, Schwartz A, et al. Increased pregnancy loss rate in thyroid antibody negative women with TSH levels between 2.5 and 5.0 in the first trimester of pregnancy. *J Clin Endocrinol Metab* 95(9):44–48, 2010.

Nelson L. Primary ovarian insufficiency. *N Engl J Med* 360(6):606–14, 2009.

Ness RB, Grisso JA, et al. Risk of ovarian cancer in relation to estrogen and progestin does and use characteristics of oral contraceptives. SHARE study group. Steroid hormones and reproductions. *Am J Epidemol* 152(3):233–41, 2000.

Nestler JE, Powers LP, et al. A direct effect of hyperinsulinemia on serum sex hormone-binding globulin levels in obese women with the polycystic ovary syndrome. *J Clin Endocrinol Metab* 72(1):83, 1991.

New M. Extensive clinical experience nonclassical 21-hydroxylase deficiency. *J Clin Endocrinol Metab* 91(1):4205–4214, 2006.

Newfield L, Bradlow HL, et al. Estrogen metabolism and the malignant potential of human papillomavirus immortalized keratinocytes. *Proc Soc Exp Biol Med* 217(3):322, 1998.

Nezhat CR, Nezhat FR, et al. *Operative Gynecologic Laparoscopy: Principles and Techniques.* New York: McGraw-Hill, 1995.

Ng EH, Ajonuma LC, et al. Adverse effects of hydrosalpinx fluid on sperm motility and survival. *Hum Reprod* 15(4):772, 2000.

Ng EH, Chan CC, et al. Comparison of endometrial and subendometrial blood flows among patients with and without hydrosalpinx shown on scanning during in vitro fertilization treatment. *Fertil Steril* 85(2):333–38, 2006.

Niebyl J. Nausea and vomiting in pregnancy. *N Engl J Med* 363(16):1544–50, 2010.

Nielsen S, Hahlin M. Expectant management of first-trimester spontaneous abortion. *Lancet* 345(8942):84, 1995.

Nielsen J, Wohlert M. Sex chromosome abnormalities found among 34,910 newborn children: resultsfrom a 13-year incidence study in Arhus, Denmark. *J Clin Endocrinol Metab* 26(4):209–23, 1990.

Nishida M, Nasu K, et al. Endometriotic cells are resistant to interferon-g-induced cell growth inhibition and apoptosis: a possible mechanism involved in the pathogenesis of endometriosis. *Mol Hum Reprod* 11(1):29, 2005.

Nisolle M, Donnez J. Endoscopic treatment of Mullerian anomalies. *Gynecol Endocrinol* 5:155, 1996.

Nisolle M, Donnez J. Peritoneal endometriosis, ovarian endometriosis, and adenomyotic nodules of the rectovaginal septum are three different entities. *Fertil Steril* 68(4):585, 1997.

Noorhasan DJ, McCulloh DH, et al. Follicle-stimulating hormone levels and medication compliance during in vitro fertilization. *Fertil Steril* 90(5):e1–3, 2008.

North American Menopause Society. Treatment of menopause-associated vasomotor symptoms: position statement of the North American Menopause Society. *Menopause* 11(1):11, 2004.

Novak ER, Woodruff JD. *Gynecologic and Obstetric Pathology.* Philadelphia: WB Saunders, 1979.

Noyes RW, Hertig AT, et al. Dating the endometrial biopsy. *Fertil Steril* 1(1):3, 1950.

Nuojua-Huttunen S, Tomas C, et al. Intrauterine insemination treatment in subfertility: an analysis of factors affecting outcome. *Hum Reprod* 14(3):698, 1999.

Nybo Andersen AM, Wohlfahrt J, et al. Maternal age and fetal loss: population based register linkage study. *BMJ.* Jun 24;320(7251):1708–12, 2000.

Oei SG, Helmerhorst FM, et al. Effectiveness of the postcoital test: randomised controlled trial. *BMJ* 317(7157):502, 1998.

REFERENCES

Ogasawara M, Aoki K, et al. Embryonic karyotype of abort uses in relation to the number of previous miscarriages. *Fertil Steril* 73(2):300, 2000.

Ohl DA, Wolf LJ, et al. Electroejaculation and assigned reproductive technologies in the treatment of anejaculatory infertility. *Fertil Steril* 76(6):1249–55, 2001.

Olson CK, Keppler-Noreuil KM, et al. In vitro fertilization is associated with an increase in major birth defects. *Fertil Steril* 84(5):1308–15, 2005.

Oktay K, Meirow D. Planning for fertility preservation before cancer treatment. *Hum Reprod* 5(1):353–543, 2001.

Oktem O, Urman B. Understanding follicle growth in vivo. *Hum Reprod* 25(12)2944–2954, 2010.

Omland AK, Abyholm T, et al. Pregnancy outcome after IVF and ICSI in unexplained, endometriosis-associated and tubal factor infertility. *Hum Reprod* 20(3):722, 2005.

Omland AK, Tanbo T, et al. Artificial insemination by husband in unexplained infertility compared with infertility associated with peritoneal endometriosis. *Hum Reprod* 13(9):2602, 1998.

Oral E, Arici A. Peritoneal growth factors and endometriosis. *Semin Reprod Endocrinol* 14:257, 1996.

Orio F, Jr., Palomba S, et al. The cardiovascular risk of young women with polycystic ovary syndrome: an observational, analytical, prospective case-control study. *J Clin Endocrinol Metab* 89(8):3696, 2004.

Oriol B, Barrio A, et al. Systematic methotrexate to treat ectopic pregnancy does not affect ovarian reserve. *Fertil Steril* (90)5:1579–82, 2008.

Otis CL, Drinkwater B, et al. American College of Sports Medicine position stand. The Female Athlete Triad. *Med Sci Sports Exerc* 29(5):i, 1997.

Pache TD, de Jong FH, et al. Association between ovarian changes assessed by transvaginal sonography and clinical and endocrine signs of the polycystic ovary syndrome. *Fertil Steril* 59(3):544, 1993.

Pagotto U, Marsicano G, et al. Normal human pituitary gland and pituitary adenomas express cannabinoid receptor type 1 and synthesize endogenous cannabinoids: first evidence for a direct role of cannabinoids on hormone modulation at the human pituitary level. *J Clin Endocrinol Metab* 86(6): 2687, 2001.

Pal L, Niklaus AL, et al. Heterogeneity in endometrial expression of aromatase in polyp-bearing uteri. *Hum Reprod* 23(1):80–4, 2008.

Pall M, Friden BE, et al. Induction of delayed follicular rupture in the human by the selective COX-2 inhibitor rofecoxib: a randomized double-blind study. *Hum Reprod* 16(7):1323, 2001.

Palmert MR, Boepple PA. Variation in the timing of puberty: clinical spectrum and genetic investigation. *J Clin Endocrinol Metab* 86(6):2364, 2001.

Panay N, Al-Azzawi F, et al. Testosterone treatment of HSDD in naturally menopausal women: the ADORE study. *Clinacteric* 13(2):121–31, 2010.

Panganiban W, Cornog JL. Endometriosis of the intestines and vermiform appendix. *Dis Colon Rectum* 15:253, 1972.

Panici PB, Bellati F, et al. Vaginoplasty using autologous in vitro cultured vaginal tissue in a patient with Mayer-von-Rokitansky-Kuster-Hauser syndrome. *Hum Reprod* 22(7):2025–8, 2007.

Papanikolaou EG, Tournaye H, et al. *Early Pregnancy Outcome Is Impaired in Early Ovarian Hyperstimulation Syndrome (OHSS) Comparing to Late OHSS*. St. Louis: American Society for Reproductive Immunology, 2004.

Parazzini F. Ablation of lesions or no treatment in minimal-mild endometriosis in infertile women: a randomized trial. Gruppo Italiano per lo Studio dell'Endometriosi. *Hum Reprod* 14(5):1332, 1999.

Parazzini F, Fedele L, et al. Postsurgical medical treatment of advanced endometriosis: results of a randomized clinical trial. *Am J Obstet Gynecol* 171(5):1205, 1994.

Parinaud J, Lesourd F. [Inhibin B is not a good marker of ovarian follicular reserve]. *Gynecol Obstet Fertil* 30(3):254, 2002.

Parsanezhad M, Azmoon M, et al. A randomized, contolled clinical trial compating the effects of aromatase inhibitor (letrozole) and gonadotropin-releasing hormone agonis (triptorelin) on uterine leiomyoma volume and hormonal status. *Fertil Steril* 93(1):192–98, 2010.

Parsanezhad ME, Alborzi S, et al. Use of dexamethasone and clomiphene citrate in the treatment of clomiphene citrate-resistant patients with polycystic ovary syndrome and normal dehydroepiandrosterone sulfate levels: a prospective, double-blind, placebo-controlled trial. *Fertil Steril* 78(5):1001, 2002.

Patton PE, Burry KA, et al. Intrauterine insemination outperforms intracervical insemination in a randomized, controlled study with frozen, donor semen. *Fertil Steril* 57(3):559–64, 1992.

Paulson J, Delgado M. The relationship between international cystits and endometriosis in patients with chronic pelvic pain. *JSLS* 11:175–181, 2007.

Pearlstein TB, Stone AB. Long-term fluoxetine treatment of late luteal phase dysphoric disorder. *J Clin Psychiatry* 55(8):332, 1994.

Pearlstone AC, Fournet N, et al. Ovulation induction in women age 40 and older: the importance of basal follicle-stimulating hormone level and chronological age. *Fertil Steril* 58(4):674, 1992.

Pellerito JS, McCarthy SM, et al. Diagnosis of uterine anomalies: relative accuracy of MR imaging, endovaginal sonography, and hysterosalpingography. *Radiology* 183(3):795, 1992.

Pellestor F, Andreo B, et al. Maternal aging and chromosomal abnormalities: new data drawn from in vitro unfertilized human oocytes. *Hum Genet* 112(2):195, 2003.

Pérez-Medina T, Bajo-Arenas J, et al. Endometrial polyps and their implication in the pregnancy rates of patients undergoing intrauterine insemination: a prospective, randomized study. *Hum Reprod* 22(6) 1632–1635, 2005.

Perimenis P, Markou S, et al. Effect of subinguinal varicocelectomy on sperm parameters and pregnancy rate: a two-group study. *Eur Urology* 39(3):322–25, 2001.

Phelan JP. Myomas and pregnancy. *Obstet Gynecol Clin North Am* 22(4):801–5, 1995.

Phelps P, Cakmakkaya S, et al. A simple clinical maneuver to reduce laparoscopy-induced shoulder pain. *Obstet Gynecol* 111(5):1155–60, 2008.

Phillips DR, Nathanson HG, et al. The effect of dilute vasopressin solution on blood loss during operative hysteroscopy: a randomized controlled trial. *Obstet Gynecol* 88(5):761, 1996.

Phipps WR. Polycystic ovary syndrome and ovulation induction. *Obstet Gynecol Clin North Am* 28(1):165, 2001.

Pierpoint T, McKeigue PM, et al. Mortality of women with polycystic ovary syndrome at long-term follow-up. *J Clin Epidemiol* 51(7):581, 1998.

REFERENCES

Piippo S, Lenko H, et al. Use of percutaneous estrogen gel for induction of puberty in girls with Turner syndrome. *J Clin Endocrinol Metab* 89(7):3241, 2004.

Pinborg A, Wennerholm UB, et al. Why do singletons conceived after assisted reproduction technology have adverse perinatal outcome? Systematic review and meta-analysis. Hum Reprod Update. 2013 Mar-Apr;19(2):87–104. Pisarska MD, Carson SA, et al. Ectopic pregnancy. *Lancet* 351(9109):1115, 1998.

Pocock SJ, Ware JH. Translating statistical findings into plain English. *Lancet* 373(9676):1926–8, 2009.

Polson DW, Adams J, et al. Polycystic ovaries—a common finding in normal women. *Lancet* 1(8590):870, 1988.

Polyzos NP, Blockeel C, et al. Live birth rates following natural cycle IVF in women with poor ovarian response according to the Bologna criteria. *Hum Reprod.* Dec;27(12):3481–86, 2012.

Pope CS, Cook EK, et al. Influence of embryo transfer depth on in vitro fertilization and embryo transfer outcomes. *Fertil Steril* 81(1):51, 2004.

Poppe K, Glinoer D, et al. Assisted reproduction and thyroid autoimmunity: an unfortunate combination? *J Clin Endocrinol Metab* 88(9):4149, 2003.

Potlog-Nahari C, Catherino WH, et al. *Pregnancy Rates of Blastocyst-Staged Embryos Are Reduced If Transferred to an Endometrium Classified As Grade B by Transvaginal Ultrasound.* San Antonio, TX: American Society of Reproductive Medicine, 2003.

Potlog-Nahari C, Catherino WH, et al. A suboptimal endometrial pattern is associated with a reduced likelihood of pregnancy after a day 5 embryo transfer. *Fertil Steril* 83(1):235, 2005.

Practice Committee of Society for Assisted Reproductive Technology; Practice Committee of American Society for Reproductive Medicine. The role of assisted hatching in in vitro fertilization: a review of the literature. A Committee opinion. *Fertil Steril.* 2008 Nov;90(5 Suppl):S196–8.

Price TM, Allen S, et al. Lack of effect of topical finasteride suggests an endocrine role for dihydrotestosterone. *Fertil Steril* 74(2):414, 2000.

Pritts EA, Atwood AK. Luteal phase support in infertility treatment: a meta-analysis of the randomized trials. *Hum Reprod* 17(9):2287, 2002.

Pritts EA, Parker WH, et al. Fibroids and infertility: an updated systematic review of the evidence. *Fertil Steril* 91(4):1215–23, 2009.

Proctor JA, Haney AF. Recurrent first trimester pregnancy loss is associated with uterine septum but not with bicornuate uterus. *Fertil Steril* 80(5):1212, 2003.

Propst AM, Storti K, et al. Lateral cervical displacement is associated with endometriosis. *Fertil Steril* 70(3):568, 1998.

Purvin VA. Visual disturbance secondary to clomiphene citrate. *Arch Ophthalmol* 113(4):482, 1995.

Pryor JL, Howards SS. Varicocele. *Urology Clin North Am* 14(3):499–513, 1987.

Querleu D, Brasme TL, et al. Ultrasound-guided transcervical metroplasty. *Fertil Steril* 54(6):995, 1990.

Rackow B, Arici A. Options for medical treatment of myomas. *Obstet Gynecol Clin N Am* 33(1):97–113, 2006.

Raffi F, Metwally M, Amer S. The impact of excision of ovarian endometrioma on ovarian reserve: a systematic review and meta-analysis. *J Clin Endocrinol Metab.* 97(9):3146–54, 2012.

Raga F, Bauset C, et al. Reproductive impact of congenital Mullerian anomalies. *Hum Reprod* 12(10):2277, 1997.

Rahman A, Abbassy H, et al. Improved in vitro fertilization outcomes after treatment of subclinicalhypothyroidism in infertile women. *Endocrine Practice* 16(5):792–797, 2010.

Rai R, Backos M, et al. Polycystic ovaries and recurrent miscarriage—a reappraisal. *Hum Reprod* 15(3):612, 2000.

Rai R, Cohen H, et al. Randomised controlled trial of aspirin and aspirin plus heparin in pregnant women with recurrent miscarriage associated with phospholipid antibodies (or antiphospholipid antibodies). *BMJ* 314(7076):253, 1997.

Raja SN, Feehan M, et al. Prevalence and correlates of the premenstrual syndrome in adolescence. *J Am Acad Child Adolesc Psychiatry* 31(5):783, 1992.

Ramasamy R, Lin K, et al. High serum FSH levels in men with nonobstructive azoospermia does not affect success of microdissection testicular sperm extraction. *Fertil Steril.* 2009 Aug;92(2):590–3.

Ramasamy R, Schlegel PN. Microdissection testicular sperm extraction: effect of prior biopsy on success of sperm retrieval. *J Urol.* 2007 Apr;177(4):1447–9.

Ramón O, Matorras R, et al. Ultrasound-guided artificial insemination: a randomized controlled trial. *Hum Reprod* 24(5):1080–1084, 2009.

Ranke MB, Saenger P. Turner's syndrome. *Lancet* 358(9278):309, 2001.

Rarick LD, Shangold MM, et al. Cervical mucus and serum estradiol as predictors of response to progestin challenge. *Fertil Steril* 54(2):353, 1990.

Ray NF, Chan JK, et al. Medical expenditures for the treatment of osteoporotic fractures in the United States in 1995: report from the National Osteoporosis Foundation. *J Bone Miner Res* 12(1):24, 1997.

Rebar RW, Connolly HV. Clinical features of young women with hypergonadotropic amenorrhea. *Fertil Steril* 53(5):804, 1990.

Regidor PA, Schindler AE, et al. Results of long-term follow-up in treatment of endometriosis with the GnRH agonist leuprorelin acetate depot (Enantone-Gyn monthly depot). *Zentralbl Gynakol* 118(5):283, 1996.

Reid RL. Premenstrual syndrome. *Curr Probl Obstet Gynecol Fertil* 8:1, 1985.

Reindollar R, Regan M, et al. A randomized clinical trial to evaluate optimal treatment for unexplained infertility: the fast track and standard treatment (FASTT) trial. *Fertil Steril* 94(3):888–89, 2010.

Reindollar RH, Byrd JR, et al. Delayed sexual development: a study of 252 patients. *Am J Obstet Gynecol* 140(4):371, 1981.

Reindollar RH, Novak M, et al. Adult-onset amenorrhea: a study of 262 patients. *Am J Obstet Gynecol* 155(3):531, 1986.

Reis FM, Petraglia F, Taylor RN. Endometriosis: hormone regulation and clinical consequences of chemotaxis and apoptosis. Hum Reprod Update

Remohi J, Gallardo E, et al. Oocyte donation in women with recurrent pregnancy loss. *Hum Reprod* 11(9):2048, 1996.

Richman TS, Viscomi GN, et al. Fallopian tubal patency assessed by ultrasound following fluid injection. Work in progress. *Radiology* 152(2):507–10, 1984.

Rickenlund A, Carlstrom K, et al. Effects of oral contraceptives on body composition and physical performance in female athletes. *J Clin Endocrinol Metab* 89(9):4364, 2004.

REFERENCES

Rienze L, Romano S, et al. Embryo development of fresh "versus" vitrified metaphase II oocytes after ICSI: a prospective randomized sibling-oocyte study. *Hum Reprod* 25(1):66–73, 2010.

Rivera JL, Lal S, et al. Effect of acute and chronic neuroleptic therapy on serum prolactin levels in men and women of different age groups. *Clin Endocrinol (Oxf)* 5(3):273, 1976.

Rivera-Tovar AD, Frank E. Late luteal phase dysphoric disorder in young women. *Am J Psychiatry* 147(12):1634, 1990.

Roca CA, Schmidt PJ, et al. Effects of metergoline on symptoms in women with premenstrual dysphoric disorder. *Am J Psychiatry* 159(11):1876, 2002.

Rock JA, Jones HW. The clinical management of the double uterus. *Fertil Steril* 28(8):798, 1977.

Rock JA, Zacur HA. The clinical management of repeated early pregnancy wastage. *Fertil Steril* 39(2):123, 1983.

Roque M, Lattes K, et al. Fresh embryo transfer versus frozen embryo transfer in in vitro fertilization cycles: a systematic review and meta-analysis. *Fertil Steril.* 2013 Jan;99(1):156–62.

Romer T, Lober R. Hysteroscopic correction of a complete septate uterus using a balloon technique. *Hum Reprod* 12(3):478, 1997.

Ron-El R, Raziel A, et al. Birth of healthy male twins after intracytoplasmic sperm injection of frozen-thawed testicular spermatozoa from a patient with nonmosaic Klinefelter syndrome. *Fertil Steril* 74(4):832, 2000.

Rosen MP, Shen S, et al. A quantitative assessment of follicle size on oocyte developmental competence. *Fertil Steril* 90(3):684–90, 2008.

Rosenfeld CS, Wagner JS, et al. Intraovarian actions of oestrogen. *Reproduction* 122(2):215, 2001.

Rosenheim NB, Leichner PK, et al. Radiocolloids in the treatment of ovarian cancer. *Obstet Gynecol Surv* 34:708, 1979.

Rossato M, Popa FI, et al. Human sperm express cannabinoid receptor CB1 which activation inhibits motility, acrosome reaction and mitochondrial function. *J Clin Endocrinol Metab* 90:984, 2005

Rossouw JE, Anderson GL, et al. Risks and benefits of estrogen plus progestin in healthy postmenopausal women: principal results from the Women's Health Initiative randomized controlled trial. *JAMA* 288(3):321, 2002.

Rotterdam ESCHRE/ASRM–Sponsored PCOS Consensus Workshop Group, 2004.

Royar J, Becher H, et al. Low-dose oral contraceptives: protective effect on ovarian cancer risk. *Int J Cancer* 95(6):370, 2001.

Rubinek T, Hadani M, et al. Prolactin (PRL)-releasing peptide stimulates PRL secretion from human fetal pituitary cultures and growth hormone release from cultured pituitary adenomas. *J Clin Endocrinol Metab* 86(6):2826, 2001.

Rudick B, Ingles S, et al. Characterizing the influence of vitamin D levels on IVF outcomes. *Hum Reprod.* 2012 Nov;27(11):3321–7.

Ryan GL, Moss V, et al. Oral ovulation induction agents combined with low-dose gonadotropin injections and intrauterine insemination. *J Reprod Med* 50(12):943–950, 2005.

Sachdev R, Kemmann E, et al. Detrimental effect of hydrosalpinx fluid on the development and blastulation of mouse embryos in vitro. *Fertil Steril* 68(3):531, 1997.

Salat-Baroux J. [Recurrent spontaneous abortions]. *Reprod Nutr Dev* 28(6B): 1555, 1988.

Saleh A, Morris D, et al. Effects of laparoscopic ovarian drilling on adrenal steroids in polycystic ovary syndrome patients with and without hyperinsulinemia. *Fertil Steril* 75(3):501, 2001.

Sallam HN, Garcia-Velasco JA, et al. Long-term pituitary down-regulation before in vitro fertilization (IVF) for women with endometriosis. *Cochran Collaboration* 1(1):CD004635, 2006.

Sam S, Legro R, et al. Evidence for metabolic and reproductive phenotypes in mothers of women with polycystic ovary syndrome. *PNAS* 103(18):7030–35, 2006.

Sampson JA. Peritoneal endometriosis due to menstrual dissemination of endometrial tissue into the peritoneal cavity. *Am J Obstet Gynecol* 14:422, 1927.

Santoro N, Torrens J, et al. Correlates of circulating androgens in the mid-life women: the study of women's health across the nation. *J Clin Endocrinol Metab* 90(8):4836–45, 2005.

Saravelos SH, Yan J, et al. The prevalence and impact of fibroids and their treatment on the outcome of pregnancy in women with recurrent miscarriage. *Hum Reprod* 26(12):3274–3279, 2011.

Sargent IL, Wilkins T, et al. Maternal immune responses to the fetus in early pregnancy and recurrent miscarriage. *Lancet* 2(8620):1099, 1988.

Sarrel PM. Psychosexual effects of menopause: role of androgens. *Am J Obstet Gynecol* 180(3 Pt 2):S319, 1999.

Sawaya GF, Grady D, et al. Antibiotics at the time of induced abortion: the case for universal prophylaxis based on a meta-analysis. *Obstet Gynecol* 87(5 Pt 2):884, 1996.

Scheffer GJ, Broekmans FJ, et al. Antral follicle counts by transvaginal ultrasonography are related to age in women with proven natural fertility. *Fertil Steril* 72(5):845, 1999.

Schieve LA, Meikle SF, et al. Low and very low birth weight in infants conceived with use of assisted reproductive technology. *N Engl J Med* 346(10):731, 2002.

Schilcher J, Michaëlsson K, et al. Bisphosphonate use and atypical fractures of the femoral shaft. *N Engl J Med* 365(16):1551, 2011.

Schimberni M, Morgia F, Colabianchi J, et al. Natural-cycle in vitro fertilization in poor responder patients: a survey of 500 consecutive cycles. *Fertil Steril* 92(4):1297, 2009.

Schlaff W, Carson S, et al. Subcutaneous injection of depot medroxyprogesterone acetat compared with leuprolide acetate in the treatment of endometriosis-associated pain. *Fertil Steril* 85(2):314–25, 2006.

Schlaff WD, Hurst BS. Preoperative sonographic measurement of endometrial pattern predicts outcome of surgical repair in patients with severe Asherman's syndrome. *Fertil Steril* 63(2):410, 1995.

Schlaff WD, Zerhouni EA, et al. A placebo-controlled trial of a depot gonadotropin-releasing hormone analogue (leuprolide) in the treatment of uterine leiomyomata. *Obstet Gynecol* 74(6):856, 1989.

Schlechte J, Dolan K, et al. The natural history of untreated hyperprolactinemia: a prospective analysis. *J Clin Endocrinol Metab* 68(2):412, 1989.

Schlechte, JA. Approach to the patient. Long-term management of prolactionomas. *J Clin Endocrinol Metab* 92(8):2861–2865, 2007.

REFERENCES

Schlegel PN. Causes of azoospermia and their management. *Reprod Fertil Develop* 16(5):561–72, 2004.

Schlesselman JJ, Collins JA. The influence of steroids on gynecologic cancers. In *Estrogens and Progestogens in Clinical Practice*, Fraser IS, Jansen RPS, et al., eds. London: Churchill Livingstone, 1999:831.

Schmiedehausen K, Kat S, et al. Determination of velocity of tubar transport with dynamic hysterosalpingoscintigraphy. *Nuclear Med Comm* 24(1):865–870, 2003.

Schmidt PJ, Nieman LK, et al. Differential behavioral effects of gonadal steroids in women with and in those without premenstrual syndrome. *N Engl J Med* 338(4):209, 1998.

Schoor RA, Elhanbly S, et al. The role of testicular biopsy in the modern management of male infertility. *J Urol*. 2002 Jan;167(1):197–200.

Schwartz D, Mayaux MJ. Female fecundity as a function of age: results of artificial insemination in 2193 nulliparous women with azoospermic husbands. Federation CECOS. *N Engl J Med* 306(7):404, 1982.

Schwimer SR, Lebovic J. Transvaginal pelvic ultrasonography. *J Ultrasound Med* 3(8):381, 1984.

Scott RT, Elkind-Hirsch KE, et al. The predictive for in vitro fertility delivery rates is greatly impacted by the method used to select the threshold between normal and elevated basal follicle-stimulating hormone. *Fertil Steril* 89(4):868–78, 2008.

Scott RT Jr, Ferry K, et al. Comprehensive chromosome screening is highly predictive of the reproductive potential of human embryos: a prospective, blinded, nonselection study. *Fertil Steril*. 2012 Apr;97(4):870–5.

Scott RT, Opsahl MS, et al. Life table analysis of pregnancy rates in a general infertility population relative to ovarian reserve and patient age. *Hum Reprod* 10(7):1706, 1995.

Scott RT, Toner JP, et al. Follicle-stimulating hormone levels on cycle day 3 are predictive of in vitro fertilization outcome. *Fertil Steril* 51(4):651, 1989.

Scott RT Jr, Upham KM, et al. Blastocyst biopsy with comprehensive chromosome screening and fresh embryo transfer significantly increases in vitro fertilization implantation and delivery rates: a randomized controlled trial. *Fertil Steril*. 2013 [Epub ahead of print]

Scott RT Jr, Upham KM, et al. Cleavage-stage biopsy significantly impairs human embryonic implantation potential while blastocyst biopsy does not: a randomized and paired clinical trial. *Fertil Steril*. 2013 [Epub ahead of print]

Scott RT, Jr., Hofmann GE, et al. Intercycle variability of day 3 follicle-stimulating hormone levels and its effect on stimulation quality in in vitro fertilization. *Fertil Steril* 54(2):297, 1990.

Segebladh, B, Borgström A, et al. Evaluation of different add-back estradiol and progesterone treatments to gonadotropin-releasing hormone agonist treatment in patients with premenstrual dysphoric disorder. *AJOG* 201(2):139, 2009.

Segenreich E, Israilov S, et al. Evaluation of the relationship between semen parameters, pregnancy rateof wives of infertile men with varicocele, and gonadotropin-releasing hormone test before and after varicocelectomy. *Urology* 52(5):853–7, 1998.

Seifer DB, Gutmann JN, et al. Comparison of persistent ectopic pregnancy after laparoscopic salpingostomy versus salpingostomy at laparotomy for ectopic pregnancy. *Obstet Gynecol* 81(3):378, 1993.

Seifer DB, Scott RT, Jr., et al. Women with declining ovarian reserve may demonstrate a decrease in day 3 serum inhibin B before a rise in day 3 follicle-stimulating hormone. *Fertil Steril* 72(1):63, 1999.

Seki K, Kato K, et al. Parallelism in the luteinizing hormone responses to opioid and dopamine antagonists in hyperprolactinemic women with pituitary microadenoma. *J Clin Endocrinol Metab* 63(5):1225, 1986.

Semino C, Semino A, et al. Role of major histocompatibility complex class I expression and natural killer-like T cells in the genetic control of endometriosis. *Fertil Steril* 64(5):909, 1995.

Sergentanis TN, Diamantaras AA, et al. IVF and breast cancer: a systematic review and meta-analysis. *Hum Reprod Update.* 2013 Jul 24.

Shah DK, Missmer SA, et al. Effect of obesity on oocyte and embryo quality in women undergoing in vitro fertilization. *American College of Obstetricians and Gynecologists* 118(1):63–70, 2011.

Shamma FN, Lee G, et al. The role of office hysteroscopy in in vitro fertilization. *Fertil Steril* 58(6):1237, 1992.

Sharara FI, Scott RT, Jr., et al. The detection of diminished ovarian reserve in infertile women. *Am J Obstet Gynecol* 179(3 Pt 1):804, 1998.

Shebl O, Ebner T, et al. Anti muellerian hormone serum levels in women with endometriosis: a case-control study. *Gynecol Endocrinol.* 2009 Nov;25(11):713–6.

Shifren JL, Davis SR, et al. Testosterone patch for the treatment of hypoactive sexual desire disorder innaturally menopausal women: results from the INTIMATE NM1 study. *Menopause* 13(5):770–9, 2006.

Shokeir TA, Shalan HM, El-Shafei MM. Significance of endometrial polyps detected hysteroscopically in eumenorrheic infertile women. *J Obstet Gynaecol Res.* 30(2):84–9, 2004.

Shokeir T, El-Shafei M, et al. Submucous myomas and their implications in the pregnancy rates of patients with otherwise unexplained primary infertility undergoing hysteroscopic myomectomy: a randomized matched control study. *Fertil Steril.* 2010 Jul;94(2):724–9.

Shumaker SA, Legault C, et al. Conjugated equine estrogens and incidence of probable dementia and mild cognitive impairment in postmenopausal women: Women's Health Initiative Memory Study. *JAMA* 291(24):2947, 2004.

Siffroi JP, Le Bourhis C, et al. Sex chromosome mosaicism in males carrying Y chromosome long arm deletions. *Hum Reprod* 15(12):2559, 2000.

Silverberg SG, Haukkamaa M, et al. Endometrial morphology during long-term use of levonorgestrel-releasing intrauterine devices. *Int J Gynecol Pathol* 5(3):235, 1986.

Simpson J, Elias S, et al. Heritable aspects of endometriosis: genetic studies. *Am J Obstet Gynecol* 137:327, 1980.

Simpson JL, Carson SA, et al. Lack of association between antiphospholipid antibodies and first-trimester spontaneous abortion: prospective study of pregnancies detected within 21 days of conception. *Fertil Steril* 69(5):814, 1998.

Simpson JL, Elias S, et al. Heritable aspect of endometriosis, I: genetic studies. Am J Obstet Gynecol 137:327, 1980.

Sinaii N, Cleary SD, et al. Autoimmune and related diseases among women with endometriosis: a survey analysis. *Fertil Steril* 77[Suppl 1]:S7, 2002.

Sinclair AH, Berta P, et al. A gene from the human sex-determining region encodes a protein with homology to a conserved DNA-binding motif. *Nature* 19;346(6281):240–4, 1990.

Siristatidis C, Sergentanis TN, et al. Controlled ovarian hyperstimulation for IVF: impact on ovarian, endometrial and cervical cancer—a systematic review and meta-analysis. *Hum Reprod Update*. 2013 19(2):105–23.

Slayden SM, Azziz R. The role of androgen excess in acne. In Azziz R, Nestler JE, Dewailly D. *Androgen Excess Disorders in Women*. Philadelphia: Lippincott–Raven Publishers: 131, 1997.

Sluijmer AV, Lappohn RE. Clinical history and outcome of 59 patients with idiopathic hyperprolactinemia. *Fertil Steril* 58(1):72, 1992.

Smit M, Romin J, et al. Decreased sperm DNA fragmentation after surgical varicocelectomy is associatedwith increased pregnancy rate. *J of Urology* 183(1):270–4, 2010.

Smith JA, Vitale A, et al. Dry eye signs and symptoms in women with premature ovarian failure. *ArchOphthalmol* 122(2):151–156, 2004.

Smith JS, Green J, et al. Cervical cancer and use of hormonal contraceptives: a systematic review. *Lancet* 361(9364):1159, 2003.

Smotrich DB, Widra EA, et al. Prognostic value of day 3 estradiol on in vitro fertilization outcome. *Fertil Steril* 64(6):1136, 1995.

Šmuc T, Hevir N, et al. Disturbed estrogen and progesterone action in ovarian endometriosis. *Mol Cell Endocrinol* 301(1–2):59–64, 2009.

Snyder PJ. The role of androgens in women. *J Clin Endocrinol Metab* 86(3): 1006, 2001.

Soares SR, Barbosa dos Reis MM, et al. Diagnostic accuracy of sonohysterography, transvaginal sonography, and hysterosalpingography in patients with uterine cavity diseases. *Fertil Steril* 73(2):406, 2000.

Sokalska A, Timmerman D, et al. Diagnostic accuracy of transvaginal ultrasound examination for assigning a specific diagnosis to adnexal masses. *Ultrasound Obstet Gynecol* 34(4):462–70, 2009.

Somboonporn W, Davis S, et al. Testosterone for peri- and postmenopausal women. *Cochrane Database Syst Rev* 19(4), 2005.

Somigliana E, Arnold M, et al. IVF-ICSI outcome in women operated on for bilateral endometriomas. *Hum Reprod* 23(7):1526–1530, 2008.

Somigliana E, Infantino M, et al. The presence of ovarian endometriomas is associated with a reduced responsiveness to gonadotropins. *Fertil Steril* 86(1):192–96, 2006.

Somigliana E, Ragni G, et al. Does laparoscopic excision of endometriotic ovarian cysts significantly affect ovarian reserve? Insights from IVF cycles. *Hum Reprod* 18(11):2450, 2003.

Somigliana E, Vigano P, et al. Human endometrial stromal cells as a source of soluble intercellular adhesion molecule (ICAM)-1 molecules. *Hum Reprod* 11(6): 1190, 1996.

Somigliana E, Vigano P, et al. Endometriosis and unexplained recurrent spontaneous abortion: pathological states resulting from aberrant modulation of natural killer cell function? *Hum Reprod Update* 5(1):40, 1999.

Sonmezer M, Oktay K. Fertility preservation in female patients. *Hum Reprod* 10(3):251–266, 2004.

Souter I, Baltagi LM, et al. Prevalence of hyperprolactinemia and abnormal magnetic resonance imaging findings in a population with infertility. *Fertil Steril* 94(1):1159–62, 2010.

Spandorfer SD, Davis OK, et al. Relationship between maternal age and aneuploidy in in vitro fertilization pregnancy loss. *Fertil Steril* 81(5):1265, 2004.

Speildoch R, Winter T, et al. Optimal catheter placement during sonohysterography. *Obstet Gynecol* 111(1):15–21, 2008.

Speiser PW, White PC. Congenital adrenal hyperplasia. *N Engl J Med* 349(8):776, 2003.

Speroff L, Fritz MA, eds. *Clinical Gynecologic Endocrinology and Infertility* (7th ed). Philadelphia: Lippincott Williams & Wilkins, 2005.

Stagnaro-Green A, Abalovich M, et al. American Thyroid Association Taskforce on Thyroid Disease During Pregnancy and Postpartum. Guidelines of the American Thyroid Association for the diagnosis and management of thyroid disease during pregnancy and postpartum. Thyroid. 2011 Oct;21(10):1081-125.

Stahl PJ, Schlegel PN. Genetic evaluation of the azoospermic or severely oligozoospermic male. *Curr Opin Obstet Gynecol* 24(4):221–28, 2012.

Stampfer MJ, Colditz GA, et al. Postmenopausal estrogen therapy and cardiovascular disease. Ten-year follow-up from the nurses' health study. *N Engl J Med* 325(11):756, 1991.

Steege JF, Stout AL, et al. Reduced platelet tritium-labeled imipramine binding sites in women with premenstrual syndrome. *Am J Obstet Gynecol* 167(1):168, 1992.

Stefansson H, Geirsson RT, Steinthorsdottir V, et al. Genetic factors contribute to the risk of developing endometriosis. *Hum Reprod* 17:555, 2002.

Stein ZA. A woman's age: childbearing and child rearing. *Am J Epidemiol* 121 (3):327, 1985.

Steinberger E, Smith KD, et al. Testosterone levels in female partners of infertile couples. Relationship between androgen levels in the woman, the male factor, and the incidence of pregnancy. *Am J Obstet Gynecol* 133(2):133, 1979.

Steiner AZ, Chang L, et al. 3alpha-hydroxysteroid dehydrogenase type III deficiency: a novel cause of hirsutism (O-307). *J Soc Gynecol Invest* 11(2S):307, 2004.

Steiner M, Romano SJ, et al. The efficacy of fluoxetine in improving physical symptoms associated with premenstrual dysphoric disorder. *BJOG* 108(5):462, 2001.

Steiner M, Steinberg S, et al. Fluoxetine in the treatment of premenstrual dysphoria. Canadian Fluoxetine/Premenstrual Dysphoria Collaborative Study Group. *N Engl J Med* 332(23):1529, 1995.

Stephenson MD, Kutteh WH, et al. Intravenous immunoglobulin and idiopathic secondary recurrent miscarriage: a multicentered randomized placebo-controlled trial. *Hum Reprod* 25(9):2203–2209, 2010.

Stern C, Chamley L. Antiphospholipid antibodies and coagulation defects in women with implantation failure after IVF and recurrent miscarriage. *Reprod Biomed Online*. 2006 Jul;13(1):29–37.

Stewart FH, Harper CC, et al. Clinical breast and pelvic examination requirements for hormonal contraception: current practice vs evidence. *JAMA* 285(17): 2232, 2001.

Strandell A, Lindhard A. Why does hydrosalpinx reduce fertility? The importance of hydrosalpinx fluid. *Hum Reprod* 17(5):1141, 2002.

Strandell A, Lindhard A, et al. Cost-effectiveness analysis of salpingectomy prior to IVF, based on a randomized controlled trial. *Hum Reprod* 20(12):3284–3292, 2005.

Strandell A, Lindhard A, et al. Hydrosalpinx and IVF outcome: a prospective, randomized multicentre trial in Scandinavia on salpingectomy prior to IVF. *Hum Reprod* 14(11):2762, 1999.

Strandell A, Lindhard A, et al. Hydrosalpinx and IVF outcome: cumulative results after salpingectomy in a randomized controlled trial. *Hum Reprod* 16(11):2403, 2001a.

REFERENCES

Strandell A, Lindhard A, et al. Prophylactic salpingectomy does not impair the ovarian response in IVF treatment. *Hum Reprod* 16(6):1135, 2001b.

Strobelt N, Mariani E, et al. Fertility after ectopic pregnancy. Effects of surgery and expectant management. *J Reprod Med* 45(10):803, 2000.

Sun L., Peng Y, et al. FSH directly regulates bone mass. *Cell* 125(2):247–60, 2006.

Sung L, Mukherjee T, et al. Endometriosis is not detrimental to embryo implantation in oocyte recipients. *J Assist Reprod Genet* 14(3):152, 1997.

Surrey ES, Lietz AK, et al. Impact of intramural leiomyomata in patients with a normal endometrial cavity on in vitro fertilization-embryo transfer cycle outcome. *Fertil Steril* 75(2):405, 2001.

Surrey ES, Silverberg KM, et al. Effect of prolonged gonadotropin-releasing hormone agonist therapy on the outcome of in vitro fertilization-embryo transfer in patients with endometriosis. *Fertil Steril* 78(4):699, 2002.

Sussman EM, Chudnovsky A, et al. Hormonal evaluation of the infertile male: has it evolved? *Urology Clin North Am* 35(2):147–55, 2008.

Swerdloff RS, Wang C. Evaluation of male infertility. UpToDate Patient Information Web site: http://www.utdol.com. Accessed February 2005.

Syrop CH, Hammond MG. Diurnal variations in midluteal serum progesterone measurements. *Fertil Steril* 47(1):67, 1987.

Tanis BC, Van den Bosch MA, et al. Oral contraceptives and the risk of myocardial infarction. *N Engl J Med* 345(25):1787, 2001.

Tarani L, Lampariello S, et al. Pregnancy in patients with Turner's syndrome: six new cases and review of literature. *Gynecol Endocrinol* 12(2):83, 1998.

Tartagni M, Schonauer MM, et al. Intermittent low-dose finasteride is as effective as daily administration for the treatment of hirsute women. *Fertil Steril* 82(3):752, 2004.

Taylor AE, Adams JM, et al. A randomized, controlled trial of estradiol replacement therapy in women with hypergonadotropic amenorrhea. *J Clin Endocrinol Metab* 81(10):3615, 1996.

Taylor DL, Mathew RJ, et al. Serotonin levels and platelet uptake during premenstrual tension. *Neuropsychobiology* 12(1):16, 1984.

te Velde ER, Cohlen BJ. The management of infertility (editorial). *N Engl J Med* 340(3):224, 1999.

Teichmann AT, Brill K, et al. The influence of the dose of ethinylestradiol in oral contraceptives on follicle growth. *Gynecol Endocrincol* 9:229, 1995.

Telimaa S, Ronnberg L, et al. Placebo-controlled comparison of danazol and high-dose medroxyprogesterone acetate in the treatment of endometriosis after conservative surgery. *Gynecol Endocrinol* 1(4):363, 1987.

Thonneau P, Machand S, et al. Incidence and main causes of infertility in a resident population (1,850,000) of three French regions (1988–1989). *Hum Reprod* 6(6):811–16, 1991.

Thys-Jacobs S, Ceccarelli S, et al. Calcium supplementation in premenstrual syndrome: a randomized crossover trial. *J Gen Intern Med* 4(3):183, 1989.

Thys-Jacobs S, McMahon D, et al. Differences in free estradiol and sex hormone-binding globulin in women with and without premenstrual dysphoric disorder. *JCEM* 93(1):96–102, 2008.

Tian L, Shen H, et al. Insulin resistance increases the risk of spontaneous abortion after assistedreproduction technology treatment. *J Clin Endocrinol Metab* 92(4):1430–33, 2007.

Tilford CA, Kuroda-Kawaguchi T, et al. A physical map of the human Y chromosome. *Nature* 409(6822):943, 2001.

Todd AS. Endothelium and fibrinolysis. *Bibl Anat* 12:98, 1973.

Toft A. Increased levothyroxine requirements in pregnancy—why, when, and how much? *N Engl J Med* 351(3):292, 2004.

Toma SK, Stovall DW, et al. The effect of laparoscopic ablation or danocrine on pregnancy rates in patients with stage I or II endometriosis undergoing donor insemination. *Obstet Gynecol* 80(2):253, 1992.

Toner JP. Age = egg quality, FSH level = egg quantity. *Fertil Steril* 79(3):491, 2003.

Toner JP, Seifer DB. Why we may abandon basal follicle-stimulating hormone testing: a sea change in determining ovarian reserve using antimüllerian hormone. *Fertil Steril.* 2013 Jun;99(7):1825–30.

Treff NR, Scott RT Jr. Four-hour quantitative real-time polymerase chain reaction-based comprehensive chromosome screening and accumulating evidence of accuracy, safety, predictive value, and clinical efficacy. *Fertil Steril.* 2013 15;99(4):1049–53

Treloar AE, Boynton RE, et al. Variation of the human menstrual cycle through reproductive life. *Int J Fertil* 12(2)77–126, 1967.

Trio D, Strobelt N, et al. Prognostic factors for successful expectant management of ectopic pregnancy. *Fertil Steril* 63:469, 1995.

Trout SW, Seifer DB. Do women with unexplained recurrent pregnancy loss have higher day 3 serum FSH and estradiol values? *Fertil Steril* 74(2):335, 2000.

Tsoumpou I, Kyrgiou M, et al. The effect of surgical treatment for endometrioma on in vitro fertilization outcomes: a systematic review and meta-analysis. *Fertil Steril* 92(1):75–87, 2009.

Tsung-Hsien L, Chung-Hsien L, et al. Serum anti-müllerian hormone and estradiol levels as predictors of ovarian hyperstimulation syndrome in assisted reproduction technology cycles. *Hum Reprod* 23(1):160–167, 2008.

Tulandi T, Al-Took S. Laparoscopic ovarian suspension before irradiation. *Fertil Steril* 70(2):381–83, 1998.

Tulchinsky D, Hobel CJ. Plasma human chorionic gonadotropin, estrone, estradiol, estriol, progesterone, and 17 a-hydroxy-progesterone in human pregnancy. *Am J Obstet Gynecol* 117:884, 1973.

Tummon IS, Asher LJ, et al. Randomized controlled trial of superovulation and insemination for infertility associated with minimal or mild endometriosis. *Fertil Steril* 68(1):8, 1997.

Turi A, Giannubilo SR, et al. Coenzyme Q10 content in follicular fluid and its relationship with oocyte fertilization and embryo grading. *Arch Gynecol Obstet.* 2012 Apr;285(4):1173–6.

Utian WH, Shoupe D, et al. Relief of vasomotor symptoms and vaginal atrophy with lower doses of conjugated equine estrogens and medroxyprogesterone acetate. *Fertil Steril* 75(6):1065, 2001.

Uncu G, Kasapoglu I, et al. Prospective assessment of the impact of endometriomas and their removal on ovarian reserve and determinants of the rate of decline in ovarian reserve. *Hum Reprod.* 2013 Aug;28(8):2140–5.

Urman B, Yakin K. Does dehydroepiandrosterone have any benefit in fertility treatment? *Curr Opin Obstet Gynecol.* 2012 Jun;24(3):132–5.

Van den Berg MH, Van Dulmen-den Broeder E, et al. Comparison of ovarian function markers in users of hormonal contraceptives during the hormone-free interval and subsequent natural early follicular phases. *Hum Reprod* Jun;25(6):1520–27, 2010.

REFERENCES

Van der Linden M, Buckingham K, et al. Luteal support for assisted reproduction cycles. *Cochrane Database Syst Rev.* 2011

Van Leeuwen I, Branch DW, et al. First-trimester ultrasonography findings in women with a history of recurrent pregnancy loss. *Am J Obstet Gynecol* 168(1 Pt 1):111, 1993.

Van Leeuwen FE, Klip H, et al. Risk of borderline and invasive ovarian stimulation for in vitro fertilization in large Dutch cohort. *Hum Reprod* 26(12):3456–65, 2011.

Van Montfrans JM, Hoek A, et al. Predictive value of basal follicle-stimulating hormone concentrations in a general subfertility population. *Fertil Steril* 74(1):97, 2000.

Van Rumste MME, Custers IM, et al. The influence of the number of follicles on pregnancy rates in intrauterine insemination with ovarian stimulation: a meta-analysis. *Hum Reprod Update* 14(6):563–570, 2008.

Van Voorhis BJ, Sparks AE. Semen analysis: what tests are clinically useful? *Clin Obstet Gynecol* 42(4):957, 1999.

Van Voorhis BJ et al. Effect of the total motile sperm count on the efficacy and cost-effectiveness of intrauterine insemination and in vitro fertilization. *Fertil Steril* 75(4):661, 2001.

Van Waart J, Kruger TF, et al. Predictive value of normal sperm morphology in intrauterine insemination (IUI): a structured literature review. *Hum Reprod Update* 7(5):495, 2001.

Van Wely M, Van der Veen F. To assist or not to assist embryo hatching. *Hum Reprod Update* 17(4):436–437, 2011.

Vance ML. Treatment of patients with a pituitary adenoma: one clinician's experience. *Neurosurg Focus* 16(4):E1, 2004.

Vandenbroucke JP, Koster T, et al. Increased risk of venous thrombosis in oral-contraceptive users who are carriers of factor V Leiden mutation. *Lancet* 344(8935):1453, 1994.

Vandenbroucke JP, Rosing J, et al. Oral contraceptives and the risk of venous thrombosis. *N Engl J Med* 344(20):1527, 2001.

Vanderpump MP, Tunbridge WM, et al. The incidence of thyroid disorders in the community: a twenty-year follow-up of the Whickham Survey. *Clin Endocrinol (Oxf)* 43(1):55, 1995.

Vegetti W, Ragni G, et al. Laparoscopic ovarian drilling versus low-dose pure FSH in anovulatory clomiphene-resistant patients with polycystic ovarian syndrome: randomized prospective study. *Hum Reprod* 13(1):120 (abst), 1998.

Vellinga T, De Alwis S, et al. Laparoscopic Entry: The modified alwis method and more. *Obstet Gynecol* 2(3):193–198, 2009.

Vercammen EE, D'Hooghe TM. Endometriosis and recurrent pregnancy loss. *Semin Reprod Med* 18(4):363, 2000.

Vercellini P, Aimi G, et al. Laparoscopic uterosacral ligament resection for dysmenorrhea associated with endometriosis: results of a randomized, controlled trial. *Fertil Steril* 80(2):310, 2003a.

Vercellini P, De Giorgi O, et al. Menstrual characteristics in women with and without endometriosis. *Obstet Gynecol* 90:264, 1997b.

Vercellini P, Maddalena S, et al. Abdominal myomectomy for infertility: a comprehensive review. *Hum Reprod* 13:873, 1998.

Vercellini P, Somigliana E, et al. Asymmetry in distribution of diaphragmatic endometriotic lesions: evidence in favour of the menstrual reflux theory. *Hum Reprod* 22(9):2359–67, 2007.

Vercellini P, Somigliana E, et al. Blood on the corpora lutea to endometriomas. *BJOG* 116:366–371, 2009.

Verhelst J, Abs R, et al. Cabergoline in the treatment of hyperprolactinemia: a study in 455 patients. *J Clin Endocrinol Metab* 84(7):2518, 1999.

Verp MS, Simpson JL. Abnormal sexual differentiation and neoplasia. *Cancer Genet Cytogenet* 25(2):191, 1987.

Vintzileos A, Ananth C. How to write and publish an original research article. *Am J Obstet Gynecol* 202(1):344,1–6, 2010.

Volker P, Grundker C, et al. Expression of receptors for luteinizing hormone-releasing hormone in human ovarian and endometrial cancers: frequency, autoregulation, and correlation with direct antiproliferative activity of luteinizing hormone-releasing hormone analogues. *Am J Obstet Gynecol* 186(2):171, 2002.

Vollenhoven BJ, Lawrence AS, et al. Uterine fibroids: a clinical review. *Br J Obstet Gynecol* 97:285, 1990.

Waggoner W, Boots LR, et al. Total testosterone and DHEAS levels as predictors of androgen-secreting neoplasms: a populational study. *Gynecol Endocrinol* 13(6):394, 1999.

Walker AF, De Souza MC, et al. Magnesium supplementation alleviates premenstrual symptoms of fluid retention. *J Womens Health* 7(9):1157, 1998.

Walker-Bone K, Dennison E, et al. Epidemiology of osteoporosis. *Rheum Dis Clin North Am* 27(1):1, 2001.

Wallace WHB, Kelsey TW. Human ovarian reserve from conception to the menopause. *PLoS One* 5(1):e8772, 2010.

Wallach EE, Vu KK. Myomata uteri and infertility. *Obstet Gynecol Clin N Am* 22:791, 1995.

Walsh T, Croughan M, et al. Increased risk of testicular germ cell cancer among infertile men. *Arch Intern Med* 169(4):351–356, 2009.

Wamsteker K, Emanuel MH, et al. Transcervical hysteroscopic resection of submucous fibroids for abnormal uterine bleeding: results regarding the degree of intramural extension. *Obstet Gynecol* 82:736, 1993.

Wang X, Chen C, et al. Conception, early pregnancy loss, and time to clinical pregnancy: a population-based prospective study. *Fertil Steril* 79(3):577, 2003.

Wang X, Magkos F, et al. Sex differences in lipid and lipoprotein metabolism: it's not just about sexhormones. *J Clin Endocrinol Metab* 96(4):885–93, 2011.

Warburton D. De novo balanced chromosome rearrangements and extra marker chromosomes identified at prenatal diagnosis: clinical significance and distribution of breakpoints. *Am J Hum Genet* 49(5):995, 1991.

Warburton D, Fraser FC. Spontaneous abortion risks in man: data from reproductive histories collected in a medical genetics unit. *Am J Hum Genet* 16:1, 1964.

Waylen AL, Metwally M, et al. Effects of cigarette smoking upon clinical outcomes of assistedreproduction: a meta-analysis. *Hum Reprod* 15(1):31–44, 2009.

REFERENCES

Weed JC, Ray JE. Endometriosis of the bowel. *Obstet Gynecol* 69:727, 1987.

Weenen C, Laven JS, et al. Anti-müllerian hormone expression pattern in the human ovary: potentialimplications for initial and cyclic follicle recruitment. *Hum Reprod* 10(2):77–83, 2004.

Wei Q, St. Clair B, et al. Reduced expression of biomarkers associated with the implantation window inwomen with endometriosis. *Fertil Steril* 91(5):1686–91, 2008.

Weiderpass E, Adami HO, et al. Use of oral contraceptives and endometrial cancer risk (Sweden). *Cancer Causes Control* 10(4):277, 1999.

Weigel MM, Weigel RM. Nausea and vomiting of early pregnancy and pregnancy outcome. An epidemiological study. *Br J Obstet Gynecol* 96(11):1304–11, 1989.

Weng X, Odouli R, et al. Maternal caffine consumption during pregnancy and the risk of miscarriage: aprospective cohort study. *Am J Obstet Gynecol* 198(3):279e1–8, 2008.

Westhoff C, Heartwell S, et al. Initiation of oral contraceptives using a quick start compared with a conventional start: a randomized controlled trial. *Obstet Gynecol* 109(6):1270–6.

Whan LB, West MC, et al. Effects of delta-9-tetrahydrocanabinol, the primary psychoactive cannabinoid in marijuana, on human sperm function in vitro. *Fertil Steril* 85(3):653–60, 2006.

White PC, Speiser PW. Congenital adrenal hyperplasia due to 21-hydroxylase deficiency. *Endocr Rev* 21(3):245, 2000.

White Y, Woods D, et al. Oocyte formation by mitotically active germ cells purified from ovaries of reproductive-age women. *Nature* 26(1):10, 2012.

Wierman ME, Basson R, et al. Androgen therapy in women: an endocrine society clinical practiceguideline. *J Clin Endocrinol Metab* 91(10):3697–710, 2006.

Wilcox AJ, Weinberg CR, et al. Timing of sexual intercourse in relation to ovulation. Effects on the probability of conception, survival of the pregnancy, and sex of the baby. *N Engl J Med* 333(23):1517, 1995.

Wild RA, Umstot ES, et al. Androgen parameters and their correlation with body weight in one hundred thirty-eight women thought to have hyperandrogenism. *Am J Obstet Gynecol* 146(6):602, 1983.

Wild S, Pierpoint T, et al. Cardiovascular disease in women with polycystic ovary syndrome at long-term follow-up: a retrospective cohort study. *Clin Endocrinol (Oxf)* 52(5):595, 2000.

Williams RS, Littell RD, et al. Laparoscopic oophoropexy and ovarian function in the treatment ofHodgkin disease. *Cancer* 86(10):2138–42, 1999.

Wittenberger MD, Hagerman RJ, et al. The FMR1 premutation and reproduction. *Fertil Steril* 87(3):456–65, 2006.

Wong IL, Morris RS, et al. A prospective randomized trial comparing finasteride to spironolactone in the treatment of hirsute women. *J Clin Endocrinol Metab* 80(1):233, 1995.

Wright J, Lotfallah H, et al. A randomized trial of excision versus ablation for mild endometriosis. *Fertil Steril* 83(6):1830–36, 2005.

Xu B, Li Z, et al. Serum progesterone level effects on the outcome of in vitro fertilization in patients with different ovarian response: an analysis of more than 10,000 cycles. *Fertil Steril.* 2012 Jun;97(6):1321–7.

Yamamoto M, Hibi H, et al. Effect of varicocelectomy on sperm parameters and pregnancy rate in patients with subclinical varicocele: a randomized prospective controlled study. *J Urology* 155(5):1636–38, 1996.

Yanushpolsky EH, Ginsburg ES, et al. Transcervical placement of a Malecot catheter after hysteroscopic evaluation provides for easier entry into the endometrial cavity for women with histories of difficult intrauterine inseminations and/or embryo transfers: a prospective case series. *Fertil Steril.* 2000 Feb;73(2):402–5.

Yao M, Tulandi T. Current status of surgical and nonsurgical management of ectopic pregnancy. *Fertil Steril* 67:421, 1997.

Yates J, Barrett-Connor E, et al. Rapid loss of hip fracture protection after estrogen cessation: evidence from the National Osteoporosis Risk Assessment. *Obstet Gynecol* 103(3):440, 2004.

Yokoyama Y, Shimizu T, et al. Prevalence of cerebral palsy in twins, triplets and quadruplets. *Int J Epidemiol* 24(5):943, 1995.

Yoshimura Y, Wallach EE. Studies of the mechanism(s) of mammalian ovulation. *Fertil Steril* 47(1):22, 1987.

Young RL, Goldzieher JW, et al. The endocrine effects of spironolactone used as an antiandrogen. *Fertil Steril* 48(2):223, 1987.

Youssef MA, Van Wely M, et al. Can dopamine agonists reduce the incidence and severity of OHSS in IVF/ICSI treatment cycles? A systematic review and meta-analysis. *Hum Reprod Update.* 2010 Sep-Oct;16(5):459–66.

Yucelten D, Erenus M, et al. Recurrence rate of hirsutism after 3 different antiandrogen therapies. *J Am Acad Dermatol* 41(1):64, 1999.

Zhang J, Gilles JM, et al. A comparison of medical management with misoprostol and surgicalmanagement for early pregnancy failure. *N Engl J Med* 353(8):761–69, 2005.

Zini A, Boman JM, et al. Sperm DNA damage is associated with an increased risk of pregnancy loss after IVF and ICSI: systematic review and meta-analysis. *Hum Reprod* 12(1):2663–68, 2008.

Zullo F, Pellicano M, et al. A prospective randomized study to evaluate leuprolide acetate treatment before laparoscopic myomectomy: efficacy and ultrasonographic predictors. *Am J Obstet Gynecol* 178(1 Pt 1):108, 1998.

Index

Page numbers in *italics* denote figures; those followed by "t" denote tables

A

Abbe-McIndoe technique, for müllerian agenesis, 39
Abnormal uterine bleeding
  in adolescents, 33t, 34
  age group-based causes of,
    74–75
  definition of, 71
  diagnostic algorithms for,
    79–80
  endometrial biopsy of, 76
  endometrial sloughing, 72–73
  etiology of, 73t–74t, 74–75
  evaluation of, 34, 75–77
  genital tract disorders leading
    to, 74t
  history-taking, 75
  initial evaluation of, 75–76
  key points about, 479
  laboratory testing for, 75
  physical examination of, 75
  postmenopausal, 80
  premenopausal, 79
  screening for, 72t
  secondary evaluation of, 77
  sonohysterography of, 77
  systemic etiologies of, 73t
  terminology associated with,
    71, 71t
  transvaginal ultrasound of, 77
  treatment of, 34, 77–79, 79–80
Abortion
  definition of, 336
  incomplete, 357
  inevitable, 357
  missed, 358
  spontaneous
    laparoscopic ovarian cautery/
      drilling effects on, 202
    progesterone levels and, 119t
    septate uterus as cause of, 43t
  threatened, 357

Acetaminophen with codeine,
  150t
Acromegaly, 320–321
Acrosome reaction, 234–235
Acrylic olive traction device, for
  müllerian agenesis, 39
Acute respiratory distress syn-
  drome, 296
Acute vaginal bleeding, 77
Addison's disease, 368
Adnexal mass, 119
Adolescents, 478
  abnormal uterine bleeding in,
    33t, 34
  dysmenorrhea in, 34–35, 35t
Adrenal antibody test, 368
Adrenal feminizing, 28t
Adrenal gland, 92
Adrenal masculinizing, 28t
Adrenal tumor, 189
Adrenarche, 18, 24t
Adrenocorticotropic hormone
  stimulation test, 188, 194
Alcohol consumption, 279, 351
Alendronate (Fosamax), 428, 429t
Alexandrite laser, 199
Alloimmunity, 350
Alpha-blockers, 442t
Alpha-thalassemia, 381–382
Alprazolam (Xanax), 141
Ambiguous genitalia, 13f, 16. *See
  also* 46,XY
Amenorrhea
  algorithm for, *110–111*
  definition of, 105
  diagnostic algorithm for,
    105–106
  etiology of, 105
  exercise-induced, 113–116, 480
  hyperprolactinemia and, 317t
  key points about, 480
  müllerian agenesis as cause
    of, 21

539

Amenorrhea (*continued*)
oral contraceptives and, 93, 96–97
physiologic, 105
primary, 9t, 105, 107, 108t,
366t, 477
in primary ovarian insufficiency/
primary ovarian failure, 365
secondary, 105, 108–109, 366t
treatment outcomes of, 225t
American College of Obstetricians
and Gynecologists
chronic pelvic pain defined by, 143
oral contraceptives guidelines, 95t
American Society for Reproductive
Medicine, *160–161*
Amniocentesis, 390
Analysis of variance, 473, 473t
Anastrozole, 171t
Androgen excess
maternal, 6
polycystic ovary syndrome
caused by, 195, 196t
Androgen insensitivity syndrome,
7t, 8–9t, 9t, 15, 16t, 24t
Androgen replacement therapy
advantages and disadvantages
of, 400
contraindications for, 399
controversy regarding, 394
delivery of, 399–400
estrogen effects on, 400
indications for, 398–399
key points about, 486–487
overview of, 393–398
selective androgen receptor
modulators, 401
side effects of, 399
tibolone, 401
Androgen-producing neoplasia, 6
Androgens, 66
Androstenedione, 66, 394
Anembryonic pregnancy, 357
Angular pregnancy, 126, *126*
Anovulation
abnormal uterine bleeding
caused by, 73t
hyperprolactinemia and, 317t
laparoscopic ovarian cautery/drill-
ing for, 202–203, 203t–204t
polycystic ovary syndrome as
cause of, 201–203
treatment of, 201–203
Anovulatory cycles, 33t
Anterior pituitary insufficiency, 129
Antiandrogens, 198
Anticardiolipin antibody, 347
Antidepressants, 442t
Antidiuretic hormone deficiency, 131
Antifibrinolytics, 78t

Anti-ß2-glycoprotein-I antibody, 347
Antihistamines, 300t
Anti-müllerian hormone
contraceptives effect on, 260
description of, 2
diminished ovarian reserve and,
259–260, 261t
granulosa cell production of, 259
live birth rates and, 260t–261t
in müllerian agenesis, 38
production of, 259
Antiphospholipid-antibody syndrome
classification criteria for, 348
recurrent pregnancy loss associated with, 347–349, 354
treatment of, 349, 354, 355t
Antisperm antibodies, 232
Antithyroperoxidase antibodies, 332
Antral follicle, 447
Antral follicle count, 262, 447–448
Arcuate uterus, 41t, *42*
Aromatase inhibitors
endometriosis treated with, 171,
171t
fibroids treated with, 179
half-life of, 483
infertility treated with, 116, 201
luteal phase deficiency treated
with, 311
ovulation and, 219
sperm levels affected by, 250
Arrhenoblastoma, 189
Ascites, 295–296
Asherman syndrome, 109, 341–
342, 455–456
Ashkenazi Jewish disorders,
379t–381t, 380
Aspirin, 279
Assisted reproductive technologies
blastocyst scoring grade, 281
cost effectiveness of, 286
definition of, 263
egg retrieval, 263
embryo management algorithm,
282
embryo transfer, 273–274
embryology, 272–273
endometriosis and, 172–173
evaluation before using
male factor infertility, 266
ovarian reserve, 264
tubal status, 264–265
uterine cavity, 265
uterine mapping, 265
fertilization rates based on follicle
size at time of retrieval, 273
gamete intrafallopian transfer, 263
in vitro fertilization. *See* In vitro
fertilization

intracytoplasmic sperm injection, 157, 249, 264, 272
key points about, 484
live birth rate, 279, *280*
oocyte retrieval, 271, 273
ovarian response to, 447–448
postretrieval hormonal management, 273
pregnancy odds with, 288t
preimplantation genetic screening, 272
stimulation protocols and doses
 oral contraceptive–gonadotropin-releasing hormone agonist, 268–270
 oral contraceptive–gonadotropin-releasing hormone antagonist, 270–271
success rates, 276–279
superovulation induction
 gonadotropin-releasing hormone agonists, 266
 gonadotropin-releasing hormone antagonists, 267, 268t
terminology associated with, 279
zygote intrafallopian transfer, 263
Atresia
 follicle, 367
 vaginal, 12–13
Autoimmune disorders, 153
Autoimmune polyglandular syndrome, 366
Autologous vaginal tissue transplantation, for müllerian agenesis, 39
Autosomal genes, 2
Autosomal recessive inheritance, 371
Azoospermia
 description of, 225t, 238–239
 genetic testing algorithm for, *254*
 nonobstructive. *See* Nonobstructive azoospermia
 obstructive, 252

B

Bacterial vaginosis, 31
Bardet-Biedl syndrome, 244
Basal body temperature chart, 214
Bazedoxifene, 415
Beta-thalassemia, 382
Bicornuate uterus, 41t, 41–42, *42,* 341
Bipotential, 1
Birth defects, 249, 276
Bisphosphonates, 427
Blastocyst scoring grade, 281

Bleeding
 abnormal uterine. *See* Abnormal uterine bleeding
 fibroids and, 176
Blighted ovum, 357
Body surface area nomogram, *121*
Bone marrow transplantation, 66–67
Bone mineral density, 424
Bone turnover, 424–425
Brachial plexus injury, 458
BRCA1, 91
BRCA2, 91
Breakthrough bleeding, 96
Breast(s)
 delayed development of, 21
 pubertal growth of, *19*
Breast cancer, 90, 92t
Breast-feeding, 93
Bromocriptine, 325t–326t, 325–327
Bupivacaine, 362t
Buspirone (BuSpar), 141

C

Cabergoline, 297, 325t–326t, 325–327
Caffeine, 351
Calcitonin, 430t
Calcium
 exercise-induced amenorrhea treated with, 116
 supplementation of, 434t
Cancer
 endometriosis and, 152
 oral contraceptives and, 90–91, 92t
Candida, 30
Cannabinoids, 316
Carbohydrate metabolism, 89
Cardiac valvular regurgitation, 325
Carrier screening, 371–382
Case-control study, 472
Central precocious puberty, 26–27, 478
Cervical cancer, 90, 92t
Cervical mucus
 evaluation of, in female subfertility, 216
 menstrual cycle-related changes, 65, 69
Cervix, 65
Cetrorelix, 171t
Chemotherapy, 303–304
Cholecalciferol, 435t
Cholesteatoma, 51
Chorionic villus sampling, 390
Chromosome abnormalities
 fetal, 339–340, 386, 387t–388t
 parental, 337–339

Chromosome abnormalities
  (*continued*)
  recurrent pregnancy loss caused
    by, 337–340
  sex, 386
Chronic fatigue syndrome, 153t
Chronic pelvic pain
  causes of, 146–147
  definition of, 143
  diagnostic studies for, 145
  dysmenorrhea as cause of,
    147–148
  in endometriosis, 155, *174*
  history-taking, 143–144, 144t–145t
  incidence of, 143
  key points about, 481
  laboratory studies for, 145
  pelvic examination for, 144
  physical examination of, 144–145
  procedures for, 145
  treatment of, 148–149, 149t–150t
Chronic renal disease, 323
Citalopram (Celexa), 140
Clinical pregnancy rate, 279
Clomiphene citrate
  description of, 116, 148, 172t,
    200–201
  follicle-stimulating hormone
    and, 219
  luteal phase deficiency treated
    with, 311–312
  ovulation evaluations after, 215
  ovulation induction with, 217–
    218, *218*
  sperm levels affected by, 250
Clonidine, 439
CMRMN study, 200
Coagulation disorders, 33t
Coarctation of the aorta, 50
Coelomic metaplasia, 153–154
Cohort study, 472
Coital disorders, 247
Colorectal cancer, 91
Complementary and alternative
    medicine, 278–279
Complete androgen insensitivity
    syndrome, 7t, 8, 15, 22, 106t,
    108t, 477
Complete gonadal dysgenesis, 7–8
Comprehensive chromosome
    screening, 272
Condyloma acuminata, 32
Congenital adrenal hyperplasia
  corticosteroids for, 477
  11ß-hydroxylase deficiency, 6
  21-hydroxylase deficiency, 6
  3ß-hydroxysteroid dehydroge-
    nase deficiency, 6

laboratory tests for, 14
male subfertility caused by, 247
management of, 14–15
maternal, 192
nonclassic, *190*, 195
polycystic ovary syndrome
    versus, *190*
site of defect in, 5t
untreated, characteristics of, 6
Congenital bilateral absence of vas
    deferens, 240
Conjugated estrogens, 411,
    417t–418t, 430t, 432t, 456
Contraception
  emergency, 99–100
  hormonal, 101–102
  oral contraceptives. *See* Oral
    contraceptives
Contraceptive implants, 102
Copper intrauterine device, 117
Cornual pregnancy, 126
Corpus luteum, 63
Corticosteroids
  congenital adrenal hyperplasia
    treated with, 477
  lichen sclerosis treated with, 31
  Sheehan syndrome treated with,
    131
Corticotropin-releasing hormone,
    131
Cost-effective therapy, 285–287
Counsyl test, 283
Craniopharyngioma, 23, 24t
Cryptorchidism, 483
Cushing's disease, 321
Cushing's syndrome, 24t, 189
CYP11ß1 deficiency, 21
CYP21 deficiency, 21
Cyproterone acetate, 198
Cystectomy, laparoscopic, 162–163,
    466–467
Cystic fibrosis, 240, 373–375
Cystic fibrosis gene mutations, 240
Cystic fibrosis transmembrane
    conductance regulator, 239,
    373–374
Cytotrophoblasts, 117

D

Dalteparin, 349
Danazol, 167t, 171t
Dehydroepiandrosterone sulfate,
    394, 482
Delayed puberty, 21–23
Depo-subQ provera, 170–171
Dermal hyperkeratosis, 184

17,20-Desmolase deficiency, 10
Dexamethasone, 189, 191–192
Dexamethasone suppression test, 321
Diagnostic tests
    for premenstrual syndrome, 140
    for primary ovarian insuf-
        ficiency/primary ovarian
        failure, 367–369
    validity indices for, 471–472
Diethylstilbestrol-associated
    anomalies, 13
Digital rectal examination, 238
Dihydrofolate reductase, 120
Dihydrotestosterone
    degradation of, 189
    description of, 393–394
    in external genitalia development, 3
    testosterone conversion into, 9
Dilatation and curettage
    abnormal uterine bleeding
        treated with, 34
    amenorrhea after, 109t
    early pregnancy failure treated
        with, 358
    ectopic pregnancy diagnosis
        using, 119
Dimenhydrinate (Dramamine), 300t
Diminished ovarian reserve
    antral follicle count, 262
    background of, 255–256
    definition of, 255
    estradiol, 259
    follicle-stimulating hormone,
        258–259
    hormonal tests, 258
    hormones, 258–262
    implications of, 256, 257
    key points about, 483
Diode laser, 199
Dioxin, 155
Diphenhydramine (Benadryl), 300t
DNA fragmentation testing, of
    sperm, 233–234
Down syndrome, 387t
Doxycycline, 456
Doxylamine (Unisom), 300t
Droperidol (Inapsine), 301t
Dual energy x-ray absorptiometry,
    424, 426
Dubowitz disease, 378t
Dysmenorrhea
    chronic pelvic pain caused by,
        147–148
    description of, 34–35, 35t
    primary, 147
    secondary, 148
Dyspareunia, 211

E

Early pregnancy failure
    definition of, 357
    dilatation and curettage for, 358
    key points about, 485–486
    medical management of, 359–363
    misoprostol for, 359–360
    terminology associated with,
        357–358
    treatment of, 358–363
    vacuum aspiration for, 361
Early pregnancy loss, 336
Early vs. Late Intervention Trial
    with Estradiol, 407
Eccyesis, 117
Ectopic pregnancy
    angular, 126, 126
    cornual, 126
    diagnosis of, 117–119
    etiology of, 117
    in vitro fertilization as risk fac-
        tor for, 275
    incidence of, 117
    interstitial, 126, 126
    key points about, 480
    laparoscopic salpingotomy for,
        125t, 466
    location of, 117
    medical treatment of, 120, 120t,
        122t–123t, 122–124
    methotrexate for, 120, 120t,
        122t–123t
    previous history of, 120
    prognosis for, 125
    recurrence risk of, 117
    surgical treatment of, 124–125
Eflornithine, 198
Ejaculatory duct obstruction, 239,
    246
Electrolysis, 199
Electrosurgery, 463–465
11ß-Hydroxylase deficiency, 6
Embryo
    cryopreservation of, 304–305,
        308
    donation of, 389–390
    transfer of, 273–274, 449–450
Embryology
    gonads, 2
    internal genitalia, 2–3
Embryonic demise, 357
Emergency contraception, postco-
    ital, 99–100
Emotional stress, 279
Empty sella syndrome, 322
Endocan study, 165
Endocrinopathies, 247–248

Endometrial biopsy
    abnormal uterine bleeding evaluations, 76
    luteal phase deficiency evaluations, 311
Endometrial cancer
    oral contraceptives and, 90–91, 92t
    in polycystic ovary syndrome, 188
Endometriomas
    description of, 155, 158–159, 481
    laparoscopic cystectomy for, 163
Endometriosis
    algorithm for, *174*
    American Society for Reproductive Medicine classification, *160–161*
    aromatase inhibitor for, 171t, 171t
    assisted reproductive technologies, 172–173
    autoimmune disorders associated with, 153t
    cancer risks, 152
    chronic pelvic pain associated with, 155, *174*
    clinical presentation of, 155–158
    coelomic metaplasia as cause of, 153–154
    danazol for, 167t, 171t
    definition of, 151
    depo-subQ provera for, 170–171
    diagnosis of, 158–159
    dysmenorrhea secondary to, 35t
    estradiol for, 169t, 170
    expectant management of, 162
    familial disposition of, 155
    gastrointestinal involvement in, 158
    genetic predisposition of, 155
    gonadotropin-releasing hormone agonists for, 167t, 168–170, 171t
    histology for, 152t
    immunologic theory of, 154
    induction theory of, 154
    infertility associated with, 156–158, *174*, 223
    interstitial cystitis associated with, 153
    key points about, 481
    laparoscopy of, 159
    malignant neoplasms in, 152
    medical treatment of, 167–171
    menstrual irregularities associated with, 158
    minimal-mild, 157
    oral contraceptives for, 168
    pathogenesis of, 153–154
    pelvic pain associated with, 155, *174*

    pregnancy after, 156
    prevalence of, 151
    progestins for, 167, 172t
    rectovaginal, 159
    recurrent pregnancy loss and, 347
    septate uterus and, 41
    sites of, 159
    surgical management of, 162–167
    transplantation theory of, 153
    transvaginal sonography for, 158
    treatment of, 161–173, 225
    uterosacral nerve ablation for, 162
Endometrium
    decidualization of, 167
    hyperplasia of, 76, 404
    menstrual cycle-related changes, 65
    sloughing of, 72–73
    thickness of, 448
    transvaginal ultrasound assessment of, in ovulation induction, 448–449
Enoxaparin, 294, 349
Epididymis, 236
Ergocalciferol, 435t
Esterified estrogens, 417t–418t
Estradiol
    17ß-, 431t
    in diminished ovarian reserve, 259
    endometriosis treated with, 169t, 170
    libido decreases treated with, 398
    in oral contraceptives, 81
    patch delivery of, 414–415
    in polycystic ovary syndrome diagnosis, 186
Estradiol cream, 38
Estradiol valerate, 456
Estrogen
    conjugated, 411, 417t–418t, 430t, 432t, 456
    esterified, 417t–418t
    in menstrual cycle, 66
    osteoporosis prevention and, 403
    progestin and, 415
    synthetic, 417t
    transdermal, 414
Estrogen therapy
    androgens affected by, 400
    exercise-induced amenorrhea treated with, 116
    hot flashes treated with, 439, 440t
    Turner syndrome treated with, 53t–54t
    vaginal, 419t–420t
Estrogenization, 29t
Ethinyl estradiol, 432t
Ethnic-specific carrier screening, 379–382

Eugonadism, 21–22, 24t
Exercise-induced amenorrhea, 113–116, 480
External genitalia
  embryologic development of, 3
  feminization of, 3
  male, 4f
  masculinization of, 3
  sexual differentiation of, 1

F

Factor V Leiden, 345
Fallopian tube, *214*
Fasting plasma glucose, 188t
FASTT study, 286
Fecundability, 209
Fecundity
  age effects on, 255
  definition of, 209
Federal Employee Retirement
    Income Security Act, 284
Female genitalia anomalies, 12–13
Female subfertility. *See* Subfertility,
    female
Fentanyl, 150t
Ferriman-Gallwey scores, 184,
    205–206
"Fertile eunuch," 243–244
Fertility history, 235
Fertility monitors, 216
Fetus
  chromosome abnormalities of,
    339–340, 386, 387t–388t
  demise of, 357
  nonviability of, 119
  viability of, 335
Fibroids
  aromatase inhibitors for, 179
  bleeding and, 176
  classification of, 175–176
  gonadotropin-releasing hormone
    agonists for, 179–180,
    180t–181t
  infertility caused by, 177
  intramural, 176, 178t
  key points about, 481–482
  laparoscopy myomectomy for, 182
  myomectomy for, 179, 181t,
    181–182, 182t
  pain and, 177
  prevalence of, 175
  recurrence of, 182
  reproductive outcome of,
    177–179
  submucosal, 175, 177, 178t, 179
  subserosal, 176, 178t
Fibromyalgia, 153t

Financially efficient fertility care,
    283–287, 484
Finasteride, 198
First Response, Early Result preg-
    nancy test, 118
5α-Reductase deficiency
  characteristics of, 7t, 9
  gender identity affected by, 3
  laboratory tests for, 14
  male subfertility caused by, 245
Fludrocortisone, 14
Fluoxetine (Prozac), 140
Follicle
  atresia of, 367
  depletion of, 366–367
Follicle-stimulating hormone, 60,
    173t
  diminished ovarian reserve and,
    258–259, 261t
  isolated deficiency of, 244
  letrozole and, 219
  osteoclasts affected by, 424
  in polycystic ovary syndrome
    diagnosis, 186
  in puberty, 20, *20*
  recurrent pregnancy loss and, 350
  in spermatogenesis, 239t
  suppression of, 316
Follicular atresia, 61
Folliculogenesis, 60
Foreign body, 32–33
45,XO, 7, 340, 388t. *See also*
    Turner syndrome
45,X/46,XX, 49
46,Xi(Yq), 12
46,XX
  congenital adrenal hyperpla-
    sia. *See* Congenital adrenal
    hyperplasia
  differential diagnosis of, 13–14
  gonadal dysgenesis, 5t, 7, 22
  laboratory tests for, 14
  management of, 14–15
  maternal androgen excess, 6
  overview of, 5
  true hermaphroditism, 5t, 6–7
46,XY
  androgen insensitivity syndrome,
    7t, 8–9, 9t, 15, 16t, 22
  differential diagnosis of, 13–14
  5α-reductase deficiency. *See*
    5α-reductase deficiency
  gonadal dysgenesis, 7t, 7–8, 22
  laboratory tests for, 14
  Leydig cells
    function-related abnormalities,
      7t, 10
    hypoplasia of, 7t, 9
  management of, 15

46,XY (*continued*)
Müllerian duct persistence, 7t, 10
overview of, 7t
true hermaphroditism, 10–11
46,XY chromosome, 7
47,XXY, 12, 238, 387, 388t
Fragile X mental retardation gene, 368
Fragile X syndrome, 256, 366, 375–377, 384–385
Frank's vaginal dilation technique, for müllerian agenesis, 38
Free androgen index, 343
Fulguration, 463

G

Gabapentin, 442t
Galactorrhea, 317t, 485
Gamete donation, 389–390
Gamete intrafallopian transfer, 263
Gamete preservation
embryo cryopreservation, 304–305
female, 303–307
gonadotoxicity considerations, 303–304
gonadotropin-releasing hormone agonists and antagonists for, 306–307
key points about, 484–485
letrozole protocol for, 305
male, 307–308
oocyte cryopreservation, 305
oophoropexy, 306
ovarian tissue cryopreservation, 306
Gas embolus, 455
Gender identity, 3
Genetic testing
alpha-thalassemia, 381–382
amniocentesis for, 390
Ashkenazi Jewish disorders, 379t–381t, 380
autosomal recessive inheritance, 371
beta-thalassemia, 382
carrier screening, 371–382
chorionic villus sampling for, 390
cystic fibrosis, 373–375
ethnic-specific, 379–382
fragile X syndrome, 375–377
key points about, 486
maternal serum screening for, 390
non-invasive prenatal testing, 390
postnatal, 391
preconception, 389–390
in pregnancy, 390

preimplantation genetic screening/diagnosis, 272, 354, 389
Sephardic Jewish disorders, 379t, 380
sickle cell disease, 382
spinal muscular atrophy, 377–379
Germ cells
life history of, 64
mitotic division of, 59
Gestational age, ß-human chorionic gonadotropin levels and, 118t
Ginger extract, 302t
Glucocorticoids
infertility treated with, 202
polycystic ovary syndrome during pregnancy treated with, 20, 193–194
Glucose intolerance, 52
Glucose tolerance testing, 187
Gonadal dysgenesis
complete, 7–8
46,XX, 5t, 7
46,XY, 7–8
partial, 7–8
pure, 22–23
Gonadal failure, 52
Gonadectomy, 8, 477
Gonadoblastoma, 368
Gonadotoxicity, 303–304
Gonadotoxins, 245
Gonadotropin-releasing hormone
deficiency of, 24t, 243
in puberty, 20
Gonadotropin-releasing hormone agonists
commercial preparations of, 268t
endometriosis treated with, 167t, 168–170, 171t
fibroids treated with, 179–180, 180t–181t
gamete preservation using, 306–307
hypoestrogenemia induced by, 134
luteal, 269
menorrhagia treated with, 78t
microdose, 269–270
ovulation suppression using, 141
superovulation induction using, 266, 297, 312
Gonadotropin-releasing hormone antagonists
commercial preparations of, 268t
gamete preservation using, 306–307
oral contraceptives and, 270–271
superovulation induction using, 267, 268t

Gonadotropin-releasing hormone
    receptors, 266
Gonads
    embryologic development of, 2
    sexual differentiation of, 4f
    toxin exposure, 236
Goserelin, 169, 171t
Granulosa cells, 259
Growth hormone-releasing hor-
    mone, 131
Gruppo Italiano study, 165

H

HAIR-AN syndrome, 184
Harmonic scalpel, 465
Hearing loss, in Turner syndrome,
    51
Heart and Estrogen/Progestin
    Replacement Study, 407
Hemoglobin A1c, 187
Hemoglobin Barts Fetalis, 382
Hemoglobin H disease, 382
Hemoglobinopathies, 381
Hemorrhagic stroke, 88
Hermaphroditism, true
    46,XX, 5t, 6–7
    46,XY, 10–11
Hernia uteri inguinale, 10
High-dose dexamethasone suppres-
    sion test, 321
Hip fractures, 425, 427
Hirsutism
    electrolysis for, 199
    hair removal systems for, 199
    idiopathic, 189
    laboratory tests for, 213
    laser-assisted hair removal for,
        199
    in polycystic ovary syndrome,
        184, 186, 189
    prolactin receptors and, 329
HLA antigens, 352
Hormonal contraception, 101–102
Hormone replacement therapy
    administration of, 411–414,
        416t–420t
    agents for, 416t–420t
    benefits of, 406–411
    classic approach to, 405
    contraindications for, 404
    decision-making algorithm for,
        443
    indications for, 403–404
    key points about, 487
    male subfertility treated with, 250
    new formulations for, 414–415
    in perimenopause, 405

post-WHI approach to, 405
progestins, 412–413
randomized controlled trials of,
    407–410
risks of, 406–411
selective estrogen receptor
    modulators, 415
studies of, 406–411
transdermal patches for delivery
    of, 413–414
Hot flashes
    background of, 437–438
    clonidine for, 439
    decision-making algorithm for,
        443
    description of, 404
    estrogen for, 439
    etiology of, 438–439
    hormone therapy for, 443
    incidence of, 437
    key points about, 488
    treatment of, 439–440,
        440t–442t, 443
Human chorionic gonadotropin
    ß-
        ectopic pregnancy diagnosis
            using, 117–118, 127, 128
        false-positive results, 127, 127t
        ovulation induction using, 217
        pregnancy-related increases in,
            117–118
    blastocyst secretion of, 65
    commercial preparations of, 267t
    Leydig cell stimulation by, 3
    for luteal phase support during
        in vitro fertilization, 313
Human menopausal gonadotropin,
    131, 172t
Hydrocodone bitrate with acet-
    aminophen, 149t
Hydrocortisone, 14
Hydrosalpinx, 264–265, 450
21-Hydroxylase deficiency, 6, 26,
    191, 247
17-Hydroxyprogesterone, 187
3ß-Hydroxysteroid dehydrogenase
    deficiency, 6, 10
17ß-Hydroxysteroid dehydrogenase
    deficiency
    gender identity affected by, 3
    Leydig cell function affected
        by, 10
Hydroxyzine (Atarax, Vistaril), 300t
Hymen
    in children, 29t
    imperforate, 12, 22, 24t, 477
Hyperandrogenism, 199, 201
Hyperemesis in pregnancy, 299,
    300t–302t, 484

Hypergonadotropic hypogonadism, 22–23, 23t, 239t
Hyperinsulinemia, 195
Hyperlipidemia, 196
Hyperprolactinemia
    acromegaly as cause of, 320–321
    bromocriptine for, 325t–326t, 325–327
    cabergoline for, 325t–326t, 325–327
    causes of, 318t–319t
    chronic renal disease as cause of, 323
    Cushing's disease as cause of, 321
    definition of, 315
    description of, 225t, 238, 244
    empty sella syndrome as cause of, 322
    evaluation of, 323–325
    hypothalamic disease as cause of, 322
    hypothyroidism as cause of, 323
    key points about, 485
    laboratory studies for, 324t
    lactotroph hyperplasia as cause of, 322
    luteal phase insufficiency caused by, 343
    magnetic resonance imaging with enhancement for, 323–325
    management of, 324–325
    oral contraceptives in, 329
    osteoporosis and, 329
    pharmacologic agents that cause, 322–323
    pituitary tumors as cause of, 321–322
    prolactin assay for, 324
    prolactinoma as cause of, 319–320, 328
    quinagolide for, 325t–326t
    radiation therapy for, 329
    signs and symptoms of, 317–323
    stress idiopathic, 323
    transsphenoidal microsurgical resection for, 328–329
    treatment of, 325–329, 355t
Hyperreactio luteinalis, 291
Hypertension, 89
Hyperthyroidism, 343
Hypogonadism
    hypergonadotropic, 22–23, 23t, 239t
    hypogonadotropic, 23, 23t, 239t
    prevalence of, 238
    primary, 245
    testosterone replacement therapy for, 247

Hypogonadotropic hypoestrogenemia, 114
Hypogonadotropic hypogonadism, 23, 23t, 186, 239t
Hypogonadotropic syndromes, congenital, 244
Hyponatremia, 455
Hypopituitarism, 24t
Hypospadias, 247
Hypothalamic disease, 322
Hypothalamic-pituitary-ovarian axis, 33t, 306
Hypothyroidism, 153t, 323, 331–333, 343
Hysterectomy, 181t
Hysterosalpingogram, 43, 212, 451
Hysteroscopic polypectomy, 456
Hysteroscopy
    abnormal uterine bleeding evaluations, 77
    complications of, 454
    key points about, 488
    pressure and positioning for, 453–454
    resectoscope settings for, 453

I

Idiopathic hirsutism, 189
Immotile cilia syndromes, 247
Immunoglobulin G, 127
Imperforate hymen, 12, 22, 24t, 477
Implantation rate, 279
In vitro fertilization
    adjuvant therapy for, 256
    age effects on, 255
    alcohol consumption effects on, 279
    aspirin effects on, 279
    birth defects secondary to, 276
    bleeding risks, 275
    complementary and alternative medicine use during, 278–279
    definition of, 263
    description of, 157, 163, 173, 249
    donor egg, 263
    ectopic pregnancy risks, 275
    embryo transfer, 273
    emotional stress and, 279
    exercise effects on, 279t
    fertilization rates based on follicle size at time of retrieval, 273
    higher-order gestations caused by, 275
    luteal phase support in, 313
    natural cycle, 271
    offspring cancer risks, 275

oral contraceptives use in, 268
ovarian cancer risks, 275
preimplantation genetic screening, 272
procedure for, 272
progesterone levels and, 276
recurrent pregnancy loss treated with, 354
risks of, 275–276
success rates for, 276–279
Incomplete abortion, 357
Inevitable abortion, 357
Infertility. *See also* Subfertility
endometriosis-associated, 156–158, *174*
fibroids as cause of, 177
genetic causes of, 382–385
glucocorticoids for, 202
hyperprolactinemia and, 317t
polycystic ovary syndrome as cause of, 184, 201–203
treatment of, 201–203
unexplained. *See* Unexplained infertility
Ingram's modified Frank's vaginal dilation technique, for müllerian agenesis, 38
Inherited thrombophilia, 345–346, 347t
Insulin resistance, 187–188, 343
Insulin sensitizing drugs, 199–200
Insulin-like growth factor-I, 321
Intercellular adhesion molecule-1, 154
Internal genitalia
embryologic development of, 2–3
male, 4f
sexual differentiation of, 1
Interrupted puberty, 21–23
Interstitial cystitis, 153
Interstitial pregnancy, 126, *126*
Intracytoplasmic sperm injection, 157, 249, 264, 272
Intramural fibroids, 176, 178t
Intrauterine adhesions, 109, 109t, *112*, 341, 455–456
Intrauterine device, 100
copper, 117
levonorgestrel, 117
Intrauterine insemination, 223–224, 248–249, 285–286
Intrauterine pregnancy
ß-human chorionic gonadotropin levels associated with, 118
progesterone levels in, 119t
Irritable bowel syndrome, 144
Ischemic stroke, 88
Isosexual precocious puberty, 26

J

Jones metroplasty, *46*
Journal club guide, 469–477, 489

K

Kallmann syndrome, 23, 243
Kartagener syndrome, 247
Keith needle, 462
17-Ketosteroid reductase deficiency, 9
Kisspeptin neurons, 316
Klinefelter's syndrome, 12, 238, 241, 245, 387
Kronos Early Estrogen Prevention Study, 407
Kugelberg-Welander syndrome, 378t

L

Labial adhesions, 32
Lactated Ringer solution, 454
Lactotroph hyperplasia, 322
Laparoscopy
abdominal entry technique for, 458–459
access sites for, 460–461
accessory trocar insertion, 462
anesthesia for, 458
bowel preparation for, 457
complications of, 462–463
cystectomy, 162–163, 466–467
direct entry technique for, 461
ectopic pregnancy applications of, 119, 466
electrosurgery, 463–465
entry techniques for, 458–462
histamine receptor blockade for, 457
key points about, 488–489
myomectomy, 182t, 465
open entry technique for, 461–462
organ damage caused by, 462–463
ovarian cautery/drilling, for anovulation, 202–203, 203t–204t
patient preparation and positioning for, 457–458, 458t
salpingotomy, 125t, 466
trocar bleeding caused by, 462
umbilical entry via modified Alwis method for, 460
venous bleeding caused by, 463
Veress needle technique, 458–459
Laser-assisted hair removal, 199
Lasofoxifene, 415
Late pregnancy loss, 336

Lateral femoral cutaneous nerve injury, 458
Left ventricular mass index, 197
Leiomyomas, 342
Letrozole, 219, 219t–220t, 305
Leuprolide (Lupron), 141, 169, 171t, 297
Levonorgestrel intrauterine system, 78t, 101–102, 117, 167, 413
Levothyroxine, 332, 344t
Leydig cells
    diminished development of, 8
    function abnormalities of, 7t, 10
    human chorionic gonadotropin stimulation of, 3
    hypoplasia of, 7t, 9
    testosterone biosynthesis in, 10
Libido, 398
Lichen sclerosis, 31–32
Lidocaine, 362t
Likelihood ratio, 472
Linear salpingostomy, 124
Live birth rate, 279, 280
Liver tumors, 91
Longitudinal vaginal septum, 12
Low-dose dexamethasone suppression test, 321
Low-molecular-weight heparin, 349
Lubricants, 253
Luteal phase deficiency
    definition of, 309
    diagnosis of, 309–311, 353
    endometrial biopsy evaluations, 311
    etiology of, 309–310
    incidence of, 309
    key points about, 485
    progesterone for, 312–313
    recurrent pregnancy loss caused by, 342–343, 355t
    treatment of, 311–313
Luteal phase support
    in ovarian stimulation cycles, 312
    in in vitro fertilization cycles, 313
Luteinizing hormone
    isolated deficiency of, 243–244
    menstrual cycle levels of, 60, 69
    polycystic ovary syndrome and, 194–195
    in puberty, 20, 20
    in spermatogenesis, 239t
    urine detection kits for, 215
Luteinizing hormone receptor inactivation mutation, 16t
Lymphedema, 52

M

Macroadenoma, 320, 324, 328
Macroprolactin, 315
Magnesium, 141
Magnetic resonance imaging
    with enhancement, for hyperprolactinemia evaluations, 323–325
    septate uterus evaluations using, 43
Male gamete preservation, 307–308
Male sex, 4f
Male subfertility. See Subfertility, male
Mastoiditis, 51
Maternal age
    chromosomal abnormalities based on, 386t
    pregnancy and, 226t
Maternal androgen excess, 6
Maternal serum screening, 390
Mayer-Rokitansky-Kuster-Hauser syndrome, 21, 106t
McCune-Albright syndrome, 26–27, 28t
Meclizine (Bonine), 300t
Medroxyprogesterone acetate, 167, 456
Menarche
    age of onset, 59
    precocious, vaginal bleeding associated with, 33
    thelarche progression to, 18
Menometrorrhagia, 71t
Menopause, surgical, 404
Menorrhagia
    menses pattern associated with, 71t
    treatment of, 78, 78t
Menstrual cycle
    follicular phase of, 59–61
    key points about, 479
    luteal phase of, 59, 63–64
    normal, 59–60
    ovulation phase of, 59, 61–62
    parameters for, 60t
    schematic diagram of, 68
Menstrual migraines, 141–142
Metformin, 199–200
Methadone hydrochloride, 149t
Methotrexate
    contraindications for, 120t
    ectopic pregnancy treated with, 120, 120t, 122t–123t
    indications for, 120t
Methylprednisolone (Medrol), 302t
Methyltestosterone, 399
Metoclopramide (Reglan), 301t
Metroplasty
    Jones, 46
    resectoscope, 44–45, 45

Straussman, *46*
Tompkins, *46*
Metrorrhagia, 71t
Metyrapone stimulation test, 131
Microadenoma, 319–320, 324, 328
Mifepristone, 359t
Migraines, menstrual, 141–142
Minerals, 134
Miscarriage. *See also* Pregnancy loss
  age-based rates of, 335t
  ß-human chorionic gonadotro-
    pin levels and, 118
  karyotyping and, 339–340
  nonsteroidal anti-inflammatory
    drugs and, 351
  thyroid-stimulating hormone
    levels and, 344t
Misoprostol, 181, 359–360
Missed abortion, 358
Mittelschmerz, 62
Modified Alwis method, 460
Modified lithotomy position, 457
Morphine sulfate, 150t
MPA, 412–413
MTX. *See* Methotrexate
Müllerian ducts
  agenesis of, 9t, 13, 21, 24t, 37–
    39, 108t, 478
  anomaly of, 35t
  development of, 2–3, 41–42
  hypoplasia of, 13
  incomplete fusion of, 13
  isolated persistence of, 7t, 10
Multiple pregnancy, 224
Multiple sclerosis, 153t
Myocardial infarction, 88
Myomectomy, laparoscopic, 179,
    181t, 181–182, 465
Myotonic dystrophy, 245

N

Nafarelin acetate (Synarel), 141,
    169, 171t
National Osteoporosis Founda-
    tion, 487
Nausea and vomiting. *See* Hyper-
    emesis in pregnancy
Nd:YAG laser, 199
Neonatal hormone withdrawal,
    vaginal bleeding caused by, 32
Nomogram, *477*
Nonclassic congenital adrenal
    hyperplasia, *190*, 195
Nonfunctional pituitary mass, 330
Non-Hodgkin's lymphoma, 152t
Noninsulin-dependent diabetes
    mellitus, 188

Non-invasive prenatal testing, 390
Nonobstructive azoospermia
  description of, 241–242, 250
  sperm retrieval techniques for,
    252
Nonsteroidal anti-inflammatory
    drugs
  menorrhagia treated with, 78t
  primary dysmenorrhea treated
    with, 34–35, 147
Noonan's syndrome, 245
Norethindrone acetate, 170, 413
Number needed to treat, 474
Nurses' Health Study, 406–407
NuvaRing, 102

O

Obesity
  polycystic ovary syndrome and,
    184
  recurrent pregnancy loss and, 344
Obstructive azoospermia, 252
Odds ratio, 474
17-OHP, 14, 190, 191t
Oligoasthenoteratozoospermia, 240
Oligomenorrhea, 71t, 225t
Oligoovulation, 73t
Oligospermia, 225t, 242
Oligozoospermia, *254*
Oliguria, 293
Ondansetron (Zofran), 301t
Oocyte
  cryopreservation of, 305
  physiology of, 365
  retrieval of, 271, 273
Oophorectomy, 395–396
Oophoropexy, 306
Oral contraceptives
  abnormal uterine bleeding
    treated with, 34
  acne effects of, 97
  alternative route of administra-
    tion, 98
  amenorrhea and, 93, 96–97
  American College of Obstetri-
    cians and Gynecologists
    guidelines, 95t
  benefits of, 98
  breakthrough bleeding caused
    by, 96
  breast cancer and, 90, 92t
  breast-feeding and, 93
  cancer and, 90–91, 92t
  carbohydrate metabolism
    affected by, 89
  cervical cancer and, 90, 92t
  colorectal cancer and, 91

Oral contraceptives (*continued*)
contraindications, 94t
efficacy of, 83, 97
endocrine effects of, 92
endometrial cancer and, 90–91, 92t
endometriosis treated with, 168
estrogen component of, 81
fertility after cessation of, 93
gonadotropin-releasing hormone agonists and, 268–271
gonadotropin-releasing hormone antagonists and, 270–271
hemorrhagic stroke and, 88
in hyperprolactinemia, 329
hypertension and, 89
in vitro fertilization use of, 268
inadvertent use of, during pregnancy, 92
infection and, 93
ischemic stroke risks, 88
key points about, 479–480
liver tumors and, 91
menorrhagia treated with, 78t
metabolic effects of, 88–89
missed pills, 96
myocardial infarction risks, 88
for older women, 101
ovarian cancer and, 91, 92t
ovarian cysts and, 97
ovulation suppression using, 141
patient management for, 83t–88t, 94t–95t, 96
polycystic ovary syndrome treated with, 197
in postpartum period, 93
preexisting medical conditions and, 85t–87t
primary dysmenorrhea treated with, 35
problems associated with, 96–98
progestin component of, 81–82
progestin-only pill, 98–99
reproduction and, 92–94
sexually transmitted diseases and, 93
side effects of, 84t
steroid components of, 81–83
types of, 103t–104t
venous thromboembolism and, 88–89
Orchiectomy, for partial androgen insensitivity syndrome, 9
Ornithine decarboxylase, 198
Ortho-Novum, 66–67
Ospemifene, 415
Osteoporosis, postmenopausal
calcium supplementation for, 434t
definition of, 421

description of, 329
diagnosis of, 424–426
dual energy x-ray absorptiometry evaluations, 424, 426
estrogen for prevention of, 403
hip fractures associated with, 425, 427
incidence of, 421–422
key points about, 487–488
pathogenesis of, 424
predisposing factors, 422–423
prevalence of, 421–422
screening for, 422
secondary causes of, 423
treatment of
monitoring response to, 433
pharmacologic, 426–428, 427t–432t
vitamin D supplementation for, 434t
Otitis media, 51
Ovarian cancer
endometriosis and, 152
in vitro fertilization as risk factor for, 275
oral contraceptives and, 91, 92t
Ovarian cauterization, 202–203, 203t
Ovarian cysts
dysmenorrhea secondary to, 35t
oral contraceptives and, 97
precocious puberty and, 26, 27t
Ovarian drilling, 202–203, 203t–204t
Ovarian failure, 23t
Ovarian follicle depletion, 366–367
Ovarian hyperstimulation syndrome
acute respiratory distress syndrome associated with, 296
admission orders for, 294–295
algorithm for, 294
ascites associated with, 295–296
classification of, 289
complications of, 296
description of, 275
early-onset, 291
fluid replacement in, 294–295
hospital management of, 294–296
hyperreactio luteinalis versus, 291
incidence of, 289
key points about, 484
late-onset, 291
liver dysfunction associated with, 296
management of, 292–293
obstetrical outcome of, during in vitro fertilization, 298t
oliguria management in, 293
pathophysiology of, 291
prevention of, 297–298

renal impairment associated
with, 296
thromboembolic phenomena
associated with, 296
thrombosis prevention in, 295
treatment of, 293–296
Ovarian remnant syndrome, 148
Ovarian reserve
assessment of, using transvaginal
ultrasound, 447
markers of, 261t
testing of, 213, 264
Ovarian reserve factors, 350
Ovarian steroidogenesis, 66
Ovarian stimulation cycles, luteal
phase support in, 312
Ovarian tissue cryopreservation, 306
Ovaries
adult, 64–65
determinants of, 2
germ cells, *64*
polycystic-appearing, 184, 188
Oviduct, 213
Ovotestis, 6, 10
Ovulation
age of onset, 18
clomiphene citrate for induction
of, 217–218, *218*
dysfunction of, 217t–220t,
217–219
evaluation of
basal body temperature chart
for, 214
in female subfertility, 214–216
fertility monitors, 216
luteinizing hormone urine
detection kits for, 215
predictor kits for, 215–216
induction of, 217, 297, 448–449
prostaglandin's role in, 62
suppression of, for premenstrual
syndrome management, 141
timing of, 61–62
Oxycodone hydrochloride, 149t

P

P4. *See* Progesterone
Papillomatosis, 184
Paracentesis, 295
Paracervical block, 362–363
Paroxetine (Paxil), 140
Partial androgen insensitivity syn-
drome, 9, 22
Partial gonadal dysgenesis, 7–8
Pediatrics, 478
condyloma acuminata, 32
labial adhesions, 32

lichen sclerosis, 31–32
physical examination findings,
29t, 29–30
vaginal bleeding, 32–33
vulvovaginal disorders, 30–32
Pelvic adhesions, 35t
Pelvic examination, 144
Pelvic pain
chronic. *See* Chronic pelvic pain
fibroids and, 177
Perimenopause, 404–405
Peripheral precocious puberty, 26–27
Peroneal nerve injury, 458
Perrault syndrome, 7
Physiologic amenorrhea, 105
Pituitary diseases, 244
Pituitary lactotrophs, 319, 322
Pituitary mass, 330
Pituitary tumors, 321–322
Pituitary-gonadal axis, 238
Plasminogen activator inhibitor, 196
Polycystic kidney disease, 246
Polycystic ovary syndrome
in adolescents, 33t
adrenocorticotropic hormone
stimulation test for, 188
androgen excess as cause of,
195, 196t
anovulation in, 201–203
clinical evaluation of, 185–188
Cushing's syndrome versus, 189
diagnostic criteria for, 185
diagnostic studies for, 186–189
differential diagnosis of, 189–191
endometrial abnormalities in, 188
endometrial cancer in, 188
estradiol levels, 186
etiology of, 183
familial risks, 183
Ferriman-Gallwey scores, 184,
205–206
glucocorticoid replacement
for, during pregnancy, 20,
193–194
hirsutism associated with. *See*
Hirsutism
21-Hydroxylase deficiency
versus, 191
17-Hydroxyprogesterone levels,
187
hyperinsulinemia as cause of, 195
infertility caused by, 184,
201–203
inheritance risks for, 183
insulin resistance associated
with, 184
key points about, 482
lipid profile in, 188
long-term consequences of, 196t

Polycystic ovary syndrome
(*continued*)
  luteinizing hormone levels in,
    194–195
  menstrual dysfunction associated with, 183
  nonclassic congenital adrenal
    hyperplasia versus, *190*
  noninsulin-dependent diabetes
    mellitus in, 188
  obesity associated with, 184
  pathophysiology of, 194–197
  pelvic ultrasound evaluations, 188
  in pregnancy, 191–194
  prolactin levels, 187
  recurrent pregnancy loss associated with, 343
  signs and symptoms of, 183–184
  testosterone studies in, 186
  treatment of
    antiandrogens, 198
    CMRMN study, 200
    dexamethasone, 191–192
    finasteride, 198, 204t
    glucocorticoid replacement,
      193–194, 220
    goals for, 197
    insulin sensitizing drugs,
      199–200
    key points about, 204t
    laparoscopic ovarian cautery/drilling, 202–203,
      203t–204t
    metformin, 199–200, 204t
    oral contraceptives, 197
    during pregnancy, 191–194
    progestins, 197
    spironolactone, 198, 204t
    weight reduction, 197
    24-hr. urinary cortisol testing
      for, 187
    virilizing ovarian tumor versus,
      189
Polycystic-appearing ovaries, 184,
  188
Polymenorrhea, 71t
Polypectomy, 222–223, 456
Polyps, uterine, 222
Poor ovarian response, 262
Positioning, for pediatric pelvic
  examination, 29t
Postcoital emergency contraception,
  99–100
Postejaculatory urinalysis, 233
Postmenopausal Evaluation and
  Risk-Reduction with Lasofoxifene Study, 409–410
Postmenopausal osteoporosis. *See*
  Osteoporosis, postmenopausal

Postmenopausal vaginal bleeding,
  452
Postnatal genetic testing, 391
Prader-Willi syndrome, 244
Precocious puberty
  algorithm for, *25*
  central, 26–27, 478
  description of, 24–25
  diagnostic criteria for, 25–26
  evaluation of, 27
  gonadotropin-releasing
    hormone-dependent, 27, 28t
  gonadotropin-releasing hormone-
    independent, 27, 28t
  isosexual, 26
  peripheral, 26–27
  pseudo-, 27, 28t
  treatment of, 27
  true, 26
Predictive values, 471
Pregnancy
  early failure of. *See* Early pregnancy failure
  ectopic. *See* Ectopic pregnancy
  after endometriosis, 156
  genetic testing during, 390
  ß-human chorionic gonadotropin levels in, 118, 118t
  hyperemesis in, 299, 300t–302t
  interpregnancy interval, 224
  maternal age and, 226t
  multiple, 224
  polycystic ovary syndrome treatment during, 191–194
  progesterone levels in, 118, 119t
  septate uterus effects on outcome of, 41, 43, 43t
Pregnancy loss. *See also*
    Miscarriage
  early, 336
  incidence of, 357
  late, 336
  recurrent. *See* Recurrent pregnancy loss
  statistics regarding, 335, 354t
Pregnancy rate, 279
Pregnancy tests, 118
Preimplantation genetic screening/
  diagnosis, 272, 354, 389
Premature ovarian failure, 186
Premenstrual dysphoric disorder
  definition of, 133
  diagnostic criteria for, 136–137,
    481
  premenstrual syndrome versus,
    140
Premenstrual syndrome
  alprazolam for, 141
  definition of, 133

diagnosis of, 135–140
diagnostic tests for, 140
differential diagnosis of, 140
history of, 133
key points about, 481
menstrual migraines associated with, 141–142
neurotransmitters' role in, 134
ovarian steroids in, 134
ovulation suppression for, 141
pathogenesis of, 134
premenstrual dysphoric disorder versus, 140
prevalence of, 133
PRISM calendar for, 137–138, 139
serotonin reuptake inhibitors for, 140–141
symptoms of, 134–135
treatment of, 140–141
Preterm delivery, 43t
Primary amenorrhea, 9t, 105, 107, 108t, 366t, 477
Primary dysmenorrhea, 34–35, 147
Primary hypogonadism, 245
Primary ovarian insufficiency/primary ovarian failure
characteristics of, 366
definition of, 365
diagnostic tests for, 367–369
etiology of, 366–367
incidence of, 365–366
key points about, 486
ovarian follicle depletion as cause of, 366–367
treatment of, 369–370
PRISM calendar, 137–138, 139
Prochlorperazine (Compazine), 301t
Progesterone
ectopic pregnancy diagnosis using, 118–119
in vitro fertilization and, 276
luteal phase deficiency treated with, 312–313
in menstrual cycle, 63, 63, 64t, 66
mid-luteal phase level of, 310
natural, 412–413
replacement therapy, 64t
vaginal gel, 413
Progestin(s)
androgenic activity of, 83t
endometriosis treated with, 167, 172t
estrogen and, 415
hormone replacement therapy, 412–413
hot flashes treated with, 442t
polycystic ovary syndrome treated with, 197

primary ovarian insufficiency treated with, 369
side effects of, 89
synthetic, 81, 82
Progestin withdrawal test, 110, 480
Progestin-only pill, 98–99
Progestogen, 440t–441t
Prolactin
big-big, 315, 315t
characteristics of, 315t
elevated levels of, 244. See also Hyperprolactinemia
in female subfertility evaluations, 213
functions of, 316
physiology of, 316
in polycystic ovary syndrome evaluations, 187
in spermatogenesis, 239t
Prolactin receptors, 329
Prolactinomas, 24t, 319–320, 328
Prolactin-releasing peptide, 316
Prolactin-secreting pituitary adenoma, 244
Prolactin-secreting pituitary tumor, 239t
Promethazine (Phenergan), 301t
Prostaglandin E2, 61, 259
Protamine sulfate, 349
Protein C resistance, 345
Prothrombin G20210A, 345
Pseudoprecocious puberty, 27, 28t
Pubertal disorders
frequency of, 23t–24t
hypergonadotropic hypogonadism, 22–23, 23t
hypogonadotropic hypogonadism, 23, 23t
irreversible, 24t
ovarian failure, 23t
precocious puberty. See Precocious puberty
reversible, 23t–24t
Puberty
definition of, 17
delayed, 21–23
development-related aberrations, 21–23
in girls, 19
interrupted, 21–23
key points about, 477–478
mechanisms underlying, 20
onset of, 17, 18
physical changes during, 18–20, 18–20
precocious. See Precocious puberty
Tanner staging of, 20
in Turner syndrome, 52–53

Pubic hair
  delayed development of, *21*
  normal development of, *19*
Pure gonadal dysgenesis, 22–23

Q

Quality of evidence, 471t

R

Radiation therapy, for hyperprolac-
    tinemia, 329
Raloxifene (Evista), 415, 430t
Raloxifene Use for the Heart, 409
RANK ligand inhibitor, 430t
Reactive oxygen species, 235
Reciprocal translocation, 338, 339t
Rectoabdominal palpation, in
    children, 30
Rectovaginal endometriosis, 159
Recurrent pregnancy loss
  diagnosis of, 352–353
  etiology of, 337–346, 355t
    alloimmunity, 350
    antiphospholipid-
      antibody syndrome. *See*
      Antiphospholipid-antibody
      syndrome
    endocrinologic factors,
      342–345
    endometriosis, 347
    environmental factors, 351
    fetal chromosome abnormal-
      ity, 339–340
    HLA antigens, 352
    immunologic factors, 347–348
    inherited thrombophilia, 345–
      346, 347t
    insulin resistance, 343
    luteal phase deficiency, 342–
      343, 355t
    microbiologic factors, 344–345
    obesity, 344
    ovarian reserve factors, 350
    parental chromosome abnor-
      mality, 337–339
    polycystic ovary syndrome, 343
    sperm DNA damage, 352
    uterine anomalies, 341–342
    uteroplacental microthrombo-
      ses, 352
  facts about, 335–336
  history-taking, 352
  incidence of, 336–337
  key points about, 485
  physical examination for, 353
  primary, 336
  risks associated with, 336
  secondary, 336
  statistics regarding, 354t
  tests for, 352
  treatment of, 354–355
Reifenstein's syndrome, 9, 22
Renal disease, 50–51
Research article, 475–476
Resectoscope, 453
Resectoscope metroplasty, 44–45,
    45
Residual ovary syndrome, 148
Rh immune globulin, 363
Rheumatoid arthritis, 153t
Risedronate (Atelvia), 427, 429t
Robertsonian translocation, 338–
    339, 339t
Round cells, 232–233
Ruby laser, 199

S

Salpingectomy, 221, 466
Sample size, *477*
Secondary amenorrhea, 105, 108–
    109, 366t
Secondary dysmenorrhea, 148
Selective androgen receptor modu-
    lators, 401
Selective estrogen receptor modula-
    tors, 415
Selective serotonin norepinephrine
    reuptake inhibitors, 439
Selective serotonin reuptake
    inhibitors
  hot flashes treated with, 439
  premenstrual syndrome treated
    with, 140–141
Semen analysis
  abnormal, treatment for,
    248–250
  antisperm antibodies, 232
  before assisted reproductive
    technologies, 266
  description of, 230–231
  postejaculatory urinalysis, 233
  reference values for, 231t
  round cells, 232–233
  sperm morphology, 231–232,
    232t
  sperm motility, 232
  total motile count, 231, 248
Seminiferous tubules, 12
Seminoma, 8
Sensitivity, 471

Sephardic Jewish disorders, 379t, 380
Septate uterus
  diagnosis of, 42–43
  embryology of, 41–42
  histology of, 42
  hysterosalpingogram evaluation of, 43
  key points about, 478
  magnetic resonance imaging of, 43
  postoperative management of, 45–46
  pregnancy outcomes associated with, 41, 43, 43t
  prevalence of, 41t
  recurrent pregnancy loss risks, 341, 341t
  resectoscope metroplasty for, 44–45, 45
  surgery for, 43–46
  ultrasound of, 42, 42
Sertoli cells
  anti-müllerian hormone production by, 2
  diminished development of, 8
Sertoli-cell only syndrome, 245
Sertraline (Zoloft), 140
Sex chromosome abnormalities
  description of, 386
  47,XXY disorder, 12
  46,XYp-, 12
  Turner syndrome. *See* Turner syndrome
Sex hormone-binding globulin, 195, 451
Sex-determining region of Y, 2
Sex-hormone binding globulin, 393–394
Sexual differentiation
  abnormal, 6
  embryology of, 1
  facets of, 3
  key points about, 477
  timeline of, 5f
Sexual identity, 3
Sexually transmitted diseases
  oral contraceptives and, 93
  vulvovaginitis in children caused by, 30–31
Sheehan syndrome, 129–131, 481
Short stature, 52
Sickle cell disease, 382
Silver sulfadiazine, 32
Simms-Hubner test, 216
Sjögren's syndrome, 153t
Smoking, 351
Sonohysterography, 77, 451

Sonohysterosalpingography, 450
SOX9, 2
Specificity, 471
Sperm
  acrosome reaction testing, 234–235
  age-related changes in, 247
  computer-assisted analysis of, 234
  creatine kinase measurements, 235
  cryopreservation of, 308
  disorders involving, 247
  DNA fragmentation, 233–234, 352
  intracytoplasmic injection of, 249
  lubricants effect on, 253
  morphologic analysis of, 231–232, 232t
  motility of, 232, 247
  penetration assay for, 234
  retrieval techniques for, 252–253
  viability tests for, 234
  Y-chromosome microdeletions associated with isolated impairment of, 242–243
Sperm washing, 249
Spermatogenesis, 239t
Spinal muscular atrophy, 377–379
Spinnbarkeit, 65
Spironolactone, 198
Spontaneous abortion
  laparoscopic ovarian cautery/drilling effects on, 202
  progesterone levels and, 119t
  septate uterus as cause of, 43t
Statistics, 473–474
Steroid hormone biosynthesis, 207
Steroidogenic acute regulatory protein, 10
Stigma, 62
Straussman metroplasty, 46
Stress idiopathic hyperprolactinemia, 323
Stripping, 272
Subfertility. *See also* Infertility
  definition of, 209
  female
    cervical mucus evaluations, 216
    coital history, 211
    definition of, 209
    etiology of, 210t
    evaluation of, 211–217
    facts about, 209
    gonadotropins for, 220–224
    hysterosalpingogram for, 212
    imaging evaluation of, 212
    interpregnancy interval, 224
    key points about, 483
    laboratory tests for, 213

Subfertility (*continued*)
  maternal age and, 210
  multiple pregnancy risks, 224
  outcomes of, 225t
  oviduct physiology, 213–214
  ovulation evaluation in, 214–216
  ovulatory dysfunction as cause of, 217t–220t, 217–219
  physical examination for, 212
  pregnancy odds after treatment for, 226t, 288t
  salpingectomy for, 221
  transvaginal ultrasound of, 212
  treatment of, 217–224, 225t–226t, 227
  tubal disease as cause of, 221–222
  tubal reversal and, 222
  unexplained, 223–224, 225t
  uterine abnormalities as cause of, 222–223
  male
    acrosome reaction testing, 234–235
    algorithm for, *250–251*
    causes of, 229, 243–248
    diagnostic approach to, *250–251*
    digital rectal examination in, 238
    endocrinopathies as cause of, 247–248
    evaluation of, 229–239
    exogenous hormones that cause, 247
    fertility history, 235
    genetics of, 239–243
    history-taking, 235–236
    hormonal therapy for, 250
    hormones, 238, 239t
    hypothalamic diseases that cause, 243–244
    intrauterine insemination for, 248–249
    karyotypic abnormalities associated with, 241
    key points about, 483
    physical examination of, 236–238
    pituitary diseases that cause, 244
    posttesticular causes of, 246–247
    reproductive tract obstruction as cause of, 246–247
    semen analysis for. *See* Semen analysis
  sexual history, 236
  sperm-specific clinical tests, 233–235
  testicular causes of, 245
  transrectal ultrasonography for, 239
  treatment of, 248–250
  urologic evaluation for, 239
  varicocele evaluations, 237, 237t, 245, 248
  in vitro fertilization for, 249
Submucosal fibroids, 175, 177, 178t, 179
Submucosal leiomyomas, 342
Subserosal fibroids, 176, 178t
Sumatriptan/naproxen, 141
Superovulation, 227, 266–267, 268t, 289, 312
Survival motor neuron, 377
Swyer syndrome, 7–8, 9t, 16t, 22–23, 108t
Sympathetic nerve injury, 246
Systemic lupus erythematosus, 153t

T

Tanner staging of puberty, 20
Teriparatide, 430t
Testes
  chromosomal abnormalities that impair function of, 241
  in complete androgen insensitivity syndrome, 8
  determinants of, 2
  malignancies of, 247
  palpation of, 236
  size measurements of, 236
Testicular feminization. *See* Complete androgen insensitivity syndrome
Testosterone
  age-related changes in, 395
  in polycystic ovary syndrome diagnosis, 186
  in spermatogenesis, 239t
Tetrahydrofolate, 120
Thelarche, 18, 24t
Threatened abortion, 357
Thrombophilia, inherited, 345–346, 347t
Thrombosis
  oral contraceptive risks, 88
  postpartum risks, 349
  prevention of, in severe ovarian hyperstimulation syndrome, 295

Thyroid disorders, 51
Thyroid gland, 92
Thyroid-releasing hormone, 131
Thyroid-stimulating hormone, 187, 213, 238, 331, 333t, 344t
Thyroxine-binding globulin, 332
Tibolone, 401
Tompkins metroplasty, 46
Total motile count, 231, 248
Tramadol, 150t
Tranexamic acid, 78, 78t
Transdermal contraceptive patch, 102
Transdermal hormone therapy, 413–414
Transrectal ultrasonography, 239
Transscrotal ultrasonography, 239
Transsphenoidal microsurgical resection, 328–329
Transvaginal ultrasound/sonography
    abnormal uterine bleeding evaluations, 77
    ectopic pregnancy diagnosis using, 119
    embryo transfer application of, 449–450
    embryonic heart activity evaluations, 336t
    endometriosis evaluations, 158
    endometrium in ovulation induction, 448–449
    female subfertility evaluations, 212
    key points about, 488
    ovarian reserve assessment, 447
    postmenopausal vaginal bleeding evaluations, 452
    scanning principles, 445–446
    tubal patency assessments using, 450–451
    tubal pathology assessments using, 450
    uterine anomaly evaluations, 342
Transverse vaginal septum, 12, 21
Treatment
    cost-effective, 285–287
    financially efficient, 284–285
Trendelenburg position, 464
Trichloroacetic acid, 32
Triiodothyronine, 114
Trimethobenzamide (Tigan), 301t
Triploidy 69, 388t
Trisomy 13, 387t
Trisomy 16, 340
Trisomy 18, 387t
Trisomy 21, 387t
Trisomy X, 387t

Trophoblasts, 118
True hermaphroditism
    46,XX, 5t, 6–7
    46,XY, 10–11
True precocious puberty, 26
Tubal disease
    ectopic pregnancy caused by, 117
    subfertility caused by, 221–222
    transvaginal ultrasound assessment of, 450
Tubal obstruction, 225t
Tubal patency, 450–451
Tubal reversal, 222
Turner syndrome
    academic performance in, 58
    adult management of, 53–57
    characteristics of, 11–12, 22, 385, 388t
    cognitive performance in, 58
    definition of, 49
    diagnosis of, 22, 49–50
    estrogen therapy for, 53t–54t
    genetic counseling of, 57
    health care checklist for, 55t–57t
    incidence of, 9t, 108t
    karotype for, 49–50
    key points about, 478–479
    mosaic, 385
    pediatric management of, 50–52
    prepregnancy management of, 57–58
    prevalence of, 49
    puberty management in, 52–53
    short stature associated with, 52
    treatment of, 22
24-hr. urinary cortisol, 187

U

Ulnar nerve injury, 458
Ultrasound
    ectopic pregnancy diagnosis using, 119, 119t
    septate uterus diagnosis using, 42, 42
    sonohysterography, 451
    transvaginal. See Transvaginal ultrasound/sonography
Unexplained infertility
    description of, 223–224, 225t, 284
    ovarian stimulation cycles for, luteal phase support during, 312

Unfractionated heparin, 349
Unipotential, 1
Ureaplasma urealyticumas, 344
Urethral prolapse, 33
Urogenital ridge, 41
Urogenital sinus, 42
Uterine anomalies
    female subfertility caused by,
        222–223
    polyps, 222
    prevalence of, 41t
    recurrent pregnancy loss caused
        by, 341–342
    septate uterus. *See* Septate
        uterus
Uterine artery embolization, 177
Uterine bleeding, abnormal. *See*
    Abnormal uterine bleeding
Uterine cavity, 265
Uterine mapping, 265
Uterine polyps, 342
Uteroplacental microthromboses, 352
Uterosacral nerve ablation, 162

V

Vacuum aspiration, 361
Vagina
    acute bleeding, 77
    agenesis of, 106t
    atresia of, 12–13
    in children, 29t
    estrogen therapy via, 419t–420t
    menstrual cycle-related changes,
        65
Vaginal bleeding
    in children, 32–33
    description of, 66–67
    postmenopausal, 452
Vaginal ring, 102
Vaginal septum
    longitudinal, 12
    transverse, 12, 21
Vanishing testis syndrome, 245
Varicocele, 237, 237t, 245, 248
Varicocelectomy, 234
Vas deferens
    congenital bilateral absence
        of, 240
    physical examination of, 236
Vasectomy, 246, 246t
Vasopressin, 181
Vecchietti operation, for müllerian
    agenesis, 39
Venlafaxine (Effexor), 140

Venous thromboembolism
    oral contraceptive risks, 88–89
    thrombophilia and, 346t
Veress needle, 458–459
Virilizing ovarian tumor, 189
Vitamin B6, 300t
Vitamin B6/doxylamine, 300t
Vitamin D
    exercise-induced amenorrhea
        treated with, 116
    supplementation of, for postmeno-
        pausal osteoporosis, 434t
Vitamin K, 116
Vitamins, 134
Vulvodynia, 148
Vulvovaginal disorders
    in children, 30–32
    condyloma acuminata, 32
    lichen sclerosis, 31
    vulvovaginitis, 30–31
Vulvovaginitis, 30–31

W

Waist-hip ratio, 195, 197
Weight loss
    anovulation treated with, 201
    polycystic ovary syndrome
        treated with, 197
Werdnig-Hoffman syndrome, 378t
Wilms' tumor suppressor gene
    mutations, 22
Wolffian ducts, 2
Women's Health Initiative, 403,
    405, 408–409, 411
Women's Health Initiative Memory
    Study, 409
Writing, of research article,
    475–476

Y

Y-chromosome microdeletion, 240,
    242–243, 383–384
Young syndrome, 246

Z

Zoledronate, 428
Zoledronic acid (Reclast), 429t
Zona pellucida, 65
Zuclomiphene, 218
Zygote intrafallopian transfer, 263